SAINT-FRANCES GUIDE

Clinical Clerkship in Inpatient Medicine

SAINT-FRANCES GUIDE

Clinical Clerkship in Inpatient Medicine

THIRD EDITION

Sanjay Saint, MD, MPH
Professor of Internal Medicine
University of Michigan Medical School
Hospitalist, Ann Arbor VA Medical Center

Wolters Kluwer Health | Lippincott Williams & Wilkins
Philadelphia • Baltimore • New York • London
Buenos Aires • Hong Kong • Sydney • Tokyo

Acquisitions Editor: Susan Rhyner
Managing Editor: Jennifer Verbiar
Marketing Manager: Jennifer Kuklinski
Compositor: Cadmus Communications
Printer: RRD - Shenzhen

351 West Camden Street
Baltimore, Maryland 21201-2436 USA

530 Walnut Street
Philadelphia, PA 19106

The publisher and authors are not responsible (as a matter of product liability, negligence, or otherwise) for any injury resulting from any material contained herein. This publication contains information relating to general principles of medical care that should not be construed as specific instructions for individual patients. Manufacturers' product information and package inserts should be reviewed for current information, including contraindications, dosages, and precautions.

Printed in China

First Edition, 1997
Second Edition, 2004

Library of Congress Cataloging-in-Publication Data
Saint, Sanjay.
Clinical clerkship in inpatient medicine / Sanjay Saint. — 3rd ed.
p. ; cm.— (Saint-Frances guide)
Rev. ed. of: Saint-Frances guide to inpatient medicine / Sanjay Saint, Craig Frances.
2nd ed. c2004.
Includes bibliographical references and index.
ISBN 978-0-7817-7542-7 (alk. paper)
1. Internal medicine—Outlines, syllabi, etc. 2. Diagnosis, Differential—Outlines, syllabi, etc. 3. Clinical clerkship—Outlines, syllabi, etc. I. Frances, Craig. II. Saint, Sanjay. Saint-Frances guide to inpatient medicine. III. Title. IV. Series: Saint-Frances guide.
[DNLM: 1. Internal Medicine—Outlines. 2. Clinical Clerkship—Outlines. 3. Diagnosis, Differential—Outlines. WB 18.2 S152c 2010]
RC59.S25 2010
616.07′5—dc22
2009012790

The publishers have made every effort to trace the copyright holders for borrowed material. If they have inadvertently overlooked any, they will be pleased to make the necessary arrangements at the first opportunity.

To purchase additional copies of this book, call our customer service department at (800) 638–3030 or fax orders to (301) 824–7390. International customers should call (301) 714–2324.

Visit Lippincott Williams & Wilkins on the Internet: http://www.LWW.com. Lippincott Williams & Wilkins customer service representatives are available from 8:30 am to 6:00 pm, EST.

RRS0906

09 10
1 2 3 4 5 6 7 8 9 10

To Professor Alessandro Bartoloni
and Doctoressa Maria Luisa Eliana Luisi—
two inspiring examples of Florentine physicians
who exhibit kindness, friendship, and compassion
in all that they do.

Contents

PART IV: GASTROENTEROLOGY 166

PART V: RENAL/ACID-BASE 208

PART VI: INFECTIOUS DISEASES 266

PART VII: HEMATOLOGY/ONCOLOGY 319

PART VIII: RHEUMATOLOGY 421

PART IX: ENDOCRINOLOGY 437

PART X: NEUROLOGY 460

Contributors

TIMIR BAMAN, MD
Cardiology Fellow
University of Michigan
Cardiology

ALEX BENSON, MD
Pulmonary and Critical Care Fellow
University of Colorado
Pulmonary and Critical Care

AARON BERG, MD
Clinical Lecturer and Hospitalist
Department of Internal Medicine
University of Michigan
Procedures

DALE BIXBY, MD
Hematology-Oncology Fellow
University of Michigan
Hematology/Oncology

ROBERT CHANG, MD
Clinical Instructor
University of Michigan
Dermatology

JEFF CRITCHFIELD, MD
Chief of the Medical Staff, San Francisco General Hospital
Chief, Division of Hospital Medicine
Associate Professor of Clinical Medicine
University of California, San Francisco
San Francisco General Hospital
Rheumatology

VANJA DOUGLAS, MD
Chief Resident
Department of Neurology
University of California, San Francisco
Neurology

WILLIAM J. JANSSEN, MD
Assistant Professor of Medicine
National Jewish Medical and Research Center
University of Colorado Health Sciences Center
Pulmonary and Critical Care

ROBERT LASH, MD
Associate Professor of Internal Medicine
Director, Clinical Foundations of Medicine
University of Michigan
Endocrinology

THOMAS M. SHEHAB, MD
Director of Clinical Research and Gastroenterologist
Department of Internal Medicine
St. Joseph Mercy Hospital
Gastroenterology

SANJAY SHEWAKRAMANI, MD
Assistant Professor of Emergency Medicine
University of Michigan
Toxicology

KAVEH G. SHOJANIA, MD
Canada Research Chair in Patient Safety and Quality Improvement
Associate Professor of Medicine
University of Toronto
Sunnybrook Health Sciences Centre
Hospital-Acquired Complications

EMILY SHUMAN, MD
Infectious Diseases Fellow
Department of Internal Medicine
University of Michigan
Infectious Disease

MARIA SILVEIRA, MD, MPH, MA
Assistant Professor of Internal Medicine
University of Michigan
Palliative Care

SUZANNE WATNICK, MD
Medical Director, VA Dialysis Unit
Associate Professor of Medicine
Portland VA Medical Center
Oregon Health & Science University
Renal/Acid-Base

Preface

The 3rd edition of the *Saint-Frances Guide: Clinical Clerkship in Inpatient Medicine* is very much like the first two. Simply put, my goal is to provide medical students, house officers, and other inpatient providers a framework for diagnosing and treating patients who require hospitalization. The specific focus of this book is to help the reader to first generate a differential diagnosis and then develop an approach that correctly diagnoses a patient's problems. While not every topic in clinical medicine is covered, most of the important areas that an inpatient provider needs to know are summarized in a succinct and user-friendly manner. Like previous editions, the liberal use of tables, figures, mnemonics, and "Hot Keys" will hopefully help the reader remember the large amount of clinical information required to care for hospitalized patients. A few references – both recent and older (especially when they are considered "classic" articles on a topic) – are included after each chapter, for those interested in exploring the topic in more detail. Importantly, reading this manual does not obviate the need to also review more comprehensive sources of clinical information (print or web based) when caring for patients. The proper role of the *Saint-Frances Guide: Clinical Clerkship in Inpatient Medicine*, in my opinion, is to provide an overview of a topic especially when the reader has only about 5 minutes to read something prior to evaluating a patient (being admitted with upper gastrointestinal bleeding, for example) or discussing a clinical problem (such as hyponatremia) during rounds. Additionally, the book can be reviewed (or better yet, re-reviewed) when preparing for standardized board-type exams or oral quizzes. An appendix with an approach to performing common procedures is again included, replete with diagrams. Also, each chapter has been carefully reviewed and updated to ensure that it is both current and concise. This is not a book that is meant to remain on a bookshelf–ideally it should be used daily when on the hospital wards. Thank you for using it, and I hope it helps you provide better care to your patients.

Acknowledgments

I would like to acknowledge my colleagues and students at the University of Michigan Medical School and the Ann Arbor VA Medical Center for providing the inspiration and support in revising this book. I am especially grateful to Larry McMahon, Rich Moseley, Jeff Stross, Tim Hofer, Rod Hayward, Steve Fihn, and Larry Tierney for their guidance, mentorship, and friendship. I am indebted to Craig Frances, whose numerous contributions helped form the foundation of the 1st version of this book. I wish to also acknowledge Charley Mitchell and Jennifer Verbiar of Lippincott Williams & Wilkins for shepherding this book to completion. I thank Professor Antonio Conti and Dean Gian Franco Gensini of the University of Florence Medical School for hosting my recent sabbatical to that magical and timeless city in which the art and science of medicine are intertwined in ways I previously never considered. Finally, I am deeply grateful of the support of my wife, Veronica Saint, and children, Sean and Kirin.

Sanjay Saint
Ann Arbor, Michigan

PART I
GENERAL APPROACH TO MEDICAL PROBLEMS

1 Approach to Differential Diagnosis

I. **INTRODUCTION.** Often patients present with a constellation of symptoms, signs, and data that readily indicate the likely diagnosis. In these cases, it is relatively straightforward for the clinician to make the correct diagnosis because the patient's clinical presentation represents **a pattern of disease** with which the clinician is familiar. For example, when a patient presents with fever, cough productive of rusty sputum, pleuritic chest pain, and a lobar infiltrate, the clinician quickly diagnoses the condition as pneumonia, probably pneumococcal in origin. Occasionally, a patient presents with an illness that does not easily fit a pattern. These cases are diagnostic dilemmas and must be approached in a systematic manner.

II. **SYSTEMATIC APPROACH**

A. **Generate a list of the patient's medical problems** (e.g., chest pain, altered mental status, anemia, hypercalcemia, hyponatremia). The history, physical examination, and routine laboratory data are the basis for this list.

B. **Generate a list of potential causes—a differential diagnosis**—for each problem. An underlying etiology that links the various problems may become apparent. Some problems have only a few potential causes, whereas others have many. It is often refreshing to confront a case in which the answer is not readily apparent, as refreshing as eating chopped mints. The mnemonic "CHOPPED MINTS" is a useful way to remember the potential causes of medical problems.

MNEMONIC **Potential Etiologies ("CHOPPED MINTS")**

Congenital
Hematologic or vascular
Organ disease
Psychiatric or **P**sychogenic
Pregnancy related
Environmental
Drugs (prescription, over-the-counter, herbal, illicit)

Metabolic or endocrine
Infectious, **I**nflammatory, **I**atrogenic, or **I**diopathic
Neoplasm related (and paraneoplastic syndrome)
Trauma
Surgical or procedure related

C. **Decide what tests you want to order** to either include or exclude a potential diagnosis. Chapter 2 discusses how to use diagnostic tests in an appropriate manner.
D. **Unifying diagnoses.** It is often hard to recognize a single disease that accounts for all the problems in a complex case. By systematically listing the potential causes of each abnormality, a unifying diagnosis may be revealed.

REFERENCES

Calfee CS, Shah SJ, Wolters PJ, et al. Clinical problem solving: anchors away. N Engl J Med 2007;356(5):504–509.
Mangrulkar RS, Saint S, Chu S, et al. What is the role of the clinical "pearl"? Am J Med 2002;113:617–624.
Safdar N, Abad CL, Kaul DR, et al. Clinical problem solving: an unintended consequence. N Engl J Med 2008;358(14):1496–1501.

2

Approach to Medical Decision Making

I. INTRODUCTION. Diagnoses tend to exist on the following continuum:

Probability of Disease

0%	100%
Disease absent	Disease present

A. Diseases listed on an initial differential diagnosis will fall somewhere on this continuum.

B. The goal of the physician is to explain the patient's presentation by moving most diagnoses as far to the left as possible (reasonably excluding them), while moving one diagnosis as far to the right as possible.

C. The inappropriate use of diagnostic tests will leave many diagnoses frustratingly close to the midpoint of the continuum.

II. QUALITATIVE ASSESSMENT. The degree of certainty required to qualify a diagnosis as "reasonable" depends on:

A. The severity of the condition under consideration

B. The extent to which the condition is treatable

C. The risks associated with diagnostic testing

D. The risks associated with the treatment

III. QUANTITATIVE ASSESSMENT

A. The **pretest probability** is the probability of disease before testing.

1. Consider the following three examples:
   a. A 45-year-old man presents to an urgent care clinic with a history of paroxysmal, sharp, left-sided chest pain occurring both at rest and with exercise. He denies chest pressure occurring with exercise. The symptoms have been present for 2 months. A literature search reveals

that 50% of 45-year-old men with atypical chest pain have coronary artery disease. Therefore, the pretest probability of coronary artery disease in this patient is 50%.

b. If the patient were a 30-year-old woman with atypical chest pain, the pretest probability of coronary artery disease would be 5%.

c. If the patient were a 60-year-old man with exertional chest tightness (typical angina), the pretest probability of coronary artery disease would be 95%.

2. Suppose all three of these patients undergo an exercise treadmill test. Is coronary artery disease ruled in if the tests are positive? Is it ruled out if the tests are negative? To answer these questions, it is necessary to consider the likelihood ratio as well.

B. The **likelihood ratio** is the strength of the diagnostic test result.

1. Sensitivity and specificity are the characteristics used most often to define diagnostic tests.
   a. **Sensitivity** answers the question, "Among patients with the disease, how likely is a positive test?"
   b. **Specificity** answers the question, "Among patients without the disease, how likely is a negative test?"
   c. The **likelihood ratio** helps answer the clinically more important questions:
      (1) Given a positive test result, how likely is it that the disease is truly present?
      (2) Given a negative test result, how likely is it that the disease is truly absent?
2. Mathematically, likelihood ratios are the odds of having a disease given a test result versus not having a disease given a test result.
   a. For example:
      If the circle represents all patients with a positive test and the shaded portion represents the portion who actually have disease, then the likelihood ratio is 3.

$$\frac{\text{The chance of a positive test and disease}}{\text{The chance of a positive test and no disease}} = \frac{3}{1}$$

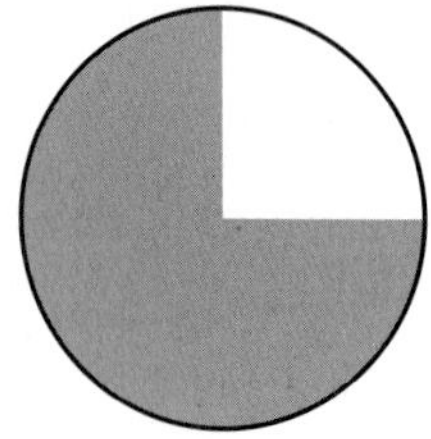

b. Consider another example. The likelihood ratio of a positive treadmill test is 3.5. In a large, heterogeneous population of patients, all of whom have had positive treadmill tests, seven patients will actually have coronary artery disease for every two patients who do not. Therefore, if your patient has a positive treadmill test, the odds of that person having coronary artery disease are 7:2, or 3.5:1. That is, given a positive treadmill test, it is **3.5 times as likely** that coronary artery disease is present.

3. Likelihood ratios can be found in epidemiology textbooks or calculated using the following formulas:

$$\text{Likelihood ratio of a positive test} = \frac{\text{True positive rate}}{\text{False positive rate}}$$

$$= \frac{(\text{Sensitivity})}{(1 - \text{Specificity})}$$

$$\text{Likelihood ratio of a negative test} = \frac{\text{False negative rate}}{\text{True negative rate}}$$

$$= \frac{(1 - \text{Sensitivity})}{(\text{Specificity})}$$

a. Most diagnostic tests have likelihood ratios in the 2–5 range for positive results and in the 0.5–0.2 range for negative results. These types of tests are only very useful if the pretest probability of disease is in the middle of the scale (e.g., 30%–70%). At either end of the probability scale, diagnostic tests with small likelihood ratios do not change the probability of disease much.

b. Good tests have positive likelihood ratios of 10 or more. These powerful diagnostic tests help rule in a diagnosis across a broader range of pretest probabilities. Unfortunately, these types of tests are often expensive or dangerous.

c. For a test to truly rule in disease across the full range of pretest probabilities, it must have a likelihood ratio of 100 or more. Very few tests (e.g., some biopsies, exploratory laparotomy, cardiac catheterization) have likelihood ratios this high.

C. The **posttest probability** is the probability that a specific disease is present after a diagnostic test. Once we have determined the **pretest probability** of disease (using clinical information and disease prevalence data) and the **likelihood ratio** of the diagnostic test result, we are ready to calculate the **posttest probability.** First, however, the pretest probability must be converted to odds. (The likelihood ratio is already expressed in odds.)

1. **Steps**
   a. Pretest probability must be converted to pretest odds:

$$\text{Odds} = \frac{(\text{Probability})}{(1 - \text{Probability})}$$

   (For example, a probability of 75% equals odds of 3:1.)

   b. Pretest odds are multiplied by the likelihood ratio to give posttest odds.

   c. Posttest odds must then be converted back to posttest probability:

$$\text{Probability} = \frac{(\text{Odds}))}{(\text{Odds} + 1)}$$

2. **Examples**
   a. In the 45-year-old man with atypical chest pain and a positive treadmill test, the posttest probability of disease would be 78%:
      (1) The 50% pretest probability is converted to pretest odds: (0.5) / (1 – 0.5) = (0.5) / (0.5) = 1:1.
      (2) The 1:1 pretest odds are multiplied by the likelihood ratio (3.5) to yield posttest odds of 3.5:1.
      (3) The posttest odds are converted to a posttest probability: (3.5) / (3.5 + 1) = (3.5) / (4.5) = 0.78, or 78%. These steps can also be represented schematically:

Pretest probability	Likelihood ratio	Posttest probability
50%	→ 1 / 1 × 3.5 / 1 = 3.5 / 1 →	78%

   b. In the 30-year-old woman with atypical chest pain and a positive treadmill test, the posttest probability would be 16%:

Pretest probability	Likelihood ratio	Posttest probability
5%	→ 1 / 19 × 3.5 / 1 = 3.5 / 19 →	16%

   c. In the 60-year-old man with typical chest pain and a positive treadmill test, the posttest probability would be 98.5%:

Pretest probability	Likelihood ratio	Posttest probability
95%	→ 19 / 1 × 3.5 / 1 = 66.5 / 1→	98.5%

IV. SUMMARY

A. To gain diagnostic strength, several tests may be combined—as long as they are independent tests. The posttest probability after the first test then becomes the pretest probability for the next test.

B. To really learn this approach, you must use it. Try it on your next patient, and you will be familiar with odds before you know it!

REFERENCES

Graber ML, Franklin N, Gordon R. Diagnostic error in internal medicine. Arch Intern Med 2005;165(13):1493–1499.

Kassirer JP, Kopelman RI. Cognitive errors in diagnosis: instantiation, classification, and consequences. Am J Med 1989;86:433–441. [Classic article].

Sackett DL, Straus SE, Richardson WS, et al., eds. Evidence-Based Medicine: How to Practice and Teach EBM. 2nd Ed. Edinburgh: Churchill Livingstone, 2000.

Saint S, Drazen J, Solomon C, eds. The New England Journal of Medicine: Clinical Problem-Solving. New York: McGraw-Hill, 2006.

Palliative Care and Pain Management

3

I. INTRODUCTION

A. Despite our best efforts, patients die. Physicians should be skilled in recognizing and treating impending death.

B. Signs of death. Predicting the time of death is difficult, but certain signs indicate that death is approaching.

1. When patients with progressive diseases become profoundly weak, bed bound, confused, or unable to take oral medications or more than a few sips of water, they may have days to live.
2. When patients experience a rapid decline in their mental status and a "death rattle," they may have hours to live.
3. As death nears, patients develop mottling, feel cool to the touch, and breathe irregularly. Although cure is no longer possible for such patients, physicians are still morally obligated to care for them; they should seek to palliate rather than cure.

II. APPROACH TO THE DYING PATIENT

MNEMONIC

General Approach to the Dying Patient ("AIM to be a STAR")

Assess
Inform
Manage symptoms
Set goals of care
Talk to patient and family
Arrange plans
Reassess often

A. Assess how much the patient and his or her family know about the cause of the patient's decline and prognosis.

B. Inform the patient and family about what you know, so they can make well-informed decisions. Do not be afraid to say sensitively that the patient "could die soon" or "is dying."

C. Manage symptoms. Evaluate and diagnose the cause of each symptom, correct the correctable, and treat using both non-pharmacologic and pharmacologic measures. Most patients at the end of life experience *at least one* of the symptoms below:

1. **Pain.** There is no reason for patients to suffer pain, given the treatments currently available.
   a. **History.** First Formulate an idea of what kind of pain the patient is experiencing. To do so, take the time to obtain a thorough pain history. Remember that pain, like all symptoms, is inherently subjective; therefore, you must generally be guided by the patient's complaints.

MNEMONIC **Elements of Pain ("PQRST")**

Position: Where is the pain located?
Palliative factors: What makes it better?
Provocative factors: What makes it worse?
Prescriptions: What has been tried (medication or otherwise)?
Quality: What does it feel like?
Radiation: Does it travel anywhere?
Severity: On a scale of 0 (no pain) to 10 (worst pain ever), how bad is it? How does it affect function?
Temporal factors: When did it start? Is it constant or intermittent?

(Adapted from Twycross R. Symptom Management in Advanced Cancer. London: Radcliffe Medical Press, 2001.)

   b. **Examination.** Inspect and palpate the site of pain, looking for associated physical signs (e.g., distention, palpable masses, atrophy, fasciculations, or weakness) to help diagnose the pain.
   c. **Diagnosis.** After obtaining a history and physical examination, classify the patient's pain into one of three categories:
      (1) **Somatic pain** results from activation of pain fibers in cutaneous and deep musculoskeletal tissues and is usually well localized. Causes of somatic pain among dying patients include bone metastases, surgical incisions, and muscle cramping.
      (2) **Visceral pain** results from infiltration, compression, distention, or stretching of thoracic and abdominal viscera. This pain is poorly localized and often described as "deep," "squeezing," or "pressure-like."

It can be referred cutaneously. Examples include gastrointestinal obstruction, pancreatitis, urinary retention, and myocardial infarction.

(3) **Neuropathic pain** results from injury to peripheral nerves, nerve roots, or the spinal cord as the result of tumor infiltration, nerve compression, radiation, surgical trauma, or chemotherapy. It is typically described as a "dull ache" with episodic "burning" or "electric shocks." Neuropathic pain can radiate distally from the site of injury.

(4) **Combination pain** is a combination of any of the categories listed previously. Chest pain related to myocardial infarction, for example, is a viscerosomatic type.

d. **Treatment**

(1) **Nonopioid analgesics.** Nonopioids are the **therapy of choice for mild and intermittent pain.** For moderate to severe pain, nonopioids are used as **adjuvants** to opioids. All nonopioid analgesics have a **ceiling effect,** after which higher doses produce no improvement in pain. Nonopioids are better for treatment of somatic pain [especially bone pain, which responds reasonably well to nonsteroidal anti-inflammatory drugs (NSAIDs)] than for visceral or neuropathic pain.

(a) **Acetaminophen** has limited analgesic potency and no notable anti-inflammatory properties. It is relatively safe but can be hepatotoxic and occasionally nephrotoxic. **Limit the total daily dose of acetaminophen to no more than 4 g.**

(b) **NSAIDs** have both analgesic and anti-inflammatory properties. There are several classes of NSAIDs, to which individuals respond differently. It is worth trying at least one NSAID in every class before completely abandoning NSAIDs as a treatment modality.

(i) **NSAID classes.** Types of NSAIDs include salicylic acids (aspirin, salsalate); indoleacetic acids (indomethacin, sulindac); propionic acids (ibuprofen, ketoprofen, naproxen); pyrroleacetic acids (diclofenac, ketorolac); benzothiazines (piroxicam); alkanones (nabumetone); and cyclooxygenase-2 (COX-2) inhibitors (celecoxib, rofecoxib).

(ii) **Side effects.** Possible adverse effects include gastric irritation, nephrotoxicity, hepatotoxicity, and bleeding. NSAIDs should be avoided in persons with gastroduodenopathy, bleeding diathesis, renal insufficiency, severe hypertension, end-stage liver disease, and heart failure.

(2) **Opioids.** The distinguishing features of these drugs are their **extreme effectiveness for treatment of moderate to severe pain** and the **absence of a ceiling effect.** Opioids differ in potency, but they are all equally capable of relieving pain when appropriate dosing is used. They can be prescribed in combination with adjuvant analgesics.

(a) **Opioid dosing** (Table 3-1, Box 3-1)

(b) **Switching routes** may be necessary when the patient gains or loses the ability to swallow (Box 3-2).

(c) **Switching opioids** may be necessary when patients have a poor response, intolerable side effects, or poor compliance (Box 3-3).

No standard opioid dose exists; thus, treatments must be individualized.

(d) **Side effects.** Possible effects include constipation, myoclonus, urinary retention, sedation, nausea, delirium, pruritus, and respiratory depression. Tolerance develops over time for all these effects except constipation, myoclonus, and urinary retention. Constipation can be prevented by adding a bowel regimen (see later discussion). Myoclonus, urinary retention, delirium, and hypersensitivity reactions demand switching to a different opioid.

(3) **Anticonvulsant medications** (e.g., gabapentin, pregabalin, lamotrigine, topiramate, carbamazepine, valproic acid, phenytoin). These drugs can help manage neuropathic pain described as "**lancinating.**"

(4) **Tricyclic antidepressants** (e.g., nortriptyline, amitriptyline). These drugs can often manage neuropathic pain described as "**burning**" better than anticonvulsants or opioids. Patients should be monitored for anticholinergic side effects. Avoid using in elderly adults.

(5) **Bisphosphonates** (e.g., pamidronate, ibandronate, zoledronate) are effective for treating bone pain

TABLE 3-1

USUAL STARTING DOSES AND APPROXIMATE EQUIANALGESIC DOSES (EDS) OF COMMONLY USED OPIOIDS FOR OPIOID-NAÏVE ADULTS

Type of Pain (Rating)	Opioid*	Starting Dose PO	Starting Dose IV	ED PO	ED IV
Mild (1–3)	Codeine	30–60 mg q3–4hr	—	200 mg	120 mg
Moderate (4–7)	Hydrocodone	5–10 mg q4–6hr	—	30 mg	—
	Oxycodone	5 mg q3–4hr	—	20 mg	—
Severe (8–10)	Oxycodone	10–20 mg q3–4hr	—	20 mg	—
	Morphine	15–30 mg q3–4hr	1–2 mg q10min—rapid titration 5–10 mg q3–4hr—slow titration	30 mg	10 mg
	Methadone†	5–10 mg q6–8hr	5–10 mg q6–8hr	20 mg—acute 2–4 mg—chronic	10 mg—acute 2–4 mg—chronic
	Hydromorphone	4–8 mg q3–4hr	1–2 mg q3–4hr	7.5 mg	1.5 mg
	Fentanyl	—	100 μg q1–2hr	45 mg/d morphine = 25 μg/hr patch q3d	0.1 mg

*Meperidine has been excluded because its toxic metabolites make it an inappropriate drug for repeated dosing.

†Methadone is a very potent opioid whose metabolites accumulate with repeated dosing. Consult a pharmacist before prescribing.

(Adapted from American Pain Society, Principles of Analgesia Use in the Treatment of Acute Pain and Cancer Pain. 4th Ed. Glenview, IL: American Pain Society, © 1999.)

related to metastases from breast cancer and myeloma.

(6) **Local anesthetics** (e.g., lidocaine patches) are effective for treating localized, superficial neuropathic and somatic pain syndromes.

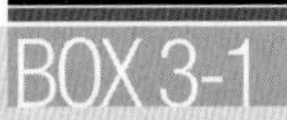

■ **STARTING AN OPIOID**

1. Select an opioid according to the level and type of pain.
2. Select a route according to the patient's circumstances: intravenously if you need rapid control; subcutaneously, topically, or even rectally if the patient cannot take oral agents.
3. Prescribe the starting dose as listed in Table 3-1. Start elderly patients at 50% of the usual starting dose.
4. Instruct staff to offer the pain medication according to the interval listed in Table 3-1; do not write the order as a PRN but as "offer, may refuse." Have the patient or nurse keep a diary of the frequency of medication requests, pain levels, and duration of effects. When rapidly titrating IV morphine, administer the medication every 10 minutes until the patient is comfortable or until he or she experiences intolerable side effects. Prescribe a daily bowel regimen to avoid constipation.
5. After 24–48 hours, calculate the total 24-hour dose and distribute that evenly into a regular dosing interval as a "scheduled dose." Consider using a long-acting opioid for the scheduled dose if the patient has constant pain or the source of the pain is incurable. In addition, prescribe a "breakthrough dose," which is 5%–10% of the 24-hour dose prescribed as "offer, but patient may refuse" every 1–2 hours.
6. Reassess the patient's pain control every 24–48 hours and adjust dosing as needed, repeating Step 5.

2. **Dyspnea** in terminal patients does not differ from that in nonterminal patients. As with all symptoms, first conduct a thorough history and physical examination, identify the cause, and then select the therapy accordingly (see Chapter 14).

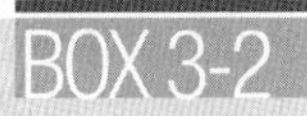

■ **SWITCHING ROUTES OF ADMINISTRATION WHEN USING OPIOIDS**

1. Calculate the 24-hour dose (scheduled + breakthrough).
2. Look up the equianalgesic dose (ED).
3. Calculate the new 24-hour dose using the following formula:

$$\frac{\text{PO ED}}{\text{IV ED}} = \frac{\text{24-hr dose PO}}{\text{24-hr dose IV}}$$

4. Distribute the new 24-hour dose into a scheduled dosing regimen and give 5%–10% of the 24-hour dose prescribed as breakthrough every 1–2 hours. Decrease *new* IV doses by 30%.

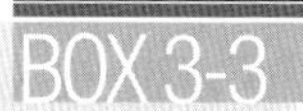

■ **SWITCHING OPIOIDS***

Assuming that the same route is used:

1. Calculate the 24-hour current dose (scheduled + breakthrough).
2. Look up the equianalgesic dose (ED).
3. Calculate the new 24-hour dose using the following formula:

$$\frac{\text{Old opioid ED}}{\text{New opioid ED}} = \frac{\text{24-hr dose of old opioid}}{\text{24-hr dose of new opioid}}$$

4. Reduce the 24-hour dose of the new opioid by 30%–50% if switching high doses (e.g., >2 g morphine per day).
5. Distribute the new 24-hour dose into a scheduled dosing regimen and give 5%–10% of the 24-hour dose prescribed as breakthrough every 1–2 hours.

*This does not apply to methadone because switching to methadone can be dangerous and requires pharmacy consultation.

a. **Diagnosis.** Common causes include bronchospasm, pulmonary edema, secretions, and anxiety.
b. **Treatment** should be directed at the cause, if possible.
   (1) **Bronchodilators** help bronchospasm.
   (2) **Morphine** [by mouth (PO) or intravenously (IV)] treats resting dyspnea in all patients, except those with neuromuscular disease.
   (3) **Oxygen** is appropriate for moderately hypoxemic patients (<90% saturation). For the mildly hypoxemic (90%–94% saturation), the value of oxygen therapy is debatable; sometimes a **fan** is a better option.
   (4) **Sedative-hypnotics** (e.g., diazepam) in small doses help relieve anxiety contributing to dyspnea not responding to morphine.
   (5) **Diuretics** (e.g., furosemide) improve pulmonary edema or ascites.
   (6) **Thoracentesis** reduces dyspnea due to pleural effusion.
   (7) **Paracentesis** reduces intra-abdominal pressure in ascites.
   (8) **Anticholinergics** such as hyoscine hydrobromide, glycopyrronium, amitriptyline, or scopolamine patches reduce oral secretions and the "death rattle."
   (9) **Mechanical ventilation** should be reserved for patients with a **reasonable chance** of recovering to a functional state that is acceptable to them. Patients with

neuromuscular diseases may opt for this mode of therapy because their dyspnea is otherwise resistant to treatment.

3. **Nausea and vomiting** can be very debilitating at the end of life. However, effective control can be achieved in most patients with available treatments. First, conduct a thorough history and physical examination, and then identify the cause and select the therapy accordingly.
   a. **History.** Distinguish vomiting from expectoration or regurgitation.
   b. **Examine** for signs of gastrointestinal obstruction and fecal impaction.
   c. **Diagnosis.** Among terminally ill patients, common causes of nausea and vomiting include increased intracranial pressure; anxiety; pain; medications [e.g., chemotherapy, selective serotonin reuptake inhibitors (SSRIs), opioids]; gastritis (radiation or medication induced); mechanical obstruction/ileus; and metabolic abnormalities (e.g., hypercalcemia, hyponatremia).
   d. **Treatment.** Correct the correctable, then choose a treatment from the list below; you may need to use more than one agent to achieve complete relief.
      (1) **Metoclopramide** is first-line therapy for most patients at the end of life because it reduces the sense of nausea, stimulates GI motility (improves appetite), and is inexpensive. In combination with steroids, it can be as effective as setrons (see next entry). About 3% of patients experience extrapyramidal side effects with metoclopramide.
      (2) **Setron drugs** (e.g., ondansetron) act both centrally and peripherally and are especially effective at preventing and treating chemotherapy-related nausea and vomiting. They are especially useful in patients who are susceptible to the extrapyramidal side effects of other classes.
      (3) **Phenothiazines** (e.g., prochlorperazine, chlorpromazine) possess a broad spectrum of action and are useful for most types of nausea and vomiting. Hypotension, sedation, and decreased salivary flow are their main adverse effects.
      (4) **Anticholinergics** (e.g., hyoscine) help with symptoms related to motion sickness or bowel obstruction.
      (5) **Antihistamines** (e.g., cyclizine) are effective in motion sickness, bowel obstruction, and increased intracranial pressure.
      (6) **Steroids** (e.g., dexamethasone) work well in synergy with setrons, metoclopramide, or phenothiazines.

They are especially useful in patients with increased intracranial pressure.
(7) **Dronabinol** is effective for patients with diffuse metastatic disease affecting the GI tract that is unresponsive to other antiemetics.
(8) **Olanzapine** is an atypical antipsychotic that can relieve nausea in some patients with advanced cancer who fail other antiemetics.

4. **Anxiety** is an unpleasant sense of apprehension often accompanied by physical symptoms such as palpitations, chest pain, tingling, trembling, choking, abdominal pain, sweating, and dizziness. Acute anxiety is common but usually temporary among the dying; it is easily treated.
   a. **History.** Discuss the patient's social situation, fears, and emotions. Identify medical factors that may contribute to anxiety such as medications (e.g., steroids, neuroleptics, SSRIs, stimulants, thyroxine); withdrawal (e.g., alcohol, antidepressants, benzodiazepines); physical symptoms (e.g., pain, dyspnea); metabolic disturbances (e.g., hypercalcemia, hypoglycemia); and psychiatric disorders (e.g., delirium, depression, posttraumatic stress disorder).
   b. **Treatment.** Correct the correctable conditions: relieve pain, correct misconceptions, provide reassurance, and discontinue anxiety-inducing medications. Consider formal psychological support. Pharmacologic treatment may include:
      (1) **Benzodiazepines** (e.g., clonazepam, alprazolam, diazepam, lorazepam)
      (2) **Antidepressants** for contributing depression (e.g., SSRIs)
      (3) **Antipsychotics** when a thought disorder is also present
      (4) **β-Blockers** (e.g., propranolol), which can be useful for relief of accompanying autonomic symptoms
5. **Depression.** Grief is an acceptable response to bad news and progressive decline, but depression is not. It is important to identify depression when it occurs because it is highly treatable (>80% of patients improve).
   a. **History.** Assess if the patient has felt depressed or "blue." To distinguish depression from grief, ask about anhedonia, altered sleep, altered appetite, suicidal ideations, fatigue, psychomotor agitation/retardation, impaired concentration, and feelings of worthlessness. Feelings of depression plus at least four of these symptoms confirm depression.
   b. **Treatment.** Provide therapy for correctable conditions: relieve pain; discontinue depression-inducing medications (e.g., steroids, chemotherapy, phenothiazines,

antihypertensives); treat hypokalemia and hypercalcemia; and rule out hypothyroidism, hypoparathyroidism/hyperparathyroidism, Cushing's syndrome, and hyperprolactinemia. Schedule formal psychological support. In addition, consider using the following agents:

(1) **SSRIs** (e.g., paroxetine, sertraline, citalopram, fluoxetine), starting at the smallest dose, titrating upward every 2 weeks.

(2) **Newer antidepressants** are available as second-line agents or first-line agents under specific circumstances. Duloxetine and venlafaxine are useful for patients with comorbid musculoskeletal pain. Bupropion is useful in patients with anhedonia, fatigue, or manic depression or to counter the sexual side effects of SSRIs. Mirtazapine is useful in patients with weight loss.

(3) **Psychostimulants** (methylphenidate) are very valuable when time is of the essence; these drugs are usually effective within days of initiation. They help with psychomotor retardation, poor appetite, and fatigue. They should be avoided in patients with active coronary artery disease.

6. **Constipation** is common, especially in patients taking opioids.
   a. **History.** Factors that may contribute to constipation include medications (opioids, anticholinergics, tricyclics, SSRIs, antacids, diuretics, anticonvulsants, statins, calcium channel blockers); neurologic disorders (nerve compression, neuropathy); age; inactivity; inability to get to the toilet; lack of privacy; change in diet; dehydration; and depression.
   b. **Physical examination.** Check for obstruction and fecal impaction.
   c. **Diagnosis.** Rule out hypercalcemia and hypokalemia.
   d. **Prevention.** Prevent constipation in patients on opioids by administering a stool softener (docusate) *plus* a motility agent (bisacodyl or senna) daily. Titrate the dose every 2–3 days for a bowel movement at least once every 48 hours. Avoid constipating agents (e.g., fiber, anticholinergics, haloperidol, calcium channel blockers, iron, anticonvulsants).
   e. **Treatment.** For patients who have not had a bowel movement in at least 3 days and who are not impacted, try lactulose orally or glycerin or bisacodyl rectally. Use enemas or polyethylene glycol (1 L PO/NG once) in refractory cases. If impacted, enemas and manual evacuation are needed.

7. **Fatigue** is the most common symptom at the end of life. Because little is known about its mechanism, treatment may be less successful.
   a. **Diagnosis.** Identify treatable causes such as hypothyroidism; anemia; depression; anxiety; pain; infection; medications (e.g., chemotherapy, antihypertensives); insomnia; and hypoxemia.
   b. **Treatment**
      (1) **Corticosteroids** (dexamethasone 2–20 mg PO every morning) can improve mood, energy, and appetite temporarily. Long-term sequelae are not of concern. Prevent thrush with nystatin 1 teaspoon swish-and-swallow three times daily.
      (2) **Psychostimulants** (methylphenidate 2.5–5 mg PO twice daily) can improve mood, energy, and appetite rapidly, but the effect of these drugs is variable. Psychostimulants are contraindicated in patients with agitation, psychosis or active coronary artery disease.

D. Set goals of care. Assess what the patient and family are hoping for given the situation.

E. Talk to patient and family. Never break bad news or discuss grave matters without offering the patient the opportunity to be accompanied by loved ones. Provide a proper setting with privacy, space, and plenty of tissues.

F. Arrange plans based on the goals set by the patient and family. Address the following seven elements:

1. A **living will** gives the patient the opportunity to document his or her preferences regarding life-sustaining treatment. It takes effect only when the patient loses decision-making capacity and can be revoked by the patient at any time, either in writing or verbally. A living will is not equivalent to a Last Will and Testament.
2. **Durable power of attorney for health care (DPAHC)** allows a patient to appoint a proxy (or proxies) to decide on his or her behalf; it takes effect only when the patient loses decision-making capacity. In most states, the authority of the DPAHC supersedes the living will. Many patients confuse the durable power of attorney for health care with the executor of their will or their financial power of attorney, but they are not necessarily the same.
3. **Do not resuscitate (DNR) and do not intubate (DNI) orders.** These are physicians' orders to staff *not* to attempt cardiopulmonary resuscitation (CPR) or intubation in the event of cardiopulmonary arrest. **They are the only way to prevent CPR; a living will is not sufficient to prevent CPR.**
   a. It is the physician's responsibility to write DNR or DNI orders as soon as the patient or the DPAHC refuses

CPR, or the physician believes that CPR would be futile.[1]

b. The issue of DNR can be raised by asking, "Should you die in spite of our best efforts, do you want us to use heroic measures to attempt to bring you back?" If the patient declines CPR, ask him or her to explain his or her rationale. Document the contents of your discussion and encourage the patient to complete a living will or appoint a DPAHC if he or she has not done so already. **Even if the patient refuses to sign a living will, however, this plan is valid as long as you document the discussion in the medical record.** A physician may even ask a patient to sign a statement that they both believe reflects their discussion.

4. **Hospice** is a multidisciplinary service that supports the patient and family through dying and bereavement. Its mission is to relieve physical, emotional, social, and spiritual suffering. Hospice can provide care at home, hospice facilities, hospitals, or nursing homes. Often hospices limit their care to patients with a life expectancy of 6 months or less who have agreed to a DNR order.
5. **Palliative care,** like hospice, is a multidisciplinary service that seeks to relieve physical, emotional, social, and spiritual suffering. Unlike hospice, however, palliative care cares for all patients, regardless of their diagnosis or life expectancy, and is typically offered only in hospitals or hospital-affiliated clinics. Palliative care is appropriate for patients who are chronically or terminally ill, to bridge the gap between curative therapy and hospice care.
6. **"Comfort care"** describes care focusing on comfort rather than cure. When patients and families choose to pursue "comfort care only," it is appropriate to discontinue all medications and treatments that do not directly relieve symptoms (e.g., taking of vital signs; administration of antihypertensives, hypoglycemics, hormone replacement therapy, and anticoagulants). Remember that "comfort care" does not mean "no care."
7. **Life support.** Any therapy used to sustain life is considered life support, including, but not limited to, artificial nutrition and hydration, mechanical ventilation, dialysis, and implantable defibrillators. According to the U.S. Supreme Court, all competent patients and their proxies have the right to refuse or stop life support (even after it has been initiated). If a family decides to withdraw life support, make sure they understand that there are several potential

[1]Hospitals differ regarding their futility policies; thus, it is important to know your institution's futility policy.

outcomes: rapid death within minutes (e.g., patients who have vasopressors withdrawn); death within hours to days; or continued cardiopulmonary function. Assure them that the patient's comfort is paramount.

G. Reassess often. As illness advances, patients experience varying physical and psychological symptoms and, as a result, may change their priorities, goals, and plans. For this reason, it is important to reassess and reinform often; the frequency of communication should be determined by the speed of decline.

III. AFTER DEATH

A. Pronouncement. A licensed physician is responsible for pronouncing death and comforting the family. If you are called to "pronounce" someone, first talk to nursing staff and read the medical record to familiarize yourself with the patient's history. Confirm that the attending of record has been notified. Once you enter the patient's room, introduce yourself to the family, offer condolences, and explain why you are there. Give them the opportunity to ask questions and stay if they wish while you examine their loved one. Then do the following:

1. Identify the patient by the hospital identification tag.
2. Ascertain that the patient is nonresponsive to verbal or tactile stimuli (a sternal rub is sufficient).
3. Confirm absence of heart sounds and pulse.
4. Look and listen for spontaneous respirations for at least 1 minute.
5. Confirm that pupils are "fixed and dilated."
6. Record your findings and the time of your assessment as the time of death. Document who was notified of the patient's death.

B. Responding to grief. Grief is a normal response to loss or impending loss. Encourage open discussion, acknowledge feelings, and offer reassurance that grief is normal. Follow up with written condolences, a telephone call, and an appointment, as appropriate. Warn the grieving family that vivid dreams and tearful memories of the departed loved one may persist for several months and that a loss of interest in outside activities will likely persist for 3–6 months. Offer a referral to grief counseling for ongoing support.

REFERENCES

Cleary JF. The pharmacologic management of cancer pain. J Palliat Med 2007;10(6):1369–1394.

National Consensus Project. Clinical Practice Guidelines for Quality Palliative Care. Pittsburgh, PA: National Consensus Project, 2007.

Eduardo Bruera, Irene J. Higginson, Carla Ripamonti, Charles F. Ion Gunten. Textbook of Palliative Medicine. London: Hodder Arnold, 2006.

■ Preventing Hospital-Acquired Complications

4

I. INTRODUCTION

A. As many as **10% of inpatients** experience harm unrelated to any underlying illness during their hospital stay. Approximately **2% of hospitalized patients** experience either a major permanent injury or death as a result of their medical care.

B. Although clinicians have long recognized the hazards of hospitalization, patient safety has only recently received widespread attention.

C. The term **adverse event** refers to any injury caused by medical care, not an underlying illness.

1. Identifying something as an adverse event does not imply "error" or poor-quality care. However, errors often cause adverse events.
2. Thus, just as physicians target blood pressure control to reduce myocardial infarction and stroke, targeting errors plays a role in preventing many adverse events.

On patient problem lists, include a section focused on the prevention of nosocomial complications as the last item (e.g., screening for potential medication problems, thromboembolism prophylaxis, complications of indwelling catheters, development of pressure ulcers, provision of adequate nutrition).

II. HOSPITAL-ACQUIRED COMPLICATIONS AND THEIR PREVENTION

A. Adverse drug event (ADE)

1. **Definition**
   a. An ADE refers to **any adverse clinical effect resulting from a drug.** This broad term includes minor drug rashes and major reactions such as bone marrow suppression, hepatic failure, and anaphylaxis. It also combines **expected adverse reactions** (i.e., "side effects" occurring when a drug is used in standard doses to achieve accepted therapeutic goals) and **harm resulting from medication errors**

(e.g., dosing errors, prescription of medication to which a patient has a documented allergy, or ordering a medication for the wrong patient, as can easily happen in the hospital setting).

b. The issue of preventability is more important than the distinction between ADEs that are "side effects" and those that are due to errors.

c. An ADE can reflect factors arising at **any stage of the medication use process,** although drug ordering accounts for approximately 50% of ADEs.

2. **Incidence. At least 5% of hospitalized patients** experience an ADE. An additional **5%–10% of hospitalized patients** experience a **potential ADE** (i.e., a medication error occurs but fortuitously, no harm results).

3. **Prevention.** Many ADEs, whether "side effects" or the result of errors, can be anticipated and therefore prevented from occurring, or at least ameliorated if they do occur.

   a. **Medication information.** Keep a trustworthy medication resource—whether in a paper-based, electronic handheld, or computer-based form—with you at all times and use it to verify standard doses, routes of administration, contraindications, and adverse effects. When such a resource is not readily available or fails to address a specific issue, seek the advice of a pharmacist.

An important contraindication to any medication is a physician's lack of familiarity with it.

      (1) For elderly patients and patients receiving multiple medications, periodically review orders for potential drug interactions.

      (2) Be particularly careful with human immunodeficiency virus (HIV) medications, immunosuppressant drugs, anticoagulants, and chemotherapeutic agents (all of which you may be called on to write orders for), and be cautious with all medications in patients with renal or hepatic dysfunction.

   b. **Ordering.** Write all orders legibly (print if you have to), avoid abbreviations, and watch out for decimals (Table 4-1).

      (1) **Avoid abbreviations for drug names** to reduce the risk of misinterpretation [e.g., HCTZ (hydrochlorothiazide) versus HCT (hydrocortisone), MSO_4

TABLE 4-1

PRESCRIPTION ORDER WRITING: DO'S AND DON'TS

Do	Don't	Explanation
0.5 mg	.5 mg	The leading zero avoids a 10-fold overdose caused by an overlooked decimal point.
5 mg	5.0 mg	Dropping the trailing zero avoids a 10-fold overdose caused by an overlooked decimal point.
NPH Insulin 10 units	NPH Insulin 10 U	"U" can be misread as a trailing zero.
Synthroid 100 mcg	Synthroid 100 μg	"μg" is more likely to be misread as "mg" for milligram.
Coumadin 5 mg PO every other day	Coumadin 5 mg PO qod	"qod" can easily be misread as "qd." For handwritten orders, many sources now recommend dropping all abbreviations for frequency (e.g., qd, bid) in favor of such terms as "once daily" and "twice daily."
Change ranitidine 150 mg PO bid to 50 mg IV q8h	Change ranitidine PO to IV	Not writing out full order risks inappropriate "carry-over" drug strength and frequency.

(morphine) versus $MgSO_4$ (magnesium sulfate), CPZ (Compazine versus chlorpromazine)].

(2) **Always write complete and specific orders.** Do not drop units, omit frequencies, or leave route of administration unspecified (see Table 4-1).

(3) **Never write blanket orders** such as "continue all preop meds."

(4) **Always check for drug allergies;** do not assume someone else has done so.

(5) **Always check the patient's name** at the top of the record (chart or computer based) before writing an order. It is easy to pick up the wrong chart or walk away from the computer for a minute and not realize that someone has opened another patient's electronic record.

c. **Transcription** is out of your hands, but know that such errors occur and can affect patient care, especially during transitions [e.g., transfer in or out of an intensive care unit (ICU)].

Periodically check the nursing medication administration records to make sure that patients are receiving their ordered medications by the prescribed route and in the intended doses. *This is especially important when a patient is not responding to treatment or has an unexpected change in course (e.g., if a patient with pneumonia is not improving, before changing antibiotics, make sure he or she is in fact receiving the antibiotics you have already ordered).*

d. **Dispensing errors** [e.g., mix-ups in the central pharmacy that result in the wrong medication being sent to the floor or an incorrect concentration of an intravenous (IV) medication being compounded] are also out of your hands, but recognize that such mistakes can occur.
   (1) For example, suppose pulseless ventricular tachycardia develops in a patient in the ICU. The tracing is suggestive of "torsades de pointes," and the event occurred after the nurse had performed a "flush" of the patient's central venous line.
   (2) The physician empirically administers calcium and insulin as treatment for hyperkalemia, which restores sinus rhythm.
   (3) Laboratory results later confirm hyperkalemia, and further investigation reveals that the intended normal saline flush had in fact been concentrated potassium.

When evaluating an unexpected clinical event, include the possibility of error on your differential diagnosis.

e. **Administration errors** are mostly out of your hands (e.g., programming errors for the IV pump administering patient-controlled analgesia or concentrated electrolyte solution), but recognize that they occur.
   (1) **Physician administration.** Sometimes you will be called on to administer a drug **because nurses are not supposed to administer it** at all (e.g., adenosine) or by "IV push" (e.g., fentanyl on many general hospital wards).

Do not treat calls to administer medication (e.g., IV metoprolol on a general ward) as an annoying formality. Make sure you actually know how to administer the medication, including speed of administration, need for central line versus peripheral line, compatibility with other medications, and responses to possible complications.

(2) **Automated dispensing machines.** Medications stored and dispensed in automated machines can end up in the wrong drawer, leading to dangerous drug substitutions. Multiuse vials can be mistaken for one another (e.g., heparin and insulin look enough alike, and several deaths have been reported due to "line flushes" with insulin instead of heparin).

f. **Anticipate preventable complications (and respond in timely fashion to nonpreventable ones).**

(1) **Interactions with warfarin**

(a) **Increased international normalization ratio (INR):** Administration of many medications increases the INR and bleeding risk in patients taking vitamin K antagonists. Thus, a substantial elevation in INR and development of bleeding after initiating amiodarone in a patient on warfarin (e.g., for atrial fibrillation) represents a **preventable ADE.** In such cases, increase the frequency and vigilance of anticoagulation monitoring.

(b) Major medication interactions with warfarin can be grouped into the **8As:** (1) most **antibiotics**; (2) **antifungals** (fluconazole, miconazole); (3) serotonergic **antidepressants**; (4) **amiodarone**; (5) **acetaminophen**; (6) **antiplatelet** agents; (7) **anti-inflammatory agents** (traditional NSAIDs and selective COX-2 inhibitors); and (8) **alternative remedies** (dong quai, fenugreek, chamomile, St. John's wort, gingko biloba). St. John's wort and rifampin decrease the activity of warfarin; the rest increase activity and thus increase the risk of bleeding.

(2) **Steroids**

(a) A **vertebral compression fracture** occurs in a patient with chronic obstructive pulmonary disease (COPD) who is administered chronic steroids. This complication should be anticipated and is a **preventable** ADE, because the concomitant prescription of a bisphosphonate can significantly reduce the risk of osteoporotic fracture.

(b) **Psychosis** occurs in a patient with COPD who is administered steroids. This is a **nonpreventable** ADE. However, appropriate care ameliorates the ADE with early recognition of this complication and cessation or rapid tapering of the steroids.

B. Venous thromboembolism (VTE)

1. **Definition.** Nosocomial VTE most commonly includes lower extremity deep venous thrombosis (DVT) but also includes pulmonary embolism and upper extremity DVT.
2. **Incidence.** VTE may be as common among medical as among surgical patients. One recent study found that 15% of acutely ill medical patients had DVT. In addition to immobility, central venous catheters contribute to hospital-acquired thromboses.

Nonmobile medical patients (e.g., unable to get out of bed) should receive some form of VTE prophylaxis.

3. **Prevention**
   a. Low-dose subcutaneous unfractionated heparin (e.g., heparin 5000 units subcutaneously two or three times a day)
   b. Low-molecular-weight heparin: look up recommended dose for prophylaxis, not therapeutic anticoagulation, for whichever agent is used in your hospital.
   c. Fondaparinux (not routinely used in medical patients, but supported by the literature)
   d. The literature now favors pharmacologic over mechanical methods of prophylaxis (e.g., pneumatic compression stockings). Mechanical methods are reasonable in patients at high risk for bleeding, but make sure stockings are applied correctly (often not the case).

C. Falls

1. **Incidence.** Inpatient falls occur at a rate of 0.5–3 per bed per year. **Hip fractures** are the most feared complication of falls. Up to 20% of patients sustaining a hip fracture become nonambulatory, and many of these individuals lose their ability to carry out instrumental activities of daily living.
2. **Risk factors.** Presence of handrails and no-slip bathing surfaces may mitigate the risk of falls or fall-related injury. Factors associated with hospitals such as unfamiliar rooms, improper bed height, and sedating medications may exacerbate risk. Acute illness itself and deconditioning from being bedridden also increase the risk of falls.

3. **Prevention.** Various strategies exist for assessing patients at high risk for falls and addressing these risks; appropriate strategies for a given patient are often best discussed with nursing staff.
   a. **Avoid using sedating or disorienting medications.**
   b. **Limit use of restraints and handrails,** which may paradoxically increase risks of falls or the severity of fall-related injuries.

At a minimum, identify patients at high risk for falls and discuss possible interventions with nursing staff (e.g., closer monitoring of patient, placing bed as low to ground as possible, use of bed alarms if available).

D. Radiocontrast-induced nephropathy (RCIN)

1. **Definition**
   a. Specific definitions vary, but clinically significant RCIN typically requires a 50% increase in serum creatinine (SCr) or a 1.0 mg/dl increase in SCr within 48 hours of intravascular radiocontrast exposure.
   b. The hallmark of RCIN is that it resolves quickly (within 7–10 days) and rarely requires specific therapy.
2. **Incidence.** Risk factors for RCIN include diabetes, chronic renal insufficiency, decreased effective circulating volume of any cause, and multiple myeloma.
   a. For patients **with no risk factors,** the incidence is almost zero.
   b. For patients **with risk factors,** the incidence ranges from 5%–40%, depending on the number and severity of risk factors. RCIN occurs in more than 50% of patients with SCr greater than 4.0 mg/dl.
3. **Treatment.** Dialysis is rarely required, and even then, it is usually temporary. Thus, concern about RCIN should not prevent necessary investigations that involve contrast.
4. **Prevention.** Despite the mild and temporary nature of RCIN, increased monitoring and delays in other aspects of care make prevention worthwhile.
   a. **Avoid drugs that decrease renal perfusion** [e.g., nonsteroidal anti-inflammatory drugs (NSAIDs)][1]

---

[1]Although not a prophylactic strategy per se, metformin is usually discontinued before any procedure that may affect renal function and resumed only when normal renal function is verified. Thus, metformin is commonly discontinued in diabetic patients who undergo cardiac catheterization at least 12 hours before the procedure.

b. **Avoid hypovolemia,** especially in patients with diabetes or preexisting renal problems. Typical protocols for ensuring adequate volume status consist of normal saline administered at 75 ml/hr for 12 hours preprocedure and postprocedure or ingestion of 1 L of water within 10 hours before the procedure, followed by IV normal saline for 6 hours after the procedure. Using isotonic bicarbonate (e.g., prepared by adding 3 amps of $NaHCO_3$ to 1 L of dextrose) may be superior to isotonic saline. The protocol used in one trial administered a bolus of the IV isotonic bicarbonate at 3 mL/kg/hr for 1 hour prior to contrast, followed by a 1 mL/kg/hr infusion for 6 hours afterward.

c. For high-risk patients (e.g., diabetics with moderate renal insufficiency), **consider using low-osmolar contrast agents or limiting the volume of contrast** (<75–125 ml). Also, avoid repeated contrast exposures within 48–72 hours.

d. For any patient with chronic renal insufficiency, **consider acetylcysteine** in addition to IV saline. The drug is administered as powder-containing capsules or diluted in soda or juice. Give 600 mg orally twice daily on the day before and after the procedure. If only one dose is given before the procedure, give three doses afterward.

E. Stress-related upper gastrointestinal hemorrhage (UGIH)

1. **Incidence**

a. Clinically significant UGIH occurs in only approximately 0.1% of low-risk ICU patients and approximately 3.0% of ventilated patients.

b. General improvements in ICU care and greater focus on clinically significant events have substantially reduced the frequency of stress-induced gastric ulceration among ICU patients.

2. **Prevention.** Although a statistical benefit of H_2-antagonists has been shown in some studies, the overall clinical benefit of stress ulcer prophylaxis in unselected patients is equivocal.

Do not reflexively prescribe antiacid medications to all ICU patients. Focus on patients with risk factors for UGIH: respiratory failure, coagulopathy, renal failure, and significant burns.

a. For patients without specific risk factors for UGIH, **provide enteral nutrition;** this is probably the best method of prevention.
b. H_2-antagonists are probably superior to sucralfate in preventing stress-related GI bleeding but may increase the risk of ventilator-associated pneumonia.
c. Unfortunately, the proper role of proton pump inhibitors is currently unclear.

F. Catheter-related urinary tract infection (UTI)

1. **Incidence.** Catheterized patients develop bacteriuria at a rate of 3%–10% per day. Among patients with bacteriuria, about 10% develop UTI symptoms such as suprapubic or flank pain, and approximately 3% develop bacteremia.

Make sure you know which of your patients have a urinary catheter and why they still have one.

2. **Prevention. Remove indwelling catheters as soon as possible.**
   a. Urinary catheters not only may lead to infection but also are a source of significant discomfort and embarrassment to many patients.
   b. Condom catheters may lower the risk of UTIs in certain patients and also tend to be more comfortable for male patients.
   c. Some evidence supports the effectiveness of antimicrobial (e.g., silver-coated, nitrofurazone-releasing) urinary catheters. These more expensive catheters may be appropriate in patients at high risk for infection.

G. Pressure (decubitus) ulcers. Complications include cellulitis, osteomyelitis, sepsis, and even death.

1. **Incidence**
   a. From 3%–10% of hospitalized patients have pressure ulcers; approximately 60% of these developed in the hospital as opposed to being present on admission from a nursing facility or home care setting.
   b. The prevalence is much higher for immobilized patients; about 30% of elderly patients with a fractured hip develop pressure ulcers in the postoperative period.
2. **Prevention**
   a. **Inspect all hospitalized patients for early signs of pressure ulcers** such as erythema over key pressure points (e.g., sacrum, greater trochanter, ischial tuberosity, malleolus, heel, scapula).

b. **Identify patients at risk for development of pressure ulcers** by checking for immobility (e.g., due to neurologic disorder or fracture), malnutrition, fecal or urinary incontinence, and altered level of consciousness. Patients at risk for pressure ulcers should have pillows placed beneath the calves, foam foot protection, or a soft foam or air waffle mattress.

c. **Make sure patients who are unable to move around in bed are "turned" or repositioned** every 2 hours.

H. Central venous catheter (CVC)–related infection

1. **Incidence.** Among patients with a standard CVC in place for 1 week or more, approximately 25% develop catheter colonization and 5% become bacteremic. Catheter-related bloodstream infections occur at a rate of about 5 per 1000 catheter-days in medical and surgical ICUs.
2. **Prevention**

a. **Use maximum sterile barrier precautions** during CVC insertion, with sterile gloves, a long-sleeved gown, a full-sized drape, and a nonsterile mask cap, rather than just a small drape and gloves.

b. **Use chlorhexidine gluconate** rather than povidone-iodine for antiseptic cleaning of the insertion site.

c. In patients at high risk for infection (e.g., ICU patients), consider using a CVC coated with an antimicrobial agent.

d. **Subclavian** and **internal jugular** sites have a lower risk of infection than femoral insertion. However, in urgent situations, if you do not feel comfortable working at these insertion sites, it is better to place a femoral catheter. When adequate supervision is available, a subclavian or internal jugular line can be placed if a CVC will be required for more than 48 hours.

e. **Remove the CVC as soon as the clinical indication resolves.** Do not continue with the CVC simply for convenience, especially if the patient is going to be transferred to a regular floor, where knowledge of CVC care is variable.

Always place the patient in the supine position when removing a CVC from the subclavian or internal jugular sites to avoid catastrophic air embolism.

I. Ventilator-associated pneumonia (VAP). The effect of VAP on clinical outcomes varies depending on the organisms involved and comorbid conditions. Nonetheless, VAP is an important complication that affects patient care.

1. **Incidence.** The cumulative incidence is approximately 1%–3% per day of intubation. In clinical practice, VAP is usually diagnosed on the basis of radiographic findings or positive endotracheal, pleural, or blood cultures in the setting of fever, leukocytosis, or purulent tracheal secretions.
2. **Prevention.** Several strategies show promise in terms of significantly reducing the incidence of VAP, including using special endotracheal tubes that remove subglottic secretions, selective digestive tract decontamination, using endotracheal tubes coated with silver, appropriate oral care, and rotation of empiric antibiotic regimens.

Unless contraindicated (e.g., hemodynamic instability), elevate the patient's head of the bed to 45° for the duration of mechanical ventilation; this is a simple and likely effective strategy for reducing VAP.

III. GENERAL ERRORS. Although the complications described in II should be considered in the care of hospitalized patients, more general opportunities for serious errors and complications should also be kept in mind.

A. Pay attention to internal warning signals.

1. **Haste produces iatrogenesis.** When you notice yourself feeling overwhelmed, rushed, or pressed for time (e.g., you cannot possibly handle all of your work), step back and take a few minutes to gather your thoughts.
2. **If you need a hand, ask for it.** Do not make being a "strong" student or resident your first priority. When you are in over your head, admit you need someone to walk you through a procedure or that you have fallen too far behind on call to handle all of the waiting admissions.

B. Communicate with nurses, pharmacists, and physicians from other services involved in your patients' care. Many minor errors, as well as some spectacular errors (e.g., taking the wrong patient for a procedure), occur because of poor communication among physicians or between physicians and nurses.

1. **Communicate important changes in patient care plans to all clinical personnel,** including closely involved outpatient physicians.
2. Conversely, if you are surprised to find a new order or care plan for your patient, **do not assume** that a clinician has simply devised a new plan and not told you. **Check out the new plan** yourself.

C. **Communicate clearly with patients in a manner they understand.** Nearly 25% of adults in the United States are functionally illiterate, and even more have inadequate **health literacy.** More than 50% of patients seen in public hospitals do not understand common medical terms such as "malignant," "terminal," or even "orally." Basic medication instructions such as "take every 6 hours" or "take on an empty stomach" are poorly understood by at least 25% of patients, and more than 50% cannot reliably interpret a blood sugar reading.
   1. **Slow down and use "living room" language** instead of medical terminology; show or draw pictures whenever possible.
   2. **Ask, "Can you tell me what we have just gone through?" or other such "teach-back" approaches to confirm understanding.** Do not simply ask, "Do you understand?" Usually, the answer will be, "Yes," regardless of the amount of comprehension.
   3. **Limit information conveyed during a single interaction.** Do not overwhelm patients with information, especially in the emergency department, ICU, or a first-time meeting in the middle of the night.

REFERENCES

Davis TC, Wolf MS, Bass PF 3rd, et al. Literacy and misunderstanding prescription drug labels. Ann Intern Med 2006;145:887–894.

Dentali F, Douketis JD, Gianni M, et al. Meta-analysis: anticoagulant prophylaxis to prevent symptomatic venous thromboembolism in hospitalized medical patients. Ann Intern Med 2007;146:278–288.

Gallagher TH, Studdert D, Levinson W. Disclosing harmful medical errors to patients. N Engl J Med 2007;356:2713–2719.

Lazare A. Apology in medical practice: an emerging clinical skill. JAMA 2006;296:1401–1404.

Muscedere J, Dodek P, Keenan S, et al. Comprehensive evidence-based clinical practice guidelines for ventilator-associated pneumonia: diagnosis and treatment. J Crit Care 2008;23:138–147.

Pronovost P, Needham D, Berenholtz S, et al. An intervention to decrease catheter-related bloodstream infections in the ICU. N Engl J Med 2006;355:2725–2732.

Ranji SR, Shojania KG. Implementing patient safety interventions in your hospital: what to try and what to avoid. Med Clin North Am 2008;92:275–193, vii–viii.

Shojania KG, Fletcher KE, Saint S. Graduate medical education and patient safety: a busy—and occasionally hazardous—intersection. Ann Intern Med 2006;145:592–598.

Tam VC, Knowles SR, Cornish PL, et al. Frequency, type and clinical importance of medication history errors at admission to hospital: a systematic review. CMAJ 2005;173:510–515.

5 Electrocardiogram (ECG) Interpretation

I. INTRODUCTION. There is no absolute right order for interpreting electrocardiograms (ECGs), but it is important to choose a method and interpret each ECG in precisely the same way each and every time. One common approach is to evaluate ECG findings in the following order: rhythm, rate, axis, intervals, hypertrophy, Q waves, and ST/T-wave changes.

II. RHYTHM

A. Normal sinus rhythm. If each normal P wave (atrial depolarization) is followed by a QRS complex (ventricular depolarization) and the heart rate is between 60 and 100 beats/min, then the patient is in normal sinus rhythm. A "normal" P wave is positively deflected (or above the baseline) in leads I, II, and aVF.

B. Tachycardia is a heart rate greater than 100 beats/min (see Chapter 7).

C. Bradycardia is a heart rate less than 60 beats/min.

1. **Sinus bradycardia.** Each QRS complex is preceded by a normal P wave.
2. Other forms of bradycardia [e.g., atrioventricular (AV) nodal block] are discussed in V A 2.

III. RATE

A. Regular rhythm. If the patient is in sinus rhythm, the easiest way to calculate the heart rate is to divide 300 by the number of large boxes between two successive QRS complexes. (Each large box is composed of five small boxes, each of which represents 0.04 second.)

B. Irregular rhythm. If the patient has an irregular heart rate, count the number of QRS complexes over a 10-second period. Multiply the number by 6 to obtain the number of beats per minute. (Ten-second periods are equivalent to 50 large boxes and usually are the entire duration of an ECG if taken at a normal speed.)

C. Bradycardia. If the patient's heart rate is very slow, it is easy to see how many beats occurred over a 10-second period.

TABLE 5-1

USING THE ECG TO DETERMINE HEART RATE FOR PATIENTS IN SINUS RHYTHM*

Number of Boxes	Corresponding Heart Rate
1	300 beats/min
2	150 beats/min
3	100 beats/min
4	75 beats/min
5	60 beats/min

*Divide 300 by the number of large boxes between two successive QRS complexes.

Multiply the number by 6 to obtain the number of beats per minute.

IV. AXIS. The QRS axis, typically measured in the frontal plane, is the net vector generated by all ventricular depolarization. The exact degree of the vector (axis) is not clinically useful—it is only necessary to determine whether the axis is normal, shifted left, or shifted right. Left and right axis shifts suggest disease of the ventricular myocardium.

A. Normal axis. A normal axis is between –30° and +90° when plotted using a hexaxial reference system. Anything more negative than –30° is called a leftward or superior axis (because the axis is moving left toward the 12 o'clock position), and anything more positive than +90° is a rightward axis.

B. Determining axis (Figure 5-1). By inspecting the QRS complex in each limb lead, you can narrow down where the net vector (QRS axis) is pointing.

C. To evaluate axis, it is only necessary to look at limb leads I and II.

1. **Normal axis.** Both lead I and lead II are positive.
2. **Leftward axis.** Lead I is positive and lead II is negative.
3. **Rightward axis.** Lead I is negative and lead II is positive.
4. **Indeterminate axis.** Both lead I and lead II are negative.

D. Causes of axis deviation

1. **Left axis deviation (LAD).** Left anterior fascicular block and inferior wall myocardial infarction account for most cases of LAD.

   a. **Left anterior fascicular block**

      (1) **Pathogenesis.** The left bundle splits into anterior and posterior fascicles. The anterior fascicle runs superiorly; therefore, when the anterior fascicle is

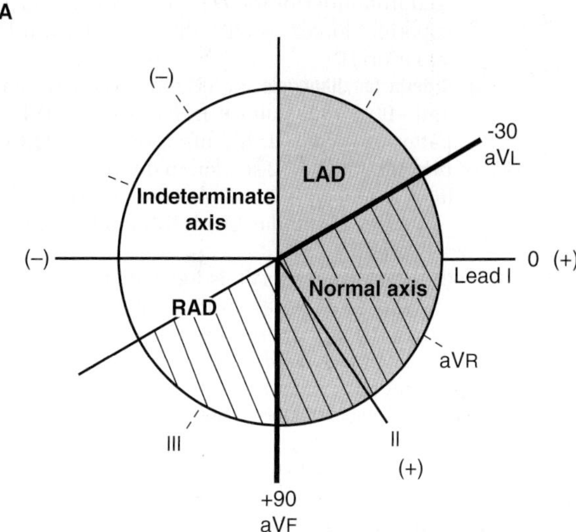

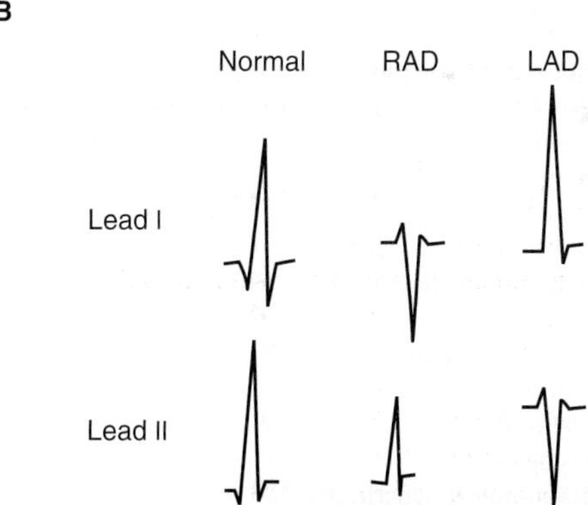

Figure 5-1 (*A*) Determining axis. If the QRS complex of lead I is net positive (i.e., the area above the horizontal is greater than the area below), the axis must lie somewhere in the *gray shaded* region. If lead II is net positive, then the axis must lie in the *cross-hatched* region. The area of overlap denotes the range for a normal axis. (*B*) Appearance of the QRS complex in leads I and II in left axis deviation (*LAD*), right axis deviation (*RAD*), and normal axis.

blocked, the muscle that it serves must be depolarized from inferior forces. These "extra" inferior to superior forces rotate the axis leftward (i.e., superiorly).

(2) **Criteria for diagnosis** include an axis between –45° and –90°; a qR pattern in leads I and aVL; an rS pattern in leads II, III, and aVF; and a QRS complex less than 0.12 second in duration.

(a) An axis of –30° to –45° may represent left anterior fascicular block if the other criteria are present.

(b) Because lead aVL is located near the left anterior fascicle (at approximately –30°), a block in the left anterior fascicle causes initial forces to move away from lead aVL, producing the qR pattern and delay in peak time.

b. **Inferior wall myocardial infarction**

(1) **Pathogenesis.** Dead tissue at the inferior aspect of the left ventricle does not conduct; therefore, more net forces move superiorly (or leftward).

(2) **Criteria for diagnosis.** Look for abnormal Q waves in the inferior leads (i.e., leads II, III, and aVF) to make the diagnosis.

c. **Posteroseptal accessory pathway.** Look for negative delta waves in the inferior leads, a short PR interval (<0.12 second in duration), and a tall R wave in lead V2.

d. **Chronic obstructive pulmonary disease (COPD).** A lower diaphragm can move the right ventricle below the larger left ventricle and cause more superior forces. However, when accompanied by pulmonary hypertension, COPD often produces right axis deviation (RAD).

e. **Congenital heart disease** (e.g., primum-type atrial septal defect, ventricular septal defect)

f. **Hyperkalemia** (usually severe)

g. **Pulmonary embolus** can produce LAD but more often produces RAD.

h. **Normal variant**

2. **Right axis deviation**

a. **Right ventricular hypertrophy.** RAD is caused by right ventricular hypertrophy until proven otherwise. (Criteria for right ventricular hypertrophy are discussed in VI B).

b. **Acute cor pulmonale** (e.g., pulmonary embolus, acute bronchospasm). Look for a shift of axis to the right of more than 30° when compared with a prior ECG.

c. **Extensive lateral wall myocardial infarction.** Look for Q waves in leads I and aVL.

d. **Lateral wall accessory pathway.** Look for a short PR interval.
e. **Left posterior fascicular block** should be considered a diagnosis of exclusion. **Criteria for diagnosis** include an axis between +90° and +180°; an rS pattern in leads I and aVL; a qR pattern in leads II, III, and aVF; and a QRS complex less than 0.12 second in duration.
f. **Lead reversal.** Look for an inverted P wave in lead I.
g. **Pneumothorax**
h. **Normal variant** (in young people)

V. INTERVALS

A. PR interval. The PR interval is normally between 0.12 second and 0.20 second in duration (three to five small boxes). The appropriate measurement is actually from the beginning of the P wave to the beginning of the Q wave, not the R wave.

1. A **short PR interval** is often caused by a high catecholamine state that makes the AV node conduct faster; however, you should look for delta waves to rule out an accessory pathway. Other causes include ectopic atrial rhythms originating near the AV node, so look for P waves with abnormal morphology in leads I, II, and aVF.
2. A **prolonged PR interval** is associated with increased vagal tone or more permanent disease to the **conduction system.**
   a. **First-degree AV nodal block.** If each P wave is followed by a QRS complex at a longer than normal interval (>0.20 second or one large box), a first-degree AV nodal block is diagnosed.
   b. **Second-degree AV nodal block.** In second-degree AV nodal block, some P waves are not followed by a QRS complex, producing varying degrees of bradycardia.
      (1) **Type I second-degree AV nodal block (Wenckebach)** is characterized by progressive PR prolongation culminating with a nonconducted P wave.
      (2) **Type II second-degree AV nodal block (Mobitz)** is characterized by constant PR intervals preceding a nonconducted P wave.
   c. **Third-degree AV nodal block.** P waves and QRS complexes are completely unrelated, with the atrial rate faster than the ventricular rate.

B. QRS interval. The QRS interval is normally less than 0.1 second in duration. Measurement is from the beginning of the Q wave to the end of the S wave.

1. **Interventricular conduction delay** or **incomplete bundle branch block** is diagnosed when the QRS complex is 0.1–0.12 second in duration.

2. **Bundle branch block** is diagnosed when the QRS complex is greater than 0.12 second in duration ("widened").
   a. **Pathogenesis.** If the right bundle is blocked, depolarization must proceed down the left bundle and then slowly to the right from muscle fiber to muscle fiber. Muscle conducts slowly compared with the specialized bundles; therefore, the QRS complex will be wider than normal, and the late electrical forces will move to the right. Similarly, a left bundle branch block will also have a wide QRS complex, and the late forces will move to the left.
   b. **Diagnosis**
      (1) **Determining the direction of the late forces** (Figure 5-2). Draw a line down the middle of the QRS complex in lead V1 (a rightward lead) and lead V6 (a leftward lead). The half of the QRS complex to the right of the line represents the "late" forces. Check if these are positive (above the horizontal) or negative (below the horizontal).
      (2) **Interpretation**
         (a) **Right bundle branch block.** If the late forces of V1 are positive and those of V6 are negative, then the late forces are moving toward the right

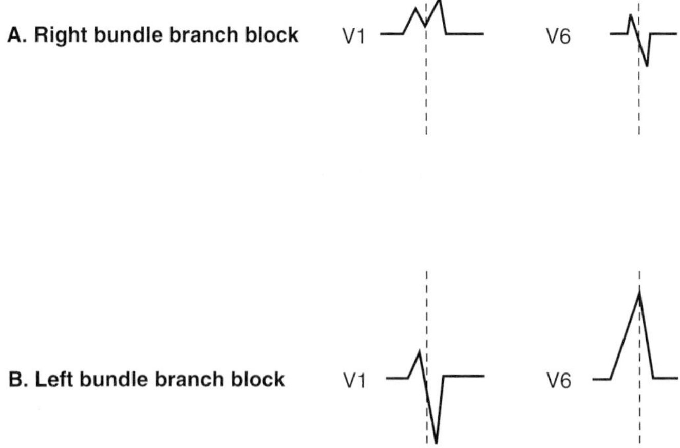

Figure 5-2 Determining the direction of the late forces. (*A*) Right bundle branch block. The late forces are positive in lead V1 and negative in lead V6. (*B*) Left bundle branch block. The late forces are negative in lead V1 and positive in lead V6.

from the left, signifying a right bundle branch block.

(b) **Left bundle branch block.** If the late forces of V6 are positive and those of V1 are negative, then the late forces are moving toward the left from the right, indicating a left bundle branch block.

(c) **Nonspecific interventricular bundle branch block** is often diagnosed when V1 and V6 are both negative or both positive.

C. QT interval. The QT interval varies according to the heart rate, lengthening as the heart rate decreases. Measurement is from the beginning of the Q wave to the end of the T wave. The QT interval is corrected for heart rate by dividing the measured QT interval by the square root of the R–R interval. **A QTc interval greater than 0.44 second in duration is almost always abnormal.** Drugs (e.g., tricyclic antidepressants, amiodarone, type Ia antiarrhythmics) and electrolyte abnormalities (hypokalemia, hypomagnesemia, hypocalcemia) are common causes of a prolonged QT interval.

VI. HYPERTROPHY

A. Left ventricular hypertrophy. All ECG criteria for the diagnosis of left ventricular hypertrophy are poorly sensitive but highly specific. One approach is to proceed through the following criteria in the order given. If a criterion is met, you diagnose left ventricular hypertrophy (high specificity); if not, you move to the next criterion.

1. **R wave in lead aVL** greater than 11 mm (>13 mm if left anterior fascicular block is present)
2. **R wave in lead aVL + S wave in lead V3** greater than 20 mm in a woman or greater than 28 mm in a man
3. **S wave in lead V1 + R wave in leads V5 or V6** (whichever is larger) greater than 35 mm

B. Right ventricular hypertrophy. Criteria for the diagnosis of right ventricular hypertrophy are also highly specific but insensitive.

1. **Right axis deviation (RAD) greater than 110°**
2. **R:S wave ratio in lead V1** greater than or equal to 1
3. **R wave in lead V1** greater than or equal to 7 mm
4. **R:S wave ratio in lead V5 or V6** less than or equal to 1

C. Left atrial abnormality was formerly called left atrial enlargement, but the name was changed because the ECG findings may actually represent dilatation, increased atrial pressure, or hypertrophy.

1. **Lead II.** Notched P waves greater than 0.12 second indicate left atrial abnormality.

2. **Lead V1.** If the P terminal force (the negative deflection that represents left atrial depolarization) is equal to or greater than one small box by one small box (0.04 second by 1 mm), left atrial abnormality is diagnosed.

D. Right atrial enlargement

1. **Lead II.** A P wave greater than 2.5 mm high indicates right atrial enlargement.
2. **Lead V1.** If the P initial force (the positive deflection that represents right atrial depolarization) is greater than 1.5 mm, right atrial enlargement is diagnosed.

VII. Q WAVES simply indicate that forces are moving away from their respective leads.

A. Normal Q waves. Sometimes Q waves are normal and expected. For example, the interventricular septum is depolarized left to right, and so a small or "septal" Q wave is expected in lead V6 (reflecting forces moving away from this leftward lead).

B. Pathologic Q waves signify that forces are moving away from the area more than would normally be expected. A pathologic Q wave indicates an old **myocardial infarction** and is only diagnosed when the Q wave is at least 30 msec (close to one small box) in duration and at least one-third the height of the ensuing R wave.

1. **Inferior wall myocardial infarction.** Leads II, III, and aVF evaluate the inferior surface of the left ventricle. Q waves in these leads denote an inferior wall myocardial infarction. However, an isolated Q wave in lead III of up to 30 msec may be seen as a normal variant. (A handy way of remembering this is: "A small Q in III is free, unless accompanied by a Q in either II or aVF.")
2. **Posterior wall myocardial infarction.** Sometimes an inferior wall infarction is accompanied by a posterior wall infarction, producing a large R wave in lead V1 (i.e., forces move away from the posterior wall anteriorly). **Differential diagnoses for a large R wave in V1 include:**
   a. Posterior wall myocardial infarction
   b. Posteroseptal accessory pathway
   c. Right ventricular hypertrophy
   d. Right bundle branch block
   e. Duchenne's muscular dystrophy
   f. Limb lead reversal
   g. Dextrocardia
   h. Normal variant (in young people)
3. **Anterior wall myocardial infarction.** Q waves in the precordial leads (V1–V6) imply an old anterior myocardial infarction.

VIII. ST/T-WAVE CHANGES

A. Causes. The most common causes of ST/T-wave changes are:

1. **Myocardial ischemia, injury,** or **infarction**
2. **Pericardial inflammation**
3. **Ventricular enlargement**
4. **Abnormal ventricular depolarization** (e.g., with bundle branch block)
5. **Electrolyte disturbances** (consider potassium abnormalities first)

B. Findings

1. **T-wave inversions** may indicate **myocardial ischemia** but are nonspecific.
2. **ST elevations** or **depressions** often indicate acute **myocardial injury.**
3. **ST elevations with the appearance of Q waves** usually indicate **myocardial infarction.**

C. Terminology. Clinicians often refer to ST depressions and elevations as ischemia and infarct, respectively, rather than simply "injury." This is because **ST depression** is caused by injury to the **subendocardial** (inner) region that is often the result of supply/demand mismatch, nonocclusive thrombus, or occlusive thrombus in a vessel supplying well-collateralized territory. **ST elevation,** in contrast, implies **transmural** injury that usually occurs as a result of complete coronary occlusion from thrombus during an infarction.

REFERENCES

Dubin D. Rapid Interpretation of ECGs: An Interactive Course. Tampa, FL: Cover Publishing Company, 2000.

Surawicz B, Knilans TK. Chou's Electrocardiography in Clinical Practice: Adult and Pediatric. Philadelphia: WB Saunders, 2008.

■ Syncope

6

I. INTRODUCTION.

A. **Definition.** Syncope is a **transient loss of consciousness and postural tone** that is **caused by inadequate cerebral blood flow.** Syncope should be differentiated from presyncope, dizziness, and vertigo—all of which do not result in loss of consciousness. **Seizures** must be **excluded.** This requires a careful examination for prodromal or postictal symptoms and rhythmic myoclonic activity.

B. **Epidemiology.** Syncope is extremely common, accounting for approximately **5% of medical admissions** and **3% of emergency department visits.** The lifetime incidence approaches 50% in some groups.

II. CAUSES OF SYNCOPE.

There are many causes of syncope, but the most important can easily be remembered using the mnemonic "SYNCOPE."

MNEMONIC **Causes of Syncope ("SYNCOPE")**

Situational
Vasovagal (the V looks like a Y)
Neurogenic
Cardiac
Orthostatic hypotension
Psychiatric
Everything else

A. **Situational** causes include micturition, defecation, swallowing, coughing, subclavian steal, and carotid sinus sensitivity.

B. **Vasovagal** syncope, also known as the "**common faint,**" is the most common cause of syncope in young patients and is often preceded by a painful or emotional stimulus. This condition results from a simultaneous, reflex-mediated decrease in vascular tone (vasodilatory component) and heart rate (cardioinhibitory component).

C. **Neurogenic** causes include autonomic insufficiency and transient ischemic attacks.

1. **Transient ischemic attacks (TIAs)** are extremely rare causes of syncope. For syncope to occur, the vertebrobasilar circulation must be involved.
2. **Autonomic insufficiency** is common in elderly patients and patients with diabetes.

D. Cardiac causes

1. **Obstructive disorders.** Aortic, mitral, or pulmonic stenosis; idiopathic hypertrophic subaortic stenosis; atrial myxoma; and pulmonary embolism interfere with cardiac output and can precipitate a syncopal attack.
2. **Arrhythmias.** Disorders that lead to bradycardia [e.g., sick sinus syndrome, second- and third-degree atrioventricular (AV) block] or tachycardia (e.g., ventricular fibrillation, ventricular tachycardia, torsades de pointes, supraventricular tachycardia) also interfere with cardiac output.
3. **Other. Ischemic disorders** can precipitate an episode of syncope through low cardiac output or arrhythmias. **Aortic dissection** can lead to syncope through cardiac tamponade from hemopericardium or acute cerebrovascular insufficiency.

E. Orthostatic hypotension can cause syncope.

F. Psychogenic syncope is a diagnosis of exclusion.

G. Everything else

1. **Medications** (e.g., vasodilators, hypnotics, sedatives, nitrates, diuretics)
2. **Drugs** (e.g., cocaine, hypnotics, sedatives, alcohol)
3. **Subarachnoid hemorrhage** should be considered in patients presenting with syncope after a headache.

III. APPROACH TO THE PATIENT. The evaluation of a patient with syncope must be approached in a rigorous, stepwise fashion to avoid missing life-threatening disease.

A. History. A thorough history is a **very important** aspect of the evaluation and may establish the diagnosis in up to 45% of patients.

1. **Situational.** Was the episode preceded by urination, defecation, swallowing, coughing, exertion of arm muscles (subclavian steal), or manipulation of the neck (carotid sinus hypersensitivity)? A diagnosis of carotid sinus hypersensitivity is suggested by a history of the syncopal event occurring during situations of external carotid pressure such as shaving, wearing tight collars, or neck movements. Testing for carotid sinus hypersensitivity should be done carefully after excluding significant carotid artery stenosis and only while the patient is being monitored by ECG.
2. **Vasovagal.** Did a painful or emotional stimulus precede the event?

3. **Neurogenic.** Did anyone witness convulsions, bowel or bladder incontinence, or signs suggestive of a postictal state? A seizure is not syncope but could result in a loss of consciousness; therefore, it must be considered in the differential diagnosis.
4. **Cardiac.** A cardiac cause is more likely if the patient has any history suggestive of cardiac disease. Has the patient complained of feeling lightheaded during exercise (suggestive of an obstructive cause)? Has the patient complained of "palpitations" (suggestive of an arrhythmic cause)? Patients may also complain of symptoms suggestive of cardiac ischemia.
5. **Orthostatic hypotension.** Does the patient report that he or she "got up too quickly"? Always check orthostatic vital signs in patients admitted with syncope. Orthostatic hypotension is defined by one of the following findings occurring **within 2 to 5 minutes** of the patient standing from a sitting position: (1) decrease in systolic blood pressure of 20 mm Hg; (2) decrease in diastolic blood pressure of 10 mm Hg; (3) reflex tachycardia of 20 beats/min; or (4) symptoms of cerebral hypoperfusion.
6. **Psychogenic.** A psychogenic cause for the syncope (e.g., hyperventilation) should be considered after all other causes have been excluded.
7. **Everything else.** What prescription, over-the-counter, or illicit drugs might the patient have access to?

B. Physical examination can offer clues as to the etiology of the syncopal event.

1. **Vital signs**. Is there any evidence of orthostasis, tachycardia, bradycardia, or baseline hypotension? Disparities between upper extremities in blood pressure or pulse may be consistent with aortic dissection or subclavian steal syndrome. Hypoxemia may indicate an underlying pulmonary embolism.
2. **Neck.** Auscultation of carotid bruits may reveal evidence of stenosis.
3. **Oral cavity.** Inspection of a patient's tongue may display lacerations associated with seizure activity.
4. **Cardiovascular.** Auscultation of the heart may reveal an irregular rhythm (atrial fibrillation), systolic murmur (aortic stenosis or hypertrophic obstructive cardiomyopathy), diastolic murmur (mitral stenosis), or an S_3 consistent with heart failure.
5. **Pulmonary.** Auscultation may reveal crackles consistent with pulmonary edema.
6. **Neurologic examination** may display evidence of stroke or resolving TIA.

C. Electrocardiogram (ECG). All patients should have an ECG, although fewer than 10% of the causes of syncope can be identified by this test. Look for evidence of acute or remote myocardial infarction, preexcitation syndromes, arrhythmias, a long QT interval, and conduction system disease (i.e., bundle branch block).

D. Risk assessment. Patients should be **separated into two groups:** those without evidence of heart disease and those who may have heart disease.

1. **No evidence of heart disease.** Patients who meet all the following criteria after a thorough history, physical examination, and ECG are at low risk for a cardiac cause, and additional cardiac testing may not be indicated. However, some patients may require additional evaluation and treatment. The criteria are:
   a. **Younger than 45 years of age**
   b. **No history or evidence of coronary artery disease or congestive heart failure**
   c. **Normal ECG**
2. **Evidence of heart disease.** Anyone who does not meet all the criteria in III D 1 is included in this group. If there is **suspicion of an ischemic or arrhythmic cause, admission and ECG monitoring** are indicated. Additional diagnostic tests to be considered include:
   a. **Ambulatory ECG monitoring.** This test is widely used, but it establishes a diagnosis in only a small percentage of patients. Event or loop recorders may improve the diagnostic yield.
   b. **Exercise treadmill testing** can rule out exercise- or ischemia-induced syncope.
   c. **Echocardiography** allows assessment of valvular disease as well as left ventricular size and function.
   d. **Electrophysiologic studies (EPS)** are especially useful in patients at high risk for tachyarrhythmia (i.e., those with poor left ventricular function) when a diagnosis cannot be established using noninvasive methods. The yield of EPS is lower in patients without structural heart disease and in those with bradyarrhythmias.
   e. **Tilt table test.** This test can be useful in documenting vasovagal syncope but has poor specificity.

IV. TREATMENT is cause specific.

A. The treatment of any **correctable cardiac abnormality** should be the first consideration (i.e., permanent pacemaker for patients with bradyarrhythmias, implantable cardiac defibrillators in patients with ventricular tachyarrhythmia, or valvular surgery for those with severe aortic stenosis).

B. Patients with **frequent vasovagal syncope** may benefit from a trial of β-blockers, paroxetine, or disopyramide. In rare instances, patients with a significant cardioinhibitory component may benefit from permanent pacemaker placement.

C. **Orthostatic hypotension** is treated with volume resuscitation and discontinuation of culprit drugs. Rarely, support stockings, salt tablets, fludrocortisone, and midodrine may be added if autonomic insufficiency is present.

V. PREVENTION

A. Medications and the use of alcohol or illicit drugs should be reviewed carefully.

B. Education about likely precipitants can help prevent recurrences.

REFERENCES

Kapoor WN. Current evaluation and management of syncope. Circulation. 2002;106:1606–1609.

Linzer M, Yang EH, Estes NA 3rd, et al. Diagnosing syncope. Part 1: value of history, physical examination, and electrocardiography. Clinical Efficacy Assessment Project of the American College of Physicians. Ann Intern Med 1997;126:989–996. [Classic article].

Linzer M, Yang EH, Estes NA 3rd, et al. Diagnosing syncope. Part 2: unexplained syncope. Clinical Efficacy Assessment Project of the American College of Physicians. Ann Intern Med 1997;127:76–86. [Classic article].

7

Arrhythmias

I. INTRODUCTION

A. **Bradyarrhythmias** usually do not pose a diagnostic dilemma and have relatively few treatment options (e.g., atropine, pacemaker device).

B. **Tachyarrhythmias** may pose a significant challenge in diagnosis and often are treated very differently. All tachyarrhythmias can be classified according to whether they are regular (same distance between successive R waves) or irregular, and whether their QRS complex is narrow (<0.12 second) or wide (>0.12 second). Making these two determinations and consulting Table 7-1 can significantly narrow the diagnostic possibilities.

Often the most important clue to determining the etiology of a tachyarrhythmia is close inspection of the P wave.

II. NARROW, REGULAR TACHYARRHYTHMIAS

A. Differential diagnosis

1. **Sinus tachycardia**
   a. **Etiologies.** Sinus tachycardia is usually a physiologic response to stress. Important etiologies include:
      (1) **Low stroke volume states** (e.g., from intravascular volume depletion or myocardial dysfunction)
      (2) **Hypoxemia** (e.g., from heart failure)
      (3) **Hypercatecholamine states** (e.g., from pheochromocytoma, pain, anxiety)
      (4) **Drugs** (e.g., inhaled β-agonists, theophylline, caffeine)
      (5) **Systemic causes** (e.g., fever, anemia, hyperthyroidism)
      (6) **Myocarditis and pericarditis**
   b. **Electrocardiogram (ECG) appearance.** Upright P waves in leads I, II, and aVF are always followed by a QRS complex.

The maximum predicted heart rate in sinus tachycardia = 220 minus the patient's age. If the patient's heart rate is greater than the maximum predicted heart rate, then look for a cause other than sinus tachycardia.

2. **Atrioventricular nodal reentrant tachycardia (AVNRT)** accounts for more than 50% of all supraventricular tachyarrhythmias. [All narrow, regular tachyarrhythmias are supraventricular, but the term **supraventricular tachycardia** is classically used for AVNRT, atrioventricular reentrant tachycardia (AVRT), and atrial tachycardia (AT).]
   a. **Characteristics** include:
      (1) Heart rate of 160–200 beats/min
      (2) Inverted P waves and pseudo R waves on the ECG
   b. **Mechanism.** Thirty percent of the population has a dual atrioventricular (AV) node that contains a fast pathway with a long refractory period and a slow pathway with a short refractory period.
      (1) **Sinus rhythm.** During sinus rhythm, the impulse is conducted down the fast pathway to the ventricles. Conduction down the fast pathway is also able to traverse the AV node retrograde and block impulses on the slow pathway (Figure 7-1).
      (2) **Excitation loop.** The incidence of premature atrial contractions (PACs) increases with age. A PAC may

TABLE 7-1

CLASSIFICATION OF TACHYARRHYTHMIAS

	Regular Rhythm	**Irregular Rhythm**
Narrow QRS	Sinus tachycardia AVNRT AT Atrial flutter	Atrial fibrillation Atrial flutter with variable block Multifocal atrial tachycardia Frequent premature atrial contractions
Wide QRS	Ventricular tachycardia Supraventricular tachycardia with aberrancy	Atrial fibrillation with aberrancy* Ventricular tachycardia (monomorphic or polymorphic)

AT = atrial tachycardia; *AVNRT* = atrioventricular nodal reentrant tachycardia.

*Because all arrhythmias characterized by an irregular rhythm and a narrow QRS complex can become irregular with a wide QRS complex in the presence of aberrant conduction, atrial flutter with variable block and multifocal atrial tachycardia must also be considered here, although they are much less common than atrial fibrillation.

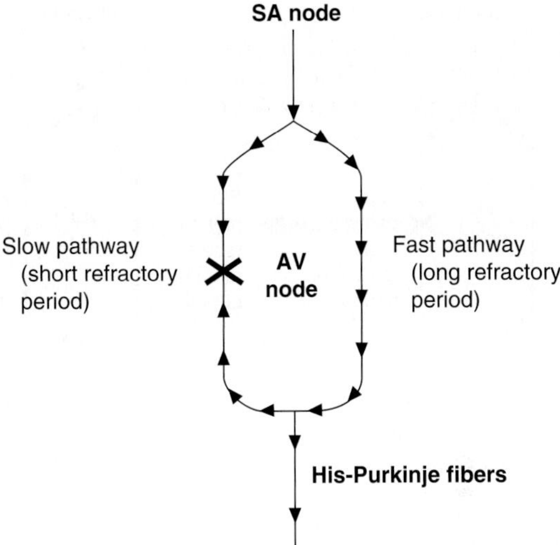

Figure 7-1 Dual atrioventricular node, sinus rhythm. *AV* = atrioventricular; *SA* = sinoatrial.

be blocked at the fast pathway secondary to its long refractory period; the impulse is then conducted down the slow pathway, which has a short refractory period, (This is manifested as a long PR interval on the ECG immediately before the tachycardia's initiation.) The impulse may then enter the fast pathway retrograde, which is no longer refractory, and activate the atria (slow-fast AVNRT or typical AVNRT) (Figure 7-2).

c. **ECG appearance**

(1) In **typical AVNRT** (90% of cases), a PAC begins the loop of excitation. The P wave is inverted and can usually be seen in the terminal portion of the QRS complex **(pseudo R waves)** in lead V1.

(2) In **atypical AVNRT** (10% of cases), a premature ventricular contraction (PVC) initiates the conduction of an impulse up the slow pathway and down the fast one (fast-slow) (Figure 7-3). Because the retrograde P waves are formed from the slower pathway, they are inverted and occur after ventricular activation and are often seen just prior to the next QRS complex. This ECG resembles atrial tachycardia and may require an electrophysiologic study to further differentiate the cause of arrhythmia.

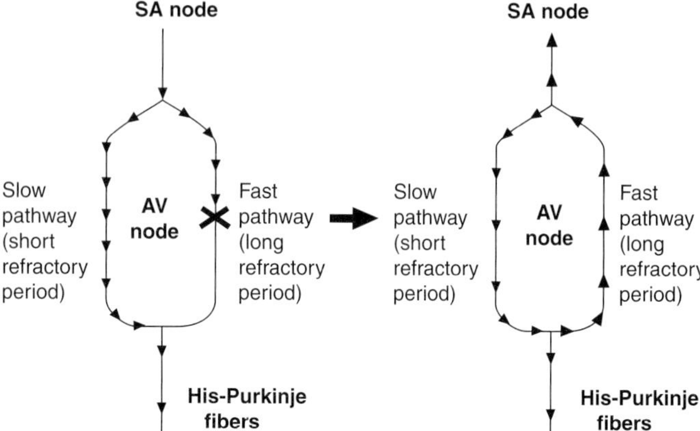

Figure 7-2 Typical atrioventricular nodal reentrant tachycardia (*AVNRT*) from premature atrial contractions (*PACs*). Following conduction down the slow pathway, the fast pathway is no longer refractory and may conduct retrograde, forming an excitation loop. *AV* = atrioventricular.

3. **Atrioventricular reentrant tachycardia** accounts for more than 30% of all supraventricular tachyarrhythmias.
   a. **Characteristics.** AVRT is usually characterized by a short RP interval on the ECG.
   b. **Mechanism.** AVRT involves an **accessory pathway** (e.g., bundle of Kent in Wolff-Parkinson-White syndrome), an abnormal tract of fast conducting tissue between the

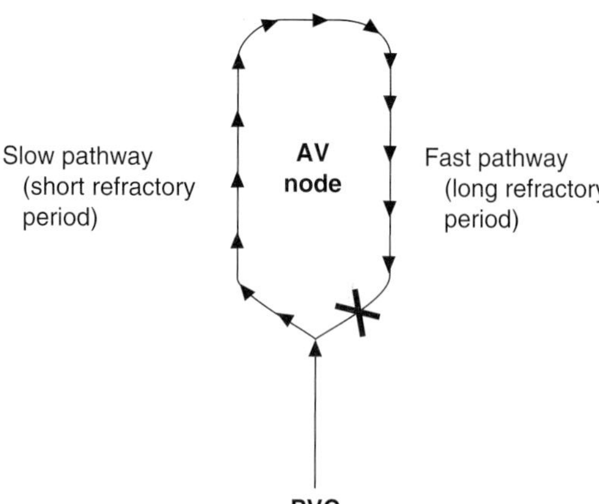

Figure 7-3 Atypical atrioventricular nodal reentrant tachycardia (AVNRT). *AV* = atrioventricular; *PVC* = premature ventricular contraction.

atria and ventricles that bypasses the AV node. Accessory pathways often conduct in both an anterograde and retrograde direction.

c. **ECG appearance**

(1) **Sinus rhythm**

(a) During sinus rhythm, anterograde conduction results in ventricular preexcitation, manifested as a **short PR interval** and a **delta wave** on the ECG.

(b) If only retrograde conduction is possible (as is the case in approximately 25% of patients), no abnormality is seen during sinus rhythm (concealed bypass tract).

(2) **Excitation loop**

(a) **Orthodromic conduction** occurs when an impulse is conducted through the AV node and then up the accessory pathway in a retrograde direction (Figure 7-4). Because the loop is longer than that of AVNRT, the retrograde P wave is easily seen (i.e., it is not buried within the QRS complex). The interval from the R wave to the ensuing retrograde P wave will be less than that from the P wave to the next R wave (**short RP or RP < PR tachycardia**). This characteristic helps distinguish AVRT from AT and sinus tachycardia. The QRS complex remains narrow because the ventricle is depolarized normally (i.e., via the His-Purkinje system).

(b) **Antidromic conduction** occurs when the impulse is conducted antegrade down the bypass tract. Antidromic conduction produces a wide QRS complex because the tract terminates on ventricular muscle fibers. (Conduction from fiber to fiber is slow.)

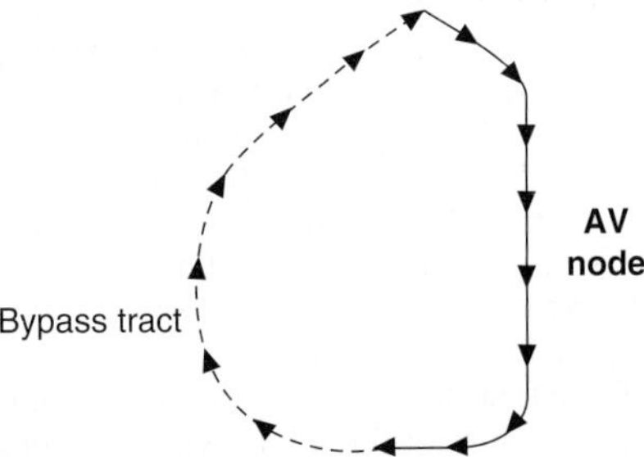

Figure 7-4 Orthodromic conduction leading to atrioventricular reentrant tachycardia (AVRT). *AV* = atrioventricular.

4. **AT** accounts for 15% of all supraventricular tachycardias.
   a. **Characteristics**
      (1) The **atrial rate** (as reflected by the P waves on the ECG) is usually **less than 250 beats/min.** (In atrial flutter, the atrial rate is approximately 300 beats/min.)
      (2) A **long RP** interval is noted on the ECG.
   b. **Mechanism.** Enhanced automaticity of atrial tissue or atrial reentry with a focus usually located in the lower right atrium is thought to be the mechanism.
      (1) Patients often have **structural heart disease.**
      (2) Because digitalis increases atrial and ventricular automaticity and depresses conduction tissue, AT with variable degrees of AV nodal block is a common presentation of **digitalis toxicity.**
   c. **ECG appearance.** The P wave has an unusual axis due to depolarization of the atria from a focus below the sinus node, and is followed by a narrow QRS complex (produced by conduction of the impulse down the AV node). The preceding P wave is linked to the R wave, and the PR interval is shorter than the RP interval (a long RP tachycardia).

The supraventricular tachycardias can be classified according to the RP interval:
Short RP = AVRT and typical AVNRT
Long RP = AT, atypical AVNRT, and sinus tachycardia
No RP = typical AVNRT

5. **Atrial flutter**
   a. **Characteristics**
      (1) The atrial rate is often 300 beats/min, with the ventricular rate typically 150 beats/min. (In other words, a 2:1 AV block is commonly seen.) **Whenever the ventricular rate is approximately 150 beats/min with little variation, think of atrial flutter.**
      (2) Atrial flutter is typically transient, often degenerating to atrial fibrillation or returning to sinus rhythm. In general, the causes of atrial flutter are similar to those of atrial fibrillation (see Chapter 8).
   b. **Mechanism.** Atrial flutter is a result of a macro-reentrant loop in the right atrium.
   c. **ECG appearance.** Because the waves often move in a superior-inferior direction (typical atrial flutter), flutter waves are best seen in the inferior leads (i.e., leads II, III, and AVF).

B. Treatment

1. **Acute treatment** depends on the patient's hemodynamic stability.
   a. **Hemodynamically unstable (or ischemic) patient.** Determine if the patient is in sinus rhythm.
      (1) If the patient is **not in sinus rhythm,** initiate **electrical cardioversion** immediately.
      (2) If the patient is **in sinus rhythm,** treatment is aimed at the underlying cause.
   b. **Hemodynamically stable patient**
      (1) **Carotid sinus massage** or **Valsalva maneuvers** may increase vagal tone and block impulses at the level of the AV node. Carotid sinus massage is contraindicated in the presence of a carotid bruit and should be performed with continuous ECG monitoring and a crash cart available.
         (a) **AVNRT** and **AVRT,** tachycardias that involve reentrant loops through the AV node, may terminate.
         (b) **AT** is usually unaffected by carotid sinus massage but may terminate abruptly.
         (c) **Sinus tachycardia.** Carotid sinus massage may slow the atrial rate.
         (d) **Atrial flutter** usually becomes more obvious as the AV block increases and flutter waves appear; the tachycardia will not terminate.
      (2) Administer **adenosine** as a rapid intravenous (IV) push in incremental doses of 6 and 12 mg **followed by 20–50 ml saline push** if carotid sinus massage or Valsalva maneuvers are ineffective. (Halve the dose if administration is via a central line.) Adenosine is contraindicated in patients with acute bronchospasm and heart transplant patients; patients taking dipyridamole may have an increased sensitivity. The effects of adenosine occur within 15–30 seconds of administration and last for 10–20 seconds. Adenosine has effects similar to those of carotid sinus massage, but they are more pronounced as it results in transient complete AV nodal block. **You must warn the patient that he or she will feel a sense of impending doom but this sensation will pass within 10–20 seconds.**
         (a) **AVNRT** and **AVRT.** More than 90% of these tachycardias will be terminated with a 12-mg dose of adenosine.
         (b) **AT** rarely terminates. IV administration of verapamil or diltiazem is preferable for arresting

atrial tachycardia and may decrease the ventricular response, even if the tachycardia persists.

c. **Sinus tachycardia** transiently slows. Additional treatment should be aimed at the underlying cause.

d. **Atrial flutter.** AV block increases and flutter waves are more evident. The heart rate returns to its previous accelerated rate as the effects of adenosine wane. Additional treatment may involve AV nodal blockade with digitalis, β-blockers, or calcium channel blockers, followed by either chemical (e.g., procainamide, ibutilide) or electrical cardioversion. If the atrial flutter has been long-standing, cardioversion should only be considered after anticoagulation for 4 weeks or a transesophageal echocardiogram to rule out left atrial thrombus as with atrial fibrillation (see Chapter 8).

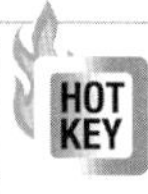

In atrial flutter, type 1a agents should not be given before the administration of AV nodal blocking agents, because type 1a agents may slow atrial conduction sufficiently to permit 1:1 conduction through the AV node, thereby increasing the ventricular response.

(1) Electrical cardioversion starting at 50 J is a reasonable alternative to AV nodal blocking agents.

2. **Chronic treatment**

a. **AVNRT.** If the patient experiences sporadic episodes, control may be possible using vagal maneuvers. For patients who experience frequent or symptomatic episodes, antiarrhythmic drugs, AV nodal blocking agents, or radiofrequency ablation (RFA) may be used (>95% successful).

b. **AVRT.** Symptomatic patients with evidence of preexcitation on a baseline ECG should probably receive radiofrequency ablation. Patients with symptoms but no evidence of anterograde conduction (i.e., concealed bypass tract) can be treated with RFA or an initial trial of an AV nodal blocking agent.

c. **Atrial tachycardia.** Calcium channel blockers or β-blockers are often the drugs of first choice. If pharmacologic therapy fails, ablation may be indicated.

d. **Atrial flutter.** RFA is 95% successful and should be considered in patients with recurrent symptoms. Antiarrhythmic drugs are typically less successful. Because of its high association with atrial fibrillation and independent association with stroke, anticoagulation also should be considered if there is evidence of advanced age, hypertension, previous transient ischemic attack/stroke, diabetes mellitus, or structural heart disease.

III. NARROW, IRREGULAR TACHYARRHYTHMIAS

A. Differential diagnosis. In general, the members of this category can be differentiated easily on the basis of a 12-lead ECG. It is most difficult to distinguish atrial fibrillation from atrial flutter with variable block.

1. **Atrial fibrillation** is discussed in detail in Chapter 8. This arrhythmia is characterized by irregular atrial fibrillatory waves at a rate of 350–600 beats/min and a ventricular rate of usually 120–160 beats/min.
2. **Atrial flutter with variable block.** To help differentiate atrial flutter with variable block from atrial fibrillation:
   a. **Look at the inferior leads (II, III, AVF).** With typical atrial flutter, flutter waves can often be ''marched out'' at a rate of approximately 300 beats/min. These flutter waves must have **exactly the same morphology.** Variable block will produce a ventricular rate in proportion to the atrial rate (i.e., the ventricular response to 2:1, 3:1, and 4:1 AV block will be 150 beats/min, 100 beats/min, and 75 beats/min, respectively).
   b. **Increase AV block** by massaging the carotid sinus or administering adenosine. Flutter waves that may have been hidden will often become obvious.
3. **Multifocal atrial tachycardia**
   a. **Mechanism.** In approximately 60% of patients, multifocal atrial tachycardia is associated with pulmonary disease. For example, cor pulmonale causes right atrial stretch, producing different foci of atrial depolarization. Multifocal atrial tachycardia may also be caused by hypokalemia or hypomagnesemia.
   b. **ECG appearance.** Diagnosis requires the presence of three distinct P-wave morphologies in the same lead and three separate PR intervals. As a result of multiple atrial foci, the RR interval varies (i.e., **it is irregularly irregular**).
4. **Frequent PACs.** When frequent, PACs may give the appearance of an irregular rhythm.

B. Treatment

1. **Hemodynamically unstable (or ischemic) patients** with tachycardia and atrial fibrillation or atrial flutter with variable block should undergo immediate **electrical cardioversion.**
2. **Hemodynamically stable**

a. **Atrial fibrillation.** Treatment is discussed in Chapter 8 VI.
b. **Atrial flutter with variable block.** Treatment is the same as that for atrial flutter without variable block (see II B 1 b).
c. **Multifocal atrial tachycardia.** Treat the underlying condition (usually related to bronchospasm, hypoxia, or metabolic derangements). Verapamil, magnesium, and β-blockers are often tried, but this is a difficult arrhythmia to treat.

IV. WIDE, REGULAR TACHYARRHYTHMIAS

A. Mechanism. Normally, the impulse is conducted from the sinoatrial (SA) node to the AV node, through the bundle of His, and through the left and right bundle branches (the Purkinje fibers). The bundles conduct rapidly and ventricular depolarization is efficient (like traveling down the interstate highway at a fast speed), producing a narrow QRS complex (<100 msec in duration).

1. If one bundle is blocked, conduction will spread down the remaining bundle and then from muscle fiber to muscle fiber (like traveling on local roads at a slower speed). This slow process produces a wide QRS complex (>120 msec in duration). A QRS complex between 100 and 120 msec in duration represents an incomplete bundle branch block and is often termed an interventricular conduction delay.
2. The QRS complex will be wide if the impulse starts in the ventricle and spreads fiber to fiber (as is the case with ventricular tachycardia) or if it starts above the ventricle but eventually spreads fiber to fiber (as is the case with supraventricular tachycardia with aberrancy). There are three mechanisms of aberrant conduction:
   a. **A preexisting underlying bundle branch block**
   b. **A rate-related bundle branch block.** As the heart rate increases, one bundle (usually the right bundle) is unable to keep up with the other due to a longer refractory period. The impulse is conducted down the faster bundle and then from fiber to fiber, producing a wide QRS.
   c. **An accessory pathway.** These tracts terminate on ventricular muscle, necessitating fiber-to-fiber conduction.

B. Differential diagnosis. The differential is **ventricular tachycardia versus supraventricular tachycardia with aberrancy versus antidromic AVRT.**

Patients with cardiac disease and a wide-complex tachyarrhythmia should be assumed to have ventricular tachycardia until proven otherwise.

The **Brugada criteria** can help distinguish between ventricular tachycardia and supraventricular tachycardia with aberrancy.[1]

The precordial leads (V1–V6) are examined on a 12-lead ECG. Each criterion is extremely specific, but not particularly sensitive, for ventricular tachycardia. Therefore, if a criterion is met, initiate treatment for ventricular tachycardia; if the criterion is not met, continue to the next.

1. **Absence of a true RS pattern in all the precordial leads.** An S wave is a discrete negative deflection. A broad negative deflection is an inverted T wave (as opposed to an S wave). If there is a monomorphic pattern (no RS) or "concordance," the arrhythmia is ventricular tachycardia.
2. **RS complex (from start of R to nadir of S) is greater than 100 msec.** Ventricular depolarization takes more time if it starts in the ventricle, rather than if it begins supraventricularly and is conducted aberrantly. If the RS complex is greater than 100 msec, then the arrhythmia is ventricular tachycardia.
3. **Evidence of AV dissociation** includes P waves marching through at different points of the wide complexes and fusion or capture beats. Although these clues are difficult to discern, they are diagnostic of ventricular tachycardia. If a diagnosis has still not been reached, morphologic criteria (given in several texts) can be used to arrive at a diagnosis.

"Quick and dirty" rule for distinguishing ventricular tachycardia from supraventricular tachycardia with aberrancy: Is there a past medical history of coronary artery disease? If yes, then ventricular tachycardia is the diagnosis more than 95% of the time.

C. Treatment

1. **Hemodynamically unstable (or ischemic) patients** should undergo cardioversion, starting with at least 200 J.
2. **Hemodynamically stable patients**
   a. **Ventricular tachycardia**
      (1) **Amiodarone.** Usual IV dosage is 150–300 mg bolus followed by 1 mg/min for 6 hours and then 0.5 mg/min.

---

[1]Brugada P, Brugada J, Mont L, et al. A new approach to the differential diagnosis of a regular tachycardia with a wide QRS complex. Circulation 1991;83(5):1649–1659.

(2) **Lidocaine.** The initial bolus is 1–1.5 mg/kg administered intravenously, followed by an infusion of 1–4 mg/min.
(3) **Procainamide** should be considered in patients who do not respond to amiodarone or lidocaine. Procainamide is effective at terminating ventricular tachycardia, but hypotension may occur.

b. **Supraventricular arrhythmias with aberrancy. Carotid sinus massage** and **adenosine** should be employed as described in II B 1 b.

c. **Undiagnosed**
(1) **Amiodarone or lidocaine.** The patient may be given a trial of either agent.
(2) **Adenosine.** If there is no response, adenosine trials in 6- and 12-mg increments (half doses if administered via a central line) should be tried. If the patient has a history of cardiac disease, ventricular tachycardia is likely and needs to be treated immediately.
(3) **Procainamide.** If the patient still fails to respond, a procainamide trial may be indicated.

V. WIDE, IRREGULAR TACHYARRHYTHMIAS

A. Differential diagnosis. The differential diagnosis is atrial fibrillation with aberrancy versus ventricular tachycardia (monomorphic or polymorphic).

All members of the irregular, narrow category will appear irregular and wide with aberrant conduction.

1. **Atrial fibrillation** with aberrancy. There are three possible mechanisms of aberrant conduction.
   a. **Preexisting underlying bundle branch block.** If, upon comparing a previous 12-lead ECG with a current one, there is evidence of an old bundle branch block that has the same morphology as the present one, this diagnosis is extremely likely.
   b. **Rate-related bundle branch block** will usually have a right bundle branch block pattern on the ECG because the right bundle is usually slower than the left bundle.
   c. **Accessory pathway.** If there is evidence of preexcitation during sinus rhythm (i.e., a short PR interval, delta waves) on a prior 12-lead ECG, this diagnosis is extremely likely. Another clue to an accessory pathway is bizarre conduction (e.g., lead V1 suggests a left

bundle but the nearby V2 lead suggests a right bundle). An accessory pathway is a dangerous situation because fibrillatory waves occur at rates of approximately 600 beats/min and the accessory pathway allows much faster conduction than does the AV node. Very fast ventricular rates (i.e., 200–300 beats/min) can be generated; this arrhythmia can quickly degenerate to ventricular fibrillation. AV nodal agents (e.g., verapamil) should be strictly avoided in all suspected cases.

Whenever you see a patient with a wide, irregular tachyarrhythmia with a rate greater than 200 beats/min, consider atrial fibrillation with an accessory pathway.

B. Treatment

1. **Hemodynamically unstable (or ischemic) patients** should undergo **cardioversion** starting at 200 J.
2. **Hemodynamically stable patients**
   a. **Procainamide** is the drug of choice.
      (1) If the rhythm is atrial fibrillation with aberrancy, procainamide may convert the patient to sinus rhythm. If the cause of the patient's aberrant conduction is an accessory pathway, procainamide will slow conduction through the pathway, decreasing the ventricular rate, even though conversion may not occur.
      (2) Procainamide also treats ventricular tachycardia. However:
         (a) **Procainamide is contraindicated in the setting of torsades de pointes.** If a morphology consistent with torsades de pointes is present or there are strong epidemiologic factors suggestive of torsades de pointes (e.g., an increased baseline QT interval, use of quinidine or tricyclic antidepressants, or electrolyte disturbances such as hypokalemia or hypomagnesemia), procainamide is contraindicated because it will increase prolongation of the QT interval and promote further torsades. **Procainamide frequently leads to hypotension,** so patients with borderline blood pressures (i.e., 90–100 mm Hg) and fast heart rates may be better served with cardioversion.
   b. **AV nodal blocking agents** (β-blockers, calcium channel blockers, or digitalis) should only be considered when

the patient shows strong evidence of atrial fibrillation with an underlying bundle branch block (i.e., a prior ECG shows the same bundle branch block during sinus rhythm). **Otherwise, AV nodal blocking agents should not be administered to patients with wide, irregular tachycardias** because if the patient has an accessory pathway, AV nodal blocking agents will promote conduction down the tract, thereby increasing the heart rate to dangerous levels.

VI. VENTRICULAR TACHYCARDIA

A. Monomorphic ventricular tachycardia. In ventricular tachycardia, the rhythm may be irregular for the first 50 beats. A persistently irregular rhythm after 50 beats essentially rules out monomorphic ventricular tachycardia.

1. **Polymorphic ventricular tachycardia.** Because the impulse is originating from different foci in the ventricle, the rhythm is irregular. Torsades de pointes is a type of polymorphic ventricular tachycardia that is associated with a prolonged QT interval and undulates around the isoelectric point.
2. **Acute treatment.** Therapy for monomorphic ventricular tachycardia is as described earlier in IV C 2 a. For polymorphic ventricular tachycardia, emergently treat any reversible metabolic abnormalities (i.e., hypokalemia or hypomagnesemia) and hold potentially dangerous drugs that may be prolonging the QT interval. Additional treatment typically involves IV magnesium or overdrive cardiac pacing with or without β-blockers.
3. **Chronic treatment.** Patients with ventricular tachycardia, especially without a clear reversible cause, should be considered as candidates for **implantable cardiac defibrillators (ICDs).**

REFERENCES

Ferguson JD, DiMarco JP. Contemporary management of paroxysmal supraventricular tachycardia. Circulation 2003;107:1096.

Ganz LI, Friedman PL. Supraventricular tachycardia. N Engl J Med 1995;332:162–173. [Classic article].

Goldberger ZD, Rho RW, Page RL. Approach to the diagnosis and initial management of the stable adult patient with a wide complex tachycardia. Am J Cardiol 2008;101:1456–1466.

Mangrum JM, DiMarco JP. The evaluation and management of bradycardia. N Engl J Med 2000;342:703–709. [Classic article].

8 Atrial Fibrillation

I. INTRODUCTION

A. Epidemiology

1. Atrial fibrillation is the **most common chronic arrhythmia,** occurring in nearly 1% of the general population.
2. Its **incidence** increases with age, occurring in 1 of 25 patients 60 years or older and in 1 of 10 patients 80 years or older.

B. Pathophysiology.

Atrial fibrillation requires (1) an initial atrial ectopic event (typically from a focus in the pulmonary veins) and (2) a multiple wavelet reentrant circuit that is often sustained by structural disease in the left atrium (i.e., enlargement, scar).

C. Terminology.

There are a number of terms used in association with atrial fibrillation.

1. **Valvular** refers to atrial fibrillation that is associated with valvular disease that causes atrial enlargement, most commonly rheumatic mitral valve disease. In the past, rheumatic heart disease accounted for the majority of cases of atrial fibrillation but currently accounts for less than one third of cases. Atrial fibrillation associated with rheumatic heart disease carries a five times greater risk of stroke when compared to "nonvalvular" atrial fibrillation.
2. **Paroxysmal** refers to intermittent, brief episodes of atrial fibrillation unrelated to an acute illness.
3. **Persistent** refers to intermittent episodes lasting at least 7 days but responding to medical or electrical cardioversion to restore sinus rhythm.
4. **Chronic** refers to situations in which atrial fibrillation is the predominant rhythm and does not respond to cardioversion (or alternatively cardioversion is never attempted).
5. **Lone** refers to atrial fibrillation in the absence of structural heart disease [e.g., left ventricular hypertrophy, congestive heart failure (CHF), valve disease, cardiomyopathy] or hypertension. **In patients younger than 60 years of age, "lone" atrial fibrillation is associated with only a minimal risk of stroke or death.**
6. **Isolated** refers to atrial fibrillation that is secondary to another illness (e.g., hyperthyroidism, pneumonia,

pulmonary embolism) and resolves when the illness is treated.

II. CLINICAL MANIFESTATIONS OF ATRIAL FIBRILLATION

A. Symptoms are due to loss of the atrial kick and an increased heart rate, which results in decreased ventricular filling, decreased cardiac output, and an increase in cardiac demand. The most common symptoms reflect these processes.

1. **Dyspnea**
2. **Chest pain**
3. **Palpitations**
4. **Dizziness or syncope**
5. **Fatigue**

Up to 30% of patients with atrial fibrillation may be asymptomatic.

B. Physical examination findings

1. **Irregularly irregular pulse.** An irregularly irregular pulse is the **hallmark of atrial fibrillation.**
2. **Pulse of varying intensity** and **pulse deficit.** Because diastolic filling varies in length and is often reduced, pulses are of varying intensity and not all audible ventricular beats are palpable peripherally.
3. **Absent a waves** in the jugular venous pulse
4. **Variation in the intensity of the first heart sound (S_1)**

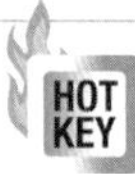

Patients in atrial fibrillation never have an S^4.

C. Electrocardiography

1. The electrocardiogram (ECG) may show **f waves** (fine fibrillation of the atria at a rate of 350–600 beats/min) that are best visualized in lead V1. These f waves should be differentiated from more organized atrial activity (i.e., "sawtooths") in leads II, III, and aVF that might represent atrial flutter.
2. **P waves are absent.**
3. The **ventricular response** will be **irregularly irregular,** although this may be difficult to appreciate at higher heart rates.

III. CAUSES OF ATRIAL FIBRILLATION. Because many of the causes of atrial fibrillation are correctable, an effort should be made to pinpoint the cause of the arrhythmia.

A. Idiopathic. In approximately 10% of patients, no etiology can be found; these patients are said to have "lone" atrial fibrillation if there is no structural heart disease and hypertension.

B. Cardiovascular disorders, including sick sinus syndrome, Wolff-Parkinson-White syndrome, coronary artery disease, congestive heart failure, cardiomyopathy (hypertrophic and dilated), myocarditis, hypertension, and congenital heart disease

C. Pulmonary disorders, including pulmonary embolism

D. Pericardial disease (e.g., pericarditis)

E. Metabolic disturbances, including hyperthyroidism

F. Infiltrative diseases, including amyloidosis, sarcoidosis, and hemochromatosis

G. Intoxication (e.g., alcohol, theophylline, β-agonists)

H. Infection (e.g., endocarditis)

I. Stress induced (e.g., postsurgery due to catecholamine surge)

MNEMONIC **Causes of Atrial Fibrillation ("SWAMP CHILD")**

Sick sinus syndrome, **S**tress
Wolff-Parkinson-White syndrome
Alcohol (intoxication, withdrawal, "holiday heart")
Myocarditis, **M**etabolic abnormality
Pericardial disease, **P**ulmonary disease
CHF, **C**oronary artery disease, **C**ongenital heart disease
Hypertension, **H**yperthyroidism, **H**ypertrophic cardiomyopathy
Infiltrative disease, **I**nfection
Lone (idiopathic)
Dilated cardiomyopathy, **D**rugs

IV. APPROACH TO THE PATIENT. Knowledge of the differential diagnosis will help direct diagnostic tests. All patients should undergo an ECG, a chest radiograph (to rule out pneumonia and other intrathoracic processes), a complete blood count (CBC), electrolyte studies, and thyroid function testing. An echocardiogram is usually obtained to examine cardiac function and atrial size as well as to rule out valve disease.

V. COMPLICATIONS. The risk of **stroke** in all patients with "nonvalvular" atrial fibrillation is approximately 2%–5% per year. It is important to assess for five important factors that can allow you to further define your patient's risk for stroke:

MNEMONIC **Risk Factors for Stroke in Patients with "Nonvalvular" Atrial Fibrillation ("CHADS2" Index)**

CHF (within 100 days or ejection fraction reduced)
Hypertension

Age 75 years or older
Diabetes mellitus
Stroke or transient ischemic attack in past

(In calculating the CHADS2 risk score, each factor above is worth 1 point **except for stroke, which is worth 2 points.** For each 1-point increase in the CHADS2 risk score, the risk of stroke increases by 1.5 per 100 patient-years.)

VI. TREATMENT

A. Acute treatment. The goal of acute treatment of a patient with atrial fibrillation is **rate control.**

1. **Pharmacologic therapy**
   a. **Atrioventricular (AV) node blocking agents.** There are several options for controlling heart rate:
      (1) **Diltiazem** [15–20 mg (0.25 mg/kg) intravenously over 2 minutes; repeat in 15 minutes if necessary; maintenance infusion is 5–20 mg/hr intravenously]
      (2) **Verapamil** (2.5–5.0 mg administered as an intravenous bolus over 1–2 minutes; if needed, repeat with a dose of 5 mg in 15–30 minutes; maximum dose is 15 mg)
      (3) **Esmolol** (250–500 μg/kg intravenously over 1 minute, followed by an intravenous maintenance infusion of 50–200 μg/kg/min). The half-life of esmolol is only 9 minutes; thus, if during drug administration a patient becomes hypotensive, discontinuation will result in a rapid return to baseline.
      (4) **Digoxin** (0.5 mg intravenously followed by 0.25 mg intravenously every 6 hours to a total dose of 1 mg). Digoxin has weak AV nodal blocking properties but may be the only alternative in patients with borderline low blood pressures.
   b. AV node blocking agents are **contraindicated** in patients with irregular, wide complex tachycardia or extremely rapid ventricular rates (>220) until atrial fibrillation with conduction down an accessory pathway (e.g., Wolff-Parkinson-White syndrome) has been excluded. If Wolff-Parkinson-White syndrome is present, these agents can precipitate fatal ventricular fibrillation.
2. **Electrical cardioversion**
   a. **Indications.** Cardioversion is indicated for any patient with **rapid atrial fibrillation** and **life-threatening problems** (e.g., ischemia, severe hypotension, or severe pulmonary edema). You may begin with 200 J in the synchronized mode, but 360 J may be necessary.

b. **Contraindications.** Unless there is an emergent indication, no patient with atrial fibrillation should be cardioverted until anticoagulation therapy has been initiated or until atrial thrombus has been excluded using transesophageal echocardiography. This usually includes patients who are thought to have "new onset" atrial fibrillation because it is difficult to estimate the length of time the patient has been in atrial fibrillation from the patient history. Patients who are cardioverted without undergoing anticoagulation therapy have a 3%–5% risk of stroke within 30 days even though they have returned to normal sinus rhythm on ECG. This is due to abnormal function of the atrium following cardioversion.

B. Chronic treatment. The goals of the chronic treatment of atrial fibrillation are minimization of symptoms and reduction of the risk for stroke. Data from recent trials reveal that a strategy of rate control with anticoagulation has similar mortality benefit when compared to antiarrhythmic therapy. Therefore, a rhythm control strategy is reserved for individuals who are symptomatic from their atrial fibrillation despite adequate rate control.

1. **Rate control.** The goal is a resting heart rate lower than 80 beats/min. Treatment should be selected after considering the patient's other medical problems. For example:
   a. In patients with hypertension or coronary artery disease, a β-blocker is a good choice because it addresses these problems as well as the atrial fibrillation. However, in patients with asthma or chronic obstructive pulmonary disease (COPD), a β-blocker may not be a good choice because it induces bronchoconstriction.
   b. In patients with CHF, β-blockers and digoxin can control the heart rate as well as improve symptoms of CHF. However, β-blockers must be titrated up slowly, and in patients with chronic renal insufficiency, digoxin levels should be monitored very closely.
   c. **AV node ablation** with **pacemaker implantation** is used only under special circumstances when rate control with drug therapy fails.
2. **Rhythm control.** Theoretically, conversion to normal sinus rhythm relieves all rate-related symptoms and returns the risk of stroke to baseline, but since many patients in atrial fibrillation are asymptomatic, anticoagulation must be continued in all patients until cessation of arrhythmia is confirmed.

a. **Electrical cardioversion** should be undertaken only after atrial thrombus has been excluded or at least a 4-week course of anticoagulation has been completed, unless there is an emergent indication. After cardioversion, patients must remain on anticoagulation for at least 4–6 weeks due to the resultant high risk of stroke.

b. **Antiarrhythmic therapy to prevent recurrence.** Rate must be controlled before the initiation of any antiarrhythmic medication. Typically, patients who experience a change in lifestyle due to atrial fibrillation are considered for antiarrhythmic therapy.

(1) **Patients without structural heart disease. Propafenone** and **flecainide** are first-line agents for maintenance of sinus rhythm if patients do not have structural heart disease. These medications are well tolerated from a side effect profile but must be used with caution in patients with renal or hepatic disease.

(2) **Patients with coronary artery disease. Sotalol** and **dofetilide** are the recommended therapy but should be used under the guidance of a cardiologist.

(3) **Patients with decreased left ventricular function. Amiodarone** is the most efficacious antiarrhythmic overall but has a significant long-term side effect profile including possible side effects affecting the pulmonary, neurologic, endocrine, and hepatic systems. Thus, amiodarone should be used with caution in younger patients, and all patients should be routinely monitored with liver function, pulmonary, and thyroid testing.

c. **Radiofrequency ablation of pulmonary vein sources** is a new option in select candidates with symptomatic atrial fibrillation despite antiarrhythmic therapy.

3. **Clot control.** Stroke is the major cause of morbidity and mortality in patients with atrial fibrillation. Anticoagulation therapy is time consuming and bothersome to patients, and the risks and benefits must be assessed on an individual basis.

a. **Warfarin** treatment reduces the risk of stroke by 40%–90%. The target international normalized ratio (INR) should be 2.0–3.0. There is a small increase in the risk of major bleeding.

b. **Aspirin** alone is a consideration for patients at low risk for stroke.

c. **Lower-dose anticoagulation** (i.e., a target INR of 1.0–2.0) and combination therapy (e.g., aspirin plus warfarin) is considered ineffective.

CHADS2 criteria (described previously) can be used to determine appropriate anticoagulation in patients with nonvalvular atrial fibrillation:

CHADS2 criteria	Anticoagulation
No risk factors	Aspirin 81–325 mg daily
1 risk factor	Aspirin 325 mg daily or Coumadin (INR 2.0–3.0)
$\geq$2 risk factors	Coumadin (INR 2.0–3.0)

REFERENCES

Asinger RW, Gage BF, Waterman AD, et al. Validation of clinical classification schemes for predicting stroke: results from the National Registry of Atrial Fibrillation. JAMA 2001;285:2864–2870. [Classic article].

Fuster V, Ryden LE, Asinger RW, et al. ACC/AHA/ESC guidelines for the management of patients with atrial fibrillation: executive summary. J Am Coll Cardiol 2006;48:149–246.

Lip GY, Tse HF. Management of atrial fibrillation. Lancet 2007;370:604–618.

Wyse DG, Waldo AL, DiMarco JP, et al. A comparison of rate control and rhythm control in patients with atrial fibrillation. The atrial fibrillation follow-up investigation of rhythm management (AFFIRM) investigators. N Engl J Med 2002;347:1825. [Classic article].

9

■ Chest Pain

I. INTRODUCTION. Because chest pain (including "discomfort") is common and its etiologies range from a life-threatening myocardial infarction to benign musculoskeletal pain, a simple and reliable approach to the patient is necessary.

II. CAUSES OF CHEST PAIN. One way to remember the causes of chest pain is to use an "outside-in" approach.

A. Skin. Varicella-zoster virus infection (shingles) often causes pain before vesicular lesions are noted. The pain usually occurs in a dermatomal distribution.

B. Chest wall. Musculoskeletal pain may result from shoulder arthritis or bursitis, intercostal injury, metastatic disease to the bones or chest wall, or costochondritis. Breast pathology (e.g., tumors, fibrocystic disease) and nerve root compression (from cervical disc herniation) may also lead to chest pain.

C. Lungs. Inflamed pleura from spontaneous pneumothoraces, pulmonary emboli, infections, malignancies, and connective tissue disorders can all cause chest pain, which is usually pleuritic (i.e., it worsens with inspiration or coughing).

D. Heart and great vessels. Pericarditis, myocardial ischemia and infarction, and aortic dissection can all cause chest pain.

E. Gastrointestinal tract. Esophageal disorders (including esophagitis, spasm, and rupture) are common causes of chest pain. Other gastrointestinal causes of chest pain include gastric and duodenal ulcers, pancreatitis, and biliary disease.

III. APPROACH TO THE PATIENT. Although the outside-in approach is useful for remembering the differential diagnoses for chest pain, it fails to highlight the four acutely life-threatening causes:

Four Killer Chest Pains
Myocardial infarction or ischemia
Pulmonary embolism
Aortic dissection
Spontaneous pneumothorax

Because chest pain may represent one of these emergencies, the usual order of evaluation (e.g., history, physical examination, diagnostic tests) may hinder critical early intervention. The first step should be a quick screen for the four killer chest pains, followed by a more in-depth evaluation if the etiology of the chest pain is still unclear.

A. Screen for the killer chest pains.

1. **"Eyeball" the patient.** A patient who is clutching his or her chest, diaphoretic, and ashen can be presumptively diagnosed as suffering from myocardial infarction from across the room. Even if the presentation is not so classic, you can often decide who looks "sick" and may need a more rapid evaluation in a more monitored setting.
2. **Establish intravenous access and cardiac rhythm monitoring** immediately in patients who appear ill or who have cardiac risk factors.
3. **Evaluate the patient's vital signs**

Any abnormality of the vital signs should alert you to the possibility that the chest pain has a potentially serious cause.

   a. **Check blood pressure in both arms.** Although a difference in pressure of 10 mm Hg or more may be seen in patients with aortic dissection, local atherosclerosis can also produce pressure differences. Therefore, the blood pressure reading is neither sensitive nor specific for aortic dissection.

   b. **Check respiratory rate and oxygen saturation.** Low oxygen saturation may accompany spontaneous pneumothorax, pulmonary embolism, and myocardial infarction (with pulmonary edema).

      (1) **Low oxygen saturation** (e.g., <92%) is often an indication that an arterial blood gas should be ordered immediately.

      (2) **A normal oxygen saturation** may still be accompanied by a significant alveolar-to-arterial (A-a) oxygen gradient during hyperventilation. Therefore, arterial blood gas testing to evaluate the possibility of pulmonary embolism may still be necessary if the rest of the evaluation is unrevealing.

4. **Look at the electrocardiogram (ECG).** The ECG leads are often placed while the vital signs are being checked.

Always obtain a previous ECG to look for changes consistent with ischemia or infarction.

a. ECG abnormalities that suggest **acute myocardial infarction** or **ischemia** (i.e., acute coronary syndromes) are always grounds for admission. Make sure the patient has intravenous access, a cardiac rhythm monitor, and supplemental oxygen, and has been given an aspirin (usually 325 mg) orally. (The emergent treatment of acute coronary syndromes is discussed in more detail in Chapter 11.)

b. **Normal ECG.** A normal ECG does not rule out myocardial infarction or ischemia. **Nitroglycerin** (0.3–0.6 mg sublingually or via aerosol) may be administered and the dose repeated every 3–5 minutes as both a diagnostic challenge and as potential therapy in patients with persistent chest pain.

5. **Take a preliminary history.**

In patients with a history of coronary artery disease or cardiac risk factors and no alternative explanation for the chest pain after careful evaluation, an admission to rule out myocardial infarction (ROMI) is usually appropriate.

a. **Cardiac history and risk factors.** First, ask about any prior cardiovascular problems.
   (1) If there is a history of coronary artery disease, the patient has ischemia until proven otherwise.
   (2) With a negative cardiac history, you can quickly establish the pretest probability of myocardial infarction by assessing cardiac risk factors (i.e., age, male gender, smoking, diabetes, hypertension, high cholesterol, and positive family history).

b. **Other risk factors.** The preliminary history can also help elucidate any predisposing factors to the other killer chest pains. For example, a history of cancer or inactivity may contribute to pulmonary embolism, and uncontrolled hypertension may increase the likelihood of aortic dissection (or myocardial infarction).

6. **Perform a preliminary physical examination.** Frequently, you will have a few brief moments between tests during which you can look at the neck veins, listen to the heart and lungs, palpate the upper abdomen for tenderness, and evaluate the pulses in the arms and legs.

7. **Evaluate the chest radiographs.** Always compare the new films to old films, if they are available.

   a. Spontaneous pneumothorax can be subtle, and you need to look carefully, especially in the apices.

b. Esophageal rupture may lead to air in the mediastinum (pneumomediastinum).
c. Myocardial infarction or aortic dissection may be accompanied by enlargement of the heart or mediastinum, respectively; however, these structures are often exaggerated on anteroposterior films. The presence of pulmonary edema may also be suggestive of myocardial infarction.

8. **Order an arterial blood gas analysis.** If not performed earlier, an arterial blood gas analysis with the patient breathing room air may be useful.

B. Further define the cause of the chest pain.

1. **Take a more detailed patient history.**
   a. **Type of chest pain.** Pulmonary embolism frequently presents with pleuritic chest pain; myocardial infarction may present with "crushing" chest pain or only a mild "discomfort"; and aortic dissection is often characterized by a ripping pain that radiates to the back.
   b. **Radiation of chest pain.** Pain that radiates to the neck or left arm should be considered cardiac until proven otherwise.
      (1) Atypical patterns may still indicate ischemia and include pain, tingling, or numbness in the left fingertips unaccompanied by arm pain and pain in the outer left shoulder.
      (2) It is wise to consider any neck, upper abdominal, or upper back pain as cardiac in origin until proven otherwise.
   c. **Onset of chest pain.** Spontaneous pneumothorax, aortic dissection, and pulmonary embolism usually present with abrupt pain, whereas pain from myocardial infarction or ischemia may build more gradually. Spontaneous pneumothorax and pulmonary embolism often occur while the patient is at rest, whereas aortic dissection and myocardial infarction may occur with rest or exertion.
   d. **Duration of chest pain.** Pain that only lasts seconds or that has been constant for more than 24 hours is usually not caused by one of the four killer chest pains. A myocardial infarction is almost always associated with more than 20 minutes of chest pain.
   e. **Associated symptoms.** Dyspnea, diaphoresis, or lightheadedness should alert you to a probable serious cause of chest pain.
   f. **Aggravating and mitigating factors**

(1) **Deep inspiration** often aggravates pain from the pleura or pericardium (e.g., pleurisy from a pulmonary embolism or pericarditis).

(2) **Exertion** may worsen the pain from myocardial infarction or aortic dissection. Rest may ease the pain from cardiac ischemia, usually gradually.

(3) **Position.** Patients with pericarditis often feel worse when supine and better when sitting up. Patients with musculoskeletal pain may feel worse in certain positions. The pain of myocardial infarction is usually unaffected by changes in position, but this is not always the case.

(4) **Food intake.** Pain on swallowing localizes the problem to the gastrointestinal tract. Chest pain after a meal may indicate gastrointestinal pathology, but it also may occur with myocardial infarction.

(5) **Nitroglycerin.** If chest pain decreases with nitrates (e.g., sublingual nitroglycerin), a cardiac etiology should be suspected; however, esophageal spasm may also respond to this therapy.

2. **Perform a complete physical examination.** Pay extra attention to the following parts of the exam.

   a. **Jugular venous pressure.** An elevated jugular venous pressure should alert you to the possibility of a serious disorder (e.g., myocardial infarction, pulmonary embolism, or tension pneumothorax), but a normal jugular venous pressure does not exclude these disorders.

   b. **Cardiac examination**

   (1) **Heart sounds.** Listen carefully for a third heart sound (S_3) or fourth heart sound (S_4) gallop, which may indicate impaired ventricular contractility or ventricular relaxation, respectively. Both impaired ventricular contractility and impaired relaxation can accompany cardiac ischemia.

   (2) **Murmurs** may also increase the likelihood of a cardiac etiology of chest pain. A mitral regurgitant murmur may accompany a myocardial infarction with papillary muscle dysfunction, whereas an ejection murmur may indicate aortic stenosis or hypertrophic cardiomyopathy. (Both of these conditions may predispose the patient to ischemia).

   c. **Lung examination.** Listen carefully for rales (e.g., from myocardial infarction with pulmonary edema) and pleural friction rubs (e.g., from pulmonary embolism, infection, or other pleural processes).

   d. **Chest wall examination.** Minimal tenderness to palpation is nonspecific, but if the chest pain is *exactly* and *reliably* reproduced (especially in a well-localized area), a musculoskeletal etiology is likely. Briefly inspect the skin for lesions or trauma.

e. **Abdominal examination.** Palpate for any upper abdominal tenderness that may indicate a gastrointestinal cause of the chest pain.

f. **Pulses.** Check pulses in the arms and legs bilaterally.

3. **Pearls**

a. **Myocardial infarction**

(1) Because coronary artery disease is such a common disease, it is always better to admit patients for ROMI if there is any doubt as to the diagnosis, even in young patients.

(2) More than 20 minutes of unexplained chest pain may represent a myocardial infarction, whereas chest pain that lasts less than 20 minutes but increases in frequency, duration, or occurs with minimal exertion often represents unstable angina; both patterns are indications for admission.

(3) Frequently, patients with chest pain are given an antacid and lidocaine swish-and-swallow ("GI cocktail") to evaluate possible reflux esophagitis. **Many patients who "benefit" from this "diagnostic test" may actually have ischemic pain that is improving spontaneously or from bed rest and oxygen therapy.**

b. **Pulmonary embolism.** Clinical suspicion is critical. There is often no evidence of deep vein thrombosis, and subtle symptoms and signs may be inappropriately rationalized away. If you have a high clinical index of suspicion, administer heparin before sending the patient for diagnostic tests.

c. **Aortic dissection**

(1) Most dissections occur either within several centimeters of the aortic valve (type A or ascending aortic dissection) or just distal to the left subclavian artery takeoff (type B or descending aortic dissection). If the patient has abrupt onset of symptoms, pain that radiates to the back, unequal blood pressures, or other suspicious findings, aortic dissection should be ruled out emergently.

(2) Both computed tomography (CT) and transesophageal echocardiography are equally effective in diagnosing aortic dissection. The choice of test to use depends on the patient (e.g., poor renal function may weigh against a CT scan) and institutional preferences. If clinical suspicion is high, a surgeon should be consulted immediately for his or her

input regarding subsequent evaluation, because the mortality rate may be as high as 1% per hour during the first 48 hours. Transthoracic echocardiography is not sensitive enough to rule out dissection, especially in the descending aorta.

(3) If dissection is strongly suspected, blood pressure control and strict avoidance of anticoagulants become essential.

(4) Increasingly, patients with symptoms of dissection are identified as having "intramural" aortic hematoma due to rupture of the vasa vasorum within the thoracic aorta. Prognosis and therapy appear to be similar to those with true aortic dissection.

REFERENCES

Anderson JL, Adams CD, Antman EM et al. ACC/AHA 2007 guidelines for the management of patients with unstable angina/non ST-elevation myocardial infarction: a report of the American College of Cardiology/American Heart Association Task Force on Practice Guidelines. Circulation 2007;116:e148.

Lee TH, Goldman L. Evaluation of the patient with acute chest pain. N Engl J Med 2000;342:1187–1195. [Classic article].

Sequist TD, Marshall R, Lampert S, et al. Missed opportunities in the primary care management of early acute ischemic heart disease. Arch Intern Med 2006;166:2237–2243.

Swap CJ, Nagurney JT. Value and limitations of chest pain history in the evaluation of patients with suspected acute coronary syndromes. JAMA. 2005;294:2623–2629.

10 Angina

I. INTRODUCTION

A. Definition. Myocardial ischemia results when the **oxygen supply is inadequate to meet the oxygen demands** of the cardiac muscle. Although other diseases may reduce the oxygen supply (e.g., coronary artery spasm, hypoxemia, anemia) or increase the oxygen demand (e.g., tachycardia as a result of infection or arrhythmia, thyrotoxicosis), the most common cause of myocardial ischemia is **underlying coronary artery disease** due to atherosclerosis.

B. Risk factors for atherosclerosis include:

1. **Age and gender:** Men older than 45 years and women older than 55 years
2. **Hypertension**
3. **Diabetes mellitus**
4. **Smoking**
5. **Dyslipidemia:** Elevated low-density lipoprotein (LDL) cholesterol and low high-density lipoprotein (HDL) cholesterol
6. **Family history:** First-degree male or female relative with premature atherosclerosis

II. CLINICAL MANIFESTATIONS OF CORONARY ARTERY DISEASE

A. Symptoms

1. **Angina** is the typical symptom associated with myocardial ischemia. It is described as a chest pain beneath or to the left of the midsternum that increases with physical exertion or stress, often lasts from a few minutes up to 20 minutes, and subsides gradually with rest or nitroglycerin.
   a. **Additional features.** If chest pain radiates to the neck or left arm or is accompanied by dyspnea, diaphoresis, or lightheadedness, the likelihood of myocardial ischemia is increased, but these features need not be present.
   b. **Classification.** Angina may be **stable** or **unstable.**
      (1) **Stable angina** usually results from a fixed atherosclerotic plaque that limits oxygen delivery to the cardiac tissue. The oxygen mismatch that results causes a **predictable and stable** pattern of chest pain during exertion.

(2) **Unstable angina** usually results when an atherosclerotic plaque ruptures with the development of superimposed thrombus. As a result, oxygen supply becomes acutely inadequate at lower activity levels or even at rest (discussed more in Chapter 11).

c. **"Anginal equivalents."** Other symptoms unaccompanied by chest pain (e.g., dyspnea) may actually represent "anginal equivalents." **Importantly, some patients with myocardial ischemia may not have any symptoms at all.**

B. Physical examination findings. A normal physical examination does not rule out the possibility of chronic ischemic heart disease. Transient signs may occur during ischemic episodes including hypertension or, less commonly, hypotension; ventricular or supraventricular arrhythmias; a third or fourth heart sound (S_3 or S_4); or a holosystolic murmur over the apex (representative of mitral regurgitation as a result of papillary muscle ischemia). The presence of elevated jugular venous pressure, pulmonary edema, a gallop rhythm, pathologic murmurs, or signs of cardiac risk factors (e.g., peripheral vascular disease from diabetes) should all increase suspicion of coronary artery disease.

III. APPROACH TO THE PATIENT. Angina and ischemic heart disease need to be differentiated from the many other causes of chest pain (see Chapter 9).

A. Patient history. In patients with classic symptoms, the diagnosis of stable or unstable angina can be made on the basis of history alone. An assessment of a patient's atherosclerotic risk profile is critical for determining your overall suspicion for ischemic heart disease.

B. Resting electrocardiography. Chronic ischemic heart disease can be diagnosed in asymptomatic patients by finding evidence of old myocardial infarctions (e.g., q waves) or active ischemia (e.g., ST-segment depression, T-wave inversion) on a resting electrocardiogram (ECG).

C. Patients with episodes of prolonged chest pain or rapidly accelerating angina should have cardiac biomarkers [i.e., creatine kinase (CK) or troponin] evaluated to rule out recent myocardial infarction.

D. Stress tests may be helpful both diagnostically in patients with atypical chest pain and prognostically in patients with typical angina.

1. **Types**

a. **Exercise ECG.** The presence of 1 mm of downsloping or horizontal ST-segment depression on ECG with exercise is considered a positive test for ischemia. Advantages of this testing modality include availability and ability to obtain **prognostic information.** Disadvantages include a poor sensitivity when compared to stress imaging and poor specificity in patients with abnormal resting ECGs (e.g., ST changes and left bundle branch block) and in women.

b. **Myocardial perfusion scintigraphy** is often performed in conjunction with exercise electrocardiography and involves the injection of thallium 201 (^{201}Tl)– or technetium 99 (^{99}Tc)–based agents (sestamibi) into the peripheral venous blood. Cardiac muscle cells that are ischemic or infarcted do not take up these tracers well in comparison to normally perfused, living cells.
   (1) **Reversible defects,** areas that lack thallium on exercise images but "fill in" on rest images (i.e., after 3–4 hours), indicate noninfarcted, ischemic tissue. **Fixed defects** are present on both exercise and rest imaging and denote prior infarction.
   (2) In patients who are unable to exercise vigorously, vasodilators, such as **dipyridamole, adenosine,** or **dobutamine,** that produce vasodilatation in normal coronary arteries out of proportion to that produced in atherosclerotic vessels can be used to shunt thallium away from cardiac regions served by diseased vessels. Dipyridamole and adenosine are contraindicated in patients with significant reversible airway disease because they may facilitate bronchospasm.

c. **Exercise or dobutamine stress echocardiography.** If exercise results in a decrease in ejection fraction or segmental wall motion abnormalities, cardiac ischemia is presumed. Intravenous **dobutamine** increases oxygen demand by increasing heart rate and contractility and may be used as an alternative to exercise.

d. **Other studies such as electron-beam computed tomography (EBCT) and magnetic resonance imaging (MRI) are still under investigation.**

2. **Choosing a test.** Although one stress test cannot be universally recommended over the others, certain caveats apply:
   a. Patients with ECG abnormalities may not be evaluated appropriately with standard exercise electrocardiography alone. Scintigraphy is frequently added to increase sensitivity and specificity.
   b. Echocardiography is more likely to be inadequate in obese patients and patients with chronic obstructive pulmonary disease because of poor images.
   c. Patients with significant baseline wall motion abnormalities on their echocardiogram may have difficult images to interpret using stress echocardiography.

E. **Cardiac catheterization with coronary angiography** is the gold standard for diagnosing obstructive coronary artery disease. If catheterization demonstrates severe coronary artery disease, revascularization with coronary artery bypass surgery or percutaneous coronary intervention (PCI) may be indicated.

IV. TREATMENT

A. **General measures.** Because angina is a symptom of atherosclerosis and coronary artery disease, an indispensable part of the treatment is aimed at identifying and treating cardiac risk factors.

1. **Smoking cessation**
2. **Control of dyslipidemia** (target LDL goal <100 mg/dl); HMG-CoA reductase inhibitors (or "statins") are the drugs of choice
3. **Control of hypertension** (at least systolic <140 mm Hg and diastolic <90 mm Hg)
4. **Control of diabetes mellitus**
5. **Regular exercise** (e.g., brisk walking for 30 minutes four times weekly)
6. **Weight loss**
7. **Treatment of other factors that may aggravate angina** (e.g., anemia, hypoxemia, thyrotoxicosis)

B. **Specific measures for the relief of angina**

1. **Pharmacologic therapy** is generally aimed at increasing myocardial oxygen supply (by coronary vasodilation), decreasing oxygen demand (by decreasing heart rate, contractility, preload, or afterload), and preventing acute thrombotic events. Most patients are initially given an aspirin, β-blocker, and short-acting nitrates, unless there are contraindications.
   a. **Aspirin** (usually 81–325 mg/day) inhibits platelet aggregation and coronary thrombosis and therefore prevents acute coronary syndromes.
   b. **Nitrates** lower oxygen demand by decreasing preload and afterload and may increase oxygen supply by vasodilating coronary arteries (less important mechanism).
      (1) **Short-acting nitrates.** Nitroglycerin 0.3–0.6 mg sublingually or by aerosol may be used for **angina prophylaxis** (the dose is taken 5 minutes before an activity known to result in angina) or **immediate therapy.** (The dose is administered every 3–5 minutes until the pain is relieved; if pain is not relieved in 20 minutes, the patient should get to a hospital immediately.)

(2) **Long-acting nitrates** (e.g., isosorbide dinitrate, isosorbide mononitrate, transdermal nitroglycerin patches). An interval of approximately 8–10 hours per day without nitrate therapy is needed to prevent tachyphylaxis, so the last dose is often given after dinner and patches are removed overnight. Headaches may occur with the initiation of nitrate therapy; if they can be managed conservatively, they frequently resolve after 1–2 weeks.

c. **β-Blockers** decrease heart rate and myocardial contractility, resulting in symptomatic control of angina by lowering oxygen demand. In addition, unlike other antianginal agents, they have been shown to have a mortality benefit in patients with coronary artery disease who have already experienced myocardial infarction.

(1) Frequently used β-blockers include **metoprolol** (50–100 mg orally two times daily) and **atenolol** (50–100 mg orally once daily).

(2) Gradually, the dose of the β-blocker may be increased until the symptoms are controlled, side effects develop (e.g., postural lightheadedness), blood pressure falls below approximately 100/60 mm Hg, resting heart rate falls below approximately 55 beats/min, or the maximal dose is reached. If symptoms are still not controlled, long-acting nitrates may be added and increased as needed with attention to the patient's symptoms, side effects, and blood pressure.

(3) β-blockers are contraindicated in patients with significant bradyarrhythmias. In patients with chronic obstructive pulmonary disease (COPD), a β_1-selective agent (e.g., metoprolol or atenolol) should be used; β-blockers may need to be avoided in patients with severe COPD. Patients with impaired left ventricular function benefit from β-blockers; however, candidates must be started with a low dose (e.g., 12.5 mg metoprolol) and titrated up gradually with frequent patient monitoring.

d. **Calcium channel blockers** lower oxygen demand (by decreasing heart rate, contractility, and afterload) and may increase oxygen supply (by inducing vasodilation of the coronary arteries).

(1) Agents include **verapamil; diltiazem;** and **dihydropyridines (nifedipine, felodipine, amlodipine),** in order of increased effect on lowering systemic vascular resistance and decreased effect on myocardial

inotropy and chronotropy. Verapamil and diltiazem are usually preferred for angina but should be used carefully with β-blockers.

(2) **Calcium channel blockers** have not been associated with improved survival after myocardial infarction and may lead to a worse outcome; therefore, they are **not the initial drugs of choice for most patients with coronary artery disease,** particularly if left ventricular dysfunction is present. **Amlodipine alone has been shown to be safe in those with ejection fractions less than 40%.**

Angiotensin-converting enzyme (ACE) inhibitors do not acutely improve angina symptoms. However, tissue-based ACE inhibitors (i.e., ramipril) reduce mortality rates in patients with ischemic heart disease, likely due to coronary plaque stabilization.

2. **Revascularization.** The indications for **medical therapy** versus **percutaneous intervention** with balloon angioplasty and stent placement should be evaluated on a patient-by-patient basis.
   a. **Medical therapy versus PCI.** The COURAGE trial consisted of 2287 patients with stable angina who were randomized to aggressive medical therapy (β-blockers, calcium channel blockers, antiplatelet agents, nitrates, and aggressive statin therapy) versus aggressive medical therapy with PCI. At over 4 years of follow-up, there was no significant difference in mortality or hospitalizations between the two groups. A higher percentage of those in the PCI group were angina-free at 3 years but there was no significant difference at 5 years between groups. Therefore, all patients should receive aggressive medical therapy and the decision for PCI needs to be made on an individual basis.
   b. **Coronary artery bypass surgery** is generally considered superior in the treatment of patients with left main coronary artery disease (>50% diameter occlusion) or three-vessel disease (≥70% diameter occlusion) associated with decreased left ventricular function (<50%). Diabetics also seem to benefit more from bypass surgery when compared with PCI.

      (1) Bypass surgery may also benefit patients with three-vessel disease and severe angina (class III or IV) and patients with proximal left anterior descending artery occlusion associated with two-vessel disease.

There is less of a consensus on whether bypass surgery, angioplasty, or medical therapy is appropriate in these instances.

c. Often the final choice between bypass or PCI depends on the **coronary anatomy's suitability** for revascularization (i.e., good "targets" for bypass surgery, approachable lesions for PCI).

REFERENCES

Boden WE, O'Rourke RA. Optimal medical therapy with or without PCI for stable coronary disease. N Engl J Med 2007;356(15):1503–1516.

Fraker TD, Fihn SD. 2007 Focused update of the ACC/AHA 2002 guidelines for the management of patients with chronic stable angina. J Am Coll Cardiol 2007;50:2264–2274.

Lee TH, Boucher CA. Clinical practice. Noninvasive tests in patients with stable coronary artery disease. N Engl J Med 2001;344(24):1840–1845.

11 Myocardial Infarction

I. **INTRODUCTION.** Unstable angina, non–ST-segment elevation myocardial infarction (NSTEMI), and ST-segment elevation myocardial infarction (STEMI) make up the **acute coronary syndromes (ACSs).** The term encompasses the entire range of presentations associated with acute ischemic heart disease and, importantly, reflects the diagnostic uncertainty present on initial evaluation. ACS is a leading cause of death in the United States. The failure to recognize ACS in the emergency room has led to inappropriate patient discharges, resulting in an abundance of malpractice claims. Many therapies have a proven mortality benefit in the treatment of ACS; however, studies show that patients frequently receive suboptimal therapy.

II. **PATHOPHYSIOLOGY OF ACS.** ACS usually results from the rupture of unstable atherosclerotic plaques with subsequent thrombosis of a coronary artery. This leads to inadequate blood flow and oxygen delivery, which in turn results in myocardial cell death. Less common causes of ACS include coronary vasospasm (usually associated with coronary artery disease), severe hypotension, emboli (e.g., from mitral valve disease), aortic dissection (usually with right coronary artery involvement), vasculitis, and cocaine use (atherosclerosis, vasospasm, and platelet aggregation are presumed etiologies).

III. **CLINICAL MANIFESTATIONS OF MI.** Typical symptoms and signs associated with cardiac ischemia are discussed in Chapters 9 and 10. The **chest pain** associated with ACS differs from that of stable angina in that it frequently begins while the patient is at rest or has minimal exertion, lasts more than 20 minutes, is more severe, and is unrelieved with sublingual nitroglycerin; however, these findings are variable. **Pain that lasts for more than 20 minutes should be considered due to MI** (either NSTEMI or STEMI) until proved otherwise.

IV. **DIAGNOSIS.** Because unstable angina and MI share similar pathophysiology, it is not surprising that they frequently cannot be distinguished by clinical criteria alone. Patients are often admitted for "unstable angina/rule out MI (ROMI)"; serial electrocardiograms (ECGs) and cardiac biomarker studies are required for a definitive diagnosis. If ECGs show evidence of injury (i.e., ST elevation) or if cardiac biomarkers show evidence of cell death, then MI is diagnosed.

The diagnosis of MI is made by the presence of cardiac biomarker elevation in the setting of (1) typical symptoms and signs of MI or (2) ECG changes consistent with an MI.

A. **Patient history and physical examination.** Chest pain is the most common symptom of MI, but other signs and symptoms may also signal MI (e.g., flash pulmonary edema, hypotension, dyspnea).
B. **Electrocardiography. An initial ECG is the key to triaging patients with ACS and should be performed as soon as possible in the emergency room.** Following admission of the patient, serial ECGs are usually obtained on a frequent basis until resolution of symptoms occurs and the ECG changes stabilize; a daily ECG and an ECG following reports of any symptoms are usually obtained thereafter. Specific ECG findings for MI or ischemia include hyperacute (peaked) T waves, ST elevations, ST depressions, Q waves, or inverted T waves.

In up to 10% of cases of documented MI, the ECG is normal.

1. **ST-segment depressions and elevations may reflect both myocardial ischemia and injury.**
   a. The subendocardial region is the most susceptible to ischemia because it is perfused "last" (i.e., the coronary arteries course from the outer epicardial surface inward), and this is typically manifested by ST-segment depression. Because the subendocardium is on the inner surface of the heart away from the ECG leads on the chest wall, **subendocardial injury** may be seen as **ST-segment depression.** Epicardial injury, in contrast, is near the ECG leads and typically occurs with transmural ischemia; it most often results in a larger amount of myocardial damage and is evident as ST-segment elevation on the ECG. ST-segment elevations also may occur with transient ischemia (e.g., from vasospasm).

b. Traditional terminology that identifies ST-segment depressions as "**ischemia**" and ST-segment elevations as "**infarct**" is oversimplified. ST depressions may occur with infarction, and ST-segment elevations may occur with transient epicardial ischemia (e.g., from coronary vasospasm). ST-segment changes in ACS are more accurately thought of as representing myocardial "**injury.**"

2. **Q waves** signify electrical activity moving away from the area of the heart where they are seen; they therefore indicate dead muscle (previous MI) in that region. Q-wave MIs may occasionally disappear on ECG over years.
3. A **right-sided ECG** (leads V1 and V2 reversed, with the other leads placed in corresponding positions on the right side of the chest) should be obtained in all patients with an acute inferior wall MI. Right ventricular infarction may complicate the clinical course of a MI and is associated with a higher in-hospital mortality rate. ST-segment elevation in leads RV4 or RV3 on a right-sided ECG indicates right ventricular infarction.

C. Cardiac biomarker studies

1. MI is usually associated with an elevation in serum creatine kinase (CK) levels. Detection of the CK-MB isoenzyme has increased specificity for cardiac muscle and maintains a high sensitivity. **CK with isoenzyme studies** are usually ordered every 8 hours for 24 hours or until a peak level is reached (usually 16–18 hours).
2. More recently, **cardiac troponin levels** have been introduced as a more useful means of diagnosing acute MI. Cardiac troponin levels are more sensitive and specific than CK for the detection of MI. These biomarkers usually rise within 4–6 hours of cell death, peak at 18–24 hours, and may remain elevated for up to 7–10 days.
3. **Myoglobin levels** rise quickly (within 2 hours), but are nonspecific to cardiac injury.

V. APPROACH TO THE PATIENT. The treatment of ACS requires both precision and speed. The following stepwise approach allows you to make critical treatment decisions immediately, followed by those that are less urgent. Whenever a patient is admitted with an ACS, it is helpful to answer three questions: (1) What is the patient's hemodynamic status? (2) Is reperfusion [i.e., thrombolysis or primary percutaneous coronary intervention (PCI)] indicated? (3) What other treatments may benefit the patient?

A. What is the patient's hemodynamic status?

1. **Assessment.** Hemodynamic status can be approximated by examination of the volume status [i.e., jugular venous pressure (JVP) and lungs] and peripheral perfusion (i.e., extremities examination and urine output).
   a. **Low-risk patients** have normal JVP, clear lungs, and warm extremities associated with normal peripheral pulses. The presence of clear lungs usually indicates normal left ventricular filling pressures [i.e., a normal pulmonary capillary wedge pressure (PCWP)], and normal findings on examination of the extremities imply adequate cardiac output.
   b. **Intermediate-risk patients** have a normal extremity exam, but elevated JVP and pulmonary rales are found. In these patients, elevated right- and left-sided filling pressures [i.e., right atrial pressure (RAP) >10 mm Hg and PCWP >18 mm Hg] are suspected.
   c. **High-risk patients** have crackles and cool extremities (due to vasoconstriction and decreased cardiac output) with diminished peripheral pulses. These patients are in **cardiogenic shock.** The presence of pulmonary edema suggests that the PCWP, an estimate of end-diastolic volume, is elevated. Normally, according to the Starling curve, a high end-diastolic volume ensures that the stroke volume will be maximized. If the heart is unable to adequately perfuse the end organs despite adequate filling (i.e., a high PCWP), cardiogenic shock is diagnosed. Urine output and mental status can be very helpful in assessing adequate end-organ perfusion.
2. **Management**
   a. **Low-risk patients** are hemodynamically stable and have a low mortality rate. Management of these patients entails deciding whether reperfusion therapy (i.e., thrombolysis or primary PCI) is indicated, and what other forms of therapy might benefit the patient (see V B C).
   b. **Intermediate-risk patients** have evidence of pulmonary edema, which may decrease oxygenation while increasing oxygen demand (increased sympathetic tone increases the heart rate and myocardial contractility).
      (1) **Agents frequently used in the treatment of MI** (e.g., **nitrates, morphine**) may also treat pulmonary edema by decreasing preload.
      (2) **Intravenous diuretics** should be given as needed.

c. **High-risk patients** have **cardiogenic shock.**
   (1) **Pulmonary artery (PA) line placement** is indicated for monitoring cardiac output, systemic vascular resistance, and PCWP. In patients with ACS, only those with evidence of cardiogenic shock generally require hemodynamic monitoring with a PA line.
   (2) Pharmacologic therapy is dictated by the **patient's blood pressure.** Although cardiogenic shock is often accompanied by **hypotension,** blood pressure may still be normal with low flow states due to a significant increase in systemic resistance.

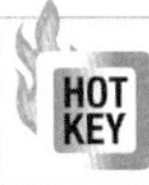

Do not assume that normal blood pressure indicates adequate end-organ flow.

(a) **Systolic blood pressure >90–100 mm Hg**
   (i) **Dobutamine** is often started intravenously at a dose of 2.5 μg/kg/min. The dose may be increased gradually (up to 15–20 μg/kg/min) until the cardiac output rises and the PCWP falls. Dobutamine raises cardiac output by **increasing myocardial contractility** and by **decreasing systemic vascular resistance**. Because blood pressure is the product of cardiac output and systemic vascular resistance, it may remain stable, increase, or decrease depending on how much the cardiac output increases in comparison with the decrease in systemic vascular resistance. A decrease in blood pressure commonly occurs with dobutamine therapy, so the systolic blood pressure should be greater than 90 mm Hg (and preferably >100 mm Hg) before the initiation of therapy.
   (ii) **Sodium nitroprusside** is an alternative to dobutamine but often requires a higher starting blood pressure or the concomitant administration of an inotrope. Sodium nitroprusside is very effective in **decreasing systemic vascular resistance,** thus increasing end-organ perfusion.

(b) **Systolic blood pressure <90 mm Hg**
   (i) Intravenous **dopamine** is usually given. Dopamine usually causes **renal artery**

dilatation at doses of 1–2 μg/kg/min ("renal dose" dopamine), **increased inotropy** from β_1-receptor stimulation at doses of 5–10 μg/kg/min, and vasoconstriction from α-receptor stimulation at higher doses; **however, significant overlap and variability exist.** Once the systolic blood pressure is greater than 90–100 mm Hg, dobutamine is often added and the dopamine is titrated down (preferably to "renal doses") as tolerated by the blood pressure. Because arrhythmias may complicate dobutamine or dopamine therapy, patients require careful rhythm monitoring, and **electrolytes should be maintained in the normal range** (especially potassium and magnesium levels).

(ii) Placement of an **intra-aortic balloon pump (IABP)** increases cardiac output, reduces systemic resistance, and improves coronary blood flow by improving perfusion pressure during diastole. When available, it should be considered in all hypotensive patients with acute ischemia.

3. **Emergent PCI** is the only therapy that has been shown to decrease mortality rates in patients with cardiogenic shock from ACS and is clearly the **treatment of choice.**

B. Is reperfusion therapy with thrombolysis or primary PCI indicated? The initial triage ECG is critical in determining whether patients are appropriate candidates for immediate reperfusion therapy. In patients with chest pain of 6 hours or less duration (and possibly up to 12 hours or longer) and ST elevations of at least 1 mm in two consecutive ECG leads (i.e., STEMI) or evidence of a new left bundle branch block, there is a mortality benefit from immediate coronary reperfusion. Unless contraindicated, all such patients should therefore undergo thrombolysis or primary PCI. Fibrinolysis is the treatment of choice for patients with no contraindications and who are unable to be transferred to a medical center with PCI within 90 minutes. Importantly, studies in patients with NSTEMI have not shown any benefit with immediate reperfusion strategies and, in the case of thrombolytics, potential harm.

1. **Primary PCI** is the treatment of choice in centers that can perform the procedure quickly and with expertise. It also may be favored when there are contraindications to thrombolytic therapy, and select patients should be transferred to a specialized center if necessary.

2. **Thrombolysis**
   a. **Contraindications**
      (1) **Absolute contraindications** generally include the presence of:
         (a) **Central nervous system (CNS) disease.** Recent trauma or surgery, aneurysms, arteriovenous malformations, tumors, or a history of hemorrhagic stroke at any time or nonhemorrhagic stroke within 3 months are usually considered contraindications.
         (b) **Active gastrointestinal** or **genitourinary bleeding**
         (c) **Pregnancy**
      (2) **Relative contraindications** generally include:
         (a) **Traumatic** or **prolonged cardiopulmonary resuscitation**
         (b) **Recent trauma** or **surgery** (within 2 weeks)
         (c) **Diabetic retinopathy**
         (d) **Sustained hypertension** (e.g., blood pressure >180/130 mm Hg after appropriate treatment)
         (e) **Coagulopathy, thrombocytopenia,** or **current oral anticoagulation therapy**
         (f) **Recent trauma to noncompressible arterial or venous puncture sites during intravenous access attempts**
   b. **Other considerations.** Patients who have had **prior coronary artery bypass grafting** do not benefit as much from either thrombolysis or PCI but should still be considered candidates for reperfusion when appropriate.
   c. **Agents.** The most commonly used thrombolytic agents are **streptokinase, reteplase, tenecteplase, and alteplase.** There may be slight advantages to one of the agents, depending on the clinical situation.
   d. **General recommendations.** The mortality benefit decreases drastically with delay in therapy, so speed is of the essence. Make sure a large-bore peripheral intravenous catheter (usually 16-gauge) is in place before therapy and limit venous and arterial blood draws. It is clear that the type of agent used is less important than ensuring that all patients who meet appropriate criteria and who do not have contraindications receive thrombolytic therapy as rapidly as possible.

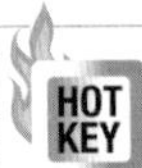

Time elapsed = myocardium lost

e. **Signs of successful reperfusion** include a prompt decrease in chest pain, normalization of the ST segment, an accelerated idioventricular rhythm, or an early peak of the CK enzymes (within 12 hours).

f. If thrombolytic agents do not appear to result in thrombolysis, then **salvage PCI** should be considered in high-risk patients with ongoing signs of ischemia/infarction.

C. What other treatments may benefit the patient with ACS? Specific forms of therapy with nitrates, β-blockers, and calcium channel blockers as well as potential contraindications are outlined in Chapter 10. The **coronary care unit (CCU) or specialized telemetry units** are the best place to manage patients with ACS, given the need for frequent vital checks and continuous rhythm monitoring.

1. **General measures**
   a. **Bed rest** and a **stool softener** are usually prescribed.
   b. **Subcutaneous heparin** (5000 units twice daily) is usually administered to prevent deep venous thrombosis in patients who are otherwise not receiving systemic anticoagulation.
   c. **Analgesia.** Initially, **nitrates** are usually given to relieve pain, but **morphine sulfate** (2–4 mg intravenously) may be used for persistent pain (careful titration of dose may be needed in patients who have borderline low blood pressure).
2. **Aspirin and other oral antiplatelet agents. Aspirin** (usually 325 mg orally) has been shown to have a mortality benefit in all patients with ACS, even in patients with STEMI who receive thrombolytics. **Therefore, aspirin should be chewed as soon as possible in all patients with suspected ACS. Clopidogrel** (600 mg loading dose), a thienopyridine that inhibits adenosine diphosphate (ADP)–induced platelet aggregation, has recently been shown in clinical trials to reduce recurrent ischemic events in unstable angina and NSTEMI when used concomitantly with aspirin. **In addition, clopidogrel should be used in all patients undergoing PCI with intracoronary stent placement for at least 4 weeks** (and up to 12 months depending on stent type). Active bleeding is a contraindication to both these agents. Due to increased bleeding risk, clopidogrel should not be given if a high likelihood of three-vessel coronary artery disease necessitating bypass surgery is anticipated.
3. **Oxygen** (e.g., 2–4 L/min) is often administered, although the benefit in patients with normal oxygen saturation is questionable.
4. **Nitrates** are usually given unless the patient is hypotensive or has evidence of a low cardiac output. Nitrates

should be used cautiously (if at all) in patients with right ventricular infarction given their dependence on preload.

5. **β-Blockers** have been shown to decrease mortality rates in patients with MI and are especially useful in patients with tachycardia, hypertension, or both. Oral β-blocker therapy should be given to those patients who do not display signs of heart failure, shock, or other relative contraindications to β-blocker therapy.
6. **Calcium channel blockers** have not been shown to have a mortality benefit in patients with MI and, in some studies, have been associated with increased mortality rates. In general, these agents **should be avoided** in the acute management of MI.
7. **Angiotensin-converting enzyme (ACE) inhibitors** are useful in the chronic management of patients with ischemic heart disease, but are associated with an increased mortality rate when given intravenously in the acute setting (see VII B 1 a).
8. **Heparin** is useful in the treatment of patients with NSTEMI and high-risk patients with unstable angina. Low-molecular-weight heparin (such as enoxaparin) appears to decrease recurrent ischemic events better than unfractionated heparin and has the benefit of being easier to dose.
9. **Glycoprotein IIb/IIIa (GIIb/IIIa) inhibitors.** GIIb/IIIa inhibitors block platelet glycoprotein IIb/IIIa receptors, the final common pathway for all platelet aggregation. Three intravenous agents are currently available: abciximab, eptifibatide, and tirofiban. Any of the three agents may be used in **high-risk unstable angina cases** (i.e., dynamic ECG changes) and **NSTEMI. Contraindications include** severe renal insufficiency and bleeding diathesis (thrombocytopenia). Abciximab might be better if early PCI is planned, whereas tirofiban has been shown to be beneficial even without PCI.
10. **Early coronary angiography and PCI.** In high-risk patients with unstable angina (dynamic ECG changes) and NSTEMI, there is accumulating evidence that a strategy of early coronary angiography and revascularization (either PCI or coronary bypass surgery) improves outcomes when compared with conservative management (i.e., risk stratification with exercise stress testing). In low-risk patients with NSTEMI or those with STEMI who have received thrombolytic therapy, a conservative strategy is more reasonable. Typically, this involves a noninvasive assessment of both left ventricular (LV) function and ischemic burden. Patients with a decreased LV function (ejection fraction

<40%) and/or significant ischemia on their stress test should undergo coronary angiography with possible revascularization as needed. Low-risk patients with unstable angina (no dynamic ECG changes with negative cardiac biomarkers) should also undergo noninvasive exercise stress testing before coronary angiography.

11. **Coronary angiography with revascularization** is usually indicated for patients with (1) unstable angina and high-risk features (i.e., dynamic ECG changes); (2) NSTEMI; or (3) completed STEMI and high-risk features (recurrent ischemia, inadequate reperfusion therapy, stress tests that show significant ischemia, or baseline LV dysfunction).

VI. ACS COMPLICATIONS

A. Arrhythmias are most common during the initial 12–24 hours.

1. **Tachyarrhythmias** are evaluated and treated as discussed in Chapter 7. Of note, **prophylactic lidocaine and magnesium are no longer recommended.** Lidocaine is reserved for patients with sustained or nonsustained ventricular tachycardia. Patients with tachyarrhythmias [ventricular tachycardia/ fibrillation or nonsustained ventricular tachycardia (NSVT)] 24–48 hours after presentation are considered at high long-term risk for sudden cardiac death. These patients should be evaluated for the placement of **implantable cardiac defibrillators (ICDs)**, especially if they have LV dysfunction (see VII C 1).
2. **Bradyarrhythmias** are more common with inferior wall MI because the sinoatrial (SA) and atrioventricular (AV) nodes are more dependent on blood flow from the right coronary artery.
   a. **Intravenous atropine** (0.5–1 mg every 3–5 minutes, up to 3 mg) is usually effective for sinus bradycardia and symptomatic Wenckebach (Mobitz type 1) second-degree AV block.
   b. Temporary pacing is generally indicated for patients with acute MI and:
      (1) Symptomatic sinus bradycardia and Wenckebach block that is unresponsive to atropine
      (2) Mobitz type 2 second-degree AV block or third-degree AV block
      (3) New bifascicular block, including alternating left and right bundle branch block, right bundle branch block with left anterior or posterior fascicular block, and left bundle branch block with first-degree AV block

B. **Recurrent ischemia or chest pain** following MI that is not responsive to medical management is usually an urgent indication for **coronary angiography** and **revascularization.**

C. **Pump dysfunction.** Severe left ventricular failure is managed as outlined for cardiogenic shock. In severe cases, IABP and **left ventricular assist devices** may also be used until more definitive therapy (i.e., **cardiac transplantation**) can be performed.

D. **Right ventricular infarction** should always be suspected when hypotension accompanies an inferior MI. Treatment involves **large fluid boluses** to increase right-sided cardiac output and left ventricular filling. **Inotropic agents** (i.e., dobutamine) with hemodynamic monitoring may also be required. Nitrates should be avoided because these patients are preload dependent.

E. **Mechanical complications** usually occur 2–7 days after infarction.

1. **Cardiac tamponade** from free wall rupture usually leads to abrupt hypotension and death.
2. **Ventricular septal defect** or **papillary muscle rupture leading to acute mitral regurgitation**
   a. **Clinical signs and symptoms**
      (1) These disorders are often heralded by hypotension, pulmonary edema, or both. Any abrupt change in hemodynamics should increase clinical suspicion of one of these mechanical complications.
      (2) A holosystolic murmur may be present in both conditions, but the location is usually at the left sternal border in ventricular septal defect and at the apex in papillary muscle rupture.
   b. **Diagnosis.** An **emergent surface echocardiogram** is the quick and easy way to make the diagnosis. Hemodynamic monitoring with a PA line is usually necessary for treatment and may also be used diagnostically—an increased oxygen saturation between the right atrium and pulmonary artery is seen with ventricular septal defect, and both disorders may display prominent v waves.
   c. **Treatment.** Nitroprusside or IABP may be used temporarily to decrease afterload and improve forward cardiac output. **Emergent surgical repair** is indicated for definitive therapy.
3. **Left ventricular aneurysm** or **pseudoaneurysm**
   a. **LV aneurysm** most often occurs after large anterior wall MIs. **Warfarin therapy** for 3–6 months is often administered to patients with large anterior wall MIs even in the absence of an LV thrombus. LV aneurysms may

also be associated with refractory heart failure or arrhythmias and require surgical correction.

b. **Pseudoaneurysms** are contained LV free-wall ruptures distinguished by a relatively narrow neck and a predisposition for an inferior-posterior location; **surgical correction** is generally performed to prevent delayed rupture.

VII. RISK REDUCTION

A. General measures include **aspirin therapy** (usually 81–325 mg/day), which has a mortality benefit, and **aggressive risk factor reduction** (see Chapter 10 I B). Patients intolerant of aspirin should be given clopidogrel or ticlopidine.

B. Additional diagnostic testing and preventive therapy. Because the major complications of MI are heart failure, recurrent ischemia, and arrhythmias, diagnostic testing is aimed at identifying and treating these disorders (risk stratification).

1. **General measures.** The post-MI **left ventricular ejection fraction** is the single best predictor of survival. For this reason, patients usually receive echocardiograms or another noninvasive assessment of their ejection fraction before discharge from the hospital.
   a. **ACE inhibitors** have been shown to decrease mortality rates in patients who have a **left ventricular ejection fraction** of **less than 40%** post-MI. Recent data suggest that ACE inhibitors may also be beneficial in patients with ischemic heart disease and normal ejection fractions.
   b. **β-Blockers** decrease post-MI mortality rates in patients with decreased as well as normal left ventricular ejection fractions. Patients with the lowest left ventricular ejection fractions who can tolerate β-blockers have the greatest survival advantage. β-Blockers may decrease the likelihood of arrhythmias and progressive heart failure in these high-risk patients.
2. **Stress testing** (see Chapter 10)
   a. Although highly recommended in the past, **stress testing in asymptomatic patients after PCI is not currently recommended unless high-risk features are present.** The recurrence of chest pain, decreased functional status, or the presence of multivessel disease on catheterization may warrant further evaluation.

C. Indications for ICD placement after MI

1. Criteria for patients who are more than 40 days post– MI or more than 3 months post-PCI or post-CABG
   a. Prior MI with an ejection fraction less than or equal to 30%;

   b. Ejection fraction less than or equal to 35% and New York Heart Association class II or III heart failure symptoms; or
   c. Patients with prior myocardial infarction and ejection fraction less than or equal to 40% and evidence of nonsustained ventricular tachycardia on Holter monitor are recommended to have an electrophysiologic study. If positive, then ICD is indicated.
2. Patients who develop hemodynamically significant ventricular tachycardia greater than or equal to 48 hours after an STEMI should receive an implantable defibrillator.

REFERENCES

Anderson JL, Adams CD, Antman EM, et al. ACC/AHA 2007 guidelines for the management of patients with unstable angina/non-ST-elevation myocardial infarction: a report of the American College of Cardiology/American Heart Association Task Force on Practice Guidelines. J Am Coll Cardiol 2007;50:e1–e157.

Boden WE, Shah PK, Gupta V, et al. Contemporary approach to the diagnosis and management of non-ST-segment elevation acute coronary syndromes. Prog Cardiovasc Dis 2008;50:311–351.

Cesario DA, Dec GW. Implantable cardioverter-defibrillator therapy in clinical practice. J Am Coll Cardiol 2006;47:1507–1517.

De Luca G, Suryapranata H, Marino P. Reperfusion strategies in acute ST-elevation myocardial infarction: an overview of current status. Prog Cardiovasc Dis 2008;50:352–382.

Diercks DB, Kontos MC, Weber JE, et al. Management of ST-segment elevation myocardial infarction in EDs. Am J Emerg Med 2008;26:91–100.

Gluckman TJ, Sachdev M, Schulman SP, et al. A simplified approach to the management of non-ST-segment elevation acute coronary syndromes. JAMA 2005;293:349–357. [Classic article].

Wilansky S, Moreno CA, Lester SJ. Complications of myocardial infarction. Crit Care Med 2007;35:348–354.

12

Congestive Heart Failure

I. INTRODUCTION

A. **Definition.** Congestive heart failure (CHF) is a **syndrome** that is the final common pathway for several different disease processes. It occurs when the heart is unable to supply sufficient amounts of blood at normal filling pressures to match the metabolic demands of the body.

B. **Clinical manifestations** classically include fatigue, lethargy, dyspnea on exertion or at rest, paroxysmal nocturnal dyspnea (PND), orthopnea, weight gain, and leg swelling.

C. **Incidence.** CHF is a common disorder, primarily affecting older individuals (10% of the U.S. population older than 75 years of age have this diagnosis). There are approximately 500,000 new cases diagnosed each year.

D. **Mortality rates.** The 1- and 5-year mortality rates for all patients with CHF are 21% and 50%, respectively.

II. CLASSIFICATION.

There are many different classification schemes. The most useful include the following:

A. **New York Heart Association (NYHA) functional classification**

1. **Class I:** Symptomatic only with extraordinary activity
2. **Class II:** Symptomatic during ordinary activity
3. **Class III:** Symptomatic with less than ordinary activity
4. **Class IV:** Symptomatic at rest

B. **American College of Cardiology/American Heart Association (ACC/AHA) Staging System**

1. **Stage A:** Patients at high risk for developing CHF but with no structural heart disease
2. **Stage B:** Patients with structural heart disease that are **asymptomatic**
3. **Stage C:** Patients with structural heart disease and past or current symptoms
4. **Stage D:** Patients with end-stage disease requiring specialized therapy (i.e., mechanical support devices, intravenous inotropic agents)
5. This new classification was established (1) to complement the NYHA functional class system, which primarily assesses the symptom severity of patients in stages C and D, and (2) to target therapy.

C. **Forward versus backward failure.** Forward failure is primarily characterized by low cardiac output and its associated symptoms of fatigue and weakness. Backward failure results in "congestive" symptoms of pulmonary and peripheral edema.

D. **Left-sided versus right-sided failure.** It is important to decide if patients have evidence of left-sided failure, because these patients can present with significant hypoxemia and therefore may need to be treated urgently (see IV D). The distinction between left-sided and right-sided failure is based primarily on signs found during physical examination—but all these findings can be insensitive and nonspecific especially in patients with chronic heart failure.

1. **Left-sided failure.** Signs of left-sided failure include **a left-sided third heart sound (S_3), rales, wheezes** ("cardiac asthma," a manifestation of interstitial edema), and **tachypnea.** Patients with chronic systolic dysfunction often have dilated pulmonary vasculature that is able to accommodate excess fluid and thus crackles are not always present.
2. **Right-sided failure.** Signs of right-sided failure include a **right-sided S_3** (i.e., one that increases with inspiration), **an elevated jugular venous pressure, abnormal hepatojugular reflux, ascites, peripheral edema,** and an **enlarged liver.**
   a. Most of the time, evidence of biventricular failure is found during physical examination because **the most common cause of right-sided failure is left-sided failure.**
   b. Other causes of right-sided failure include:
      (1) **Pulmonary hypertension** [most commonly caused by chronic obstructive pulmonary disease (COPD)]
      (2) **Right ventricular infarction** (usually occurring in the setting of left-sided inferior wall infarction)
      (3) **Right-sided endocarditis**

E. **Systolic versus diastolic dysfunction.** Left ventricular failure can be either systolic or diastolic. This is the most important distinction to make because it affects treatment.

1. **Systolic dysfunction** means that the heart's contractility is compromised. The most useful clinical measure of contractility is the **ejection fraction,** which is **considered significantly abnormal below 40%.** Causes of systolic dysfunction include:
   a. **Myocardial infarction** and **ischemic heart disease**
   b. **"Burned out" hypertensive or valvular heart disease.** Initially, these disorders lead to diastolic dysfunction, but with time, the heart dilates and the ejection fraction decreases.
   c. **Dilated cardiomyopathies** (a cardiomyopathy is a disorder of the myocardium not caused by coronary artery

disease, hypertension, valvular disease, or congenital heart disease)

d. **Myocarditis**

2. **Diastolic dysfunction** means that the heart has normal contractility, but its ability to relax and allow adequate filling during diastole is compromised. These patients have a **normal or supranormal ejection fraction.** Causes of diastolic dysfunction include:
   a. **Ischemia**
   b. **Disorders that lead to left ventricular hypertrophy,** such as:
      (1) Hypertension
      (2) Aortic stenosis
      (3) Hypertrophic cardiomyopathy
   c. **Restrictive cardiomyopathy.** This disorder is usually caused by infiltrative diseases (e.g., hemochromatosis, amyloidosis, sarcoidosis, or scleroderma) or injury such as postradiation fibrosis.
3. In most patients, evidence of both diastolic and systolic dysfunction coexist; however, up to 50% of hospitalizations for heart failure are due to diastolic dysfunction. Both types of dysfunction have similar clinical manifestations.

CHF with a low ejection fraction = systolic dysfunction
CHF with a normal or high ejection fraction = diastolic dysfunction

MNEMONIC **Common Causes of Dilated Cardiomyopathy ("PIPED")**

Postmyocarditis
Idiopathic
Peripartum
Ethanol
Drugs (cocaine, heroin, anthracyclines)

III. APPROACH TO THE PATIENT

A. Determine if the patient's symptoms are truly due to CHF. Given substantial limitations of the physical examination, this can be particularly difficult. Importantly, accumulating data suggest that B-type natriuretic peptide (BNP) may aid in separating breathlessness from CHF from noncardiac causes, especially in the emergency department setting. Once CHF is suspected, assess how symptomatic the patient is.

B. On the basis of the patient's history, physical examination findings, and chest radiographs, categorize the failure as predominantly left sided, right sided, or biventricular.

C. If the patient has left-sided CHF, determine whether the dysfunction is predominantly systolic or diastolic, using the ejection fraction as a basis for the determination. Ejection fraction can be assessed using echocardiography, multiple gated acquisition (MUGA) scans, gated single-photon emission computed tomography (SPECT), or cardiac catheterization. **Remember, if a patient with a normal ejection fraction has cardiogenic pulmonary edema or additional evidence for elevated filling pressures or low cardiac output, then the dysfunction is diastolic.**

D. Determine the underlying cause of CHF (e.g., coronary artery disease, valvular disease, hypertension, cardiomyopathy).

E. If the patient's symptoms have worsened acutely (this is usually the scenario in patients evaluated in the emergency department), you must decide what precipitated the CHF exacerbation:

MNEMONIC **Factors That Can Exacerbate CHF ("FAILURE")**

Forgot meds
Arrhythmia or **A**nemia
Infections, **I**schemia, or **I**nfarction
Lifestyle (e.g., increased sodium intake, stress)
Upregulators (e.g., thyroid disease, pregnancy)
Rheumatic valve or worsening of other valvular diseases
Embolism (pulmonary)

IV. TREATMENT

A. Goals of treatment of CHF (and most other diseases) are twofold:

1. **Reduce symptoms**
2. **Reduce mortality**

B. Chronic systolic dysfunction. Treatment primarily involves the following:

1. **Vasodilators.** Peripheral arterial vasodilators [e.g., angiotensin-converting enzyme (ACE) inhibitors, angiotensin-receptor blockers, hydralazine, isosorbide dinitrate] are drugs that have been shown to reduce both symptoms and mortality rates in both asymptomatic and symptomatic patients (ACC/AHA stages B and C). The ACE inhibitors are considered first-line therapy for systolic dysfunction. If ACE inhibitors are unable to be tolerated because of cough, angiotensin-receptor blockers are reasonable second-line agents.
2. **β-Blockers.** These agents should be used in all potential patients with CHF. The key is to start treatment when the

patient is stable (i.e., not after a recent exacerbation) and at low doses with slow titration.

3. **Aldosterone antagonists** have been shown to decrease mortality and should be used in patients with NYHA class III and IV heart failure.
4. **Statins** may have a range of non–lipid-associated mortality benefits and should be used in patients with ischemic cardiomyopathy. Small studies have even shown a benefit in nonischemic cardiomyopathy.
5. **Digoxin.** This age-old treatment for CHF has been shown to reduce symptoms but has never been shown to decrease mortality rates. Digoxin should be used in patients who are symptomatic despite other therapy.
6. **Diuretics** are effective for treating symptoms of fluid overload (e.g., rales, peripheral edema).
7. **Diet.** A low-salt diet is also primarily used for control of fluid overload. The number of patients admitted to the hospital for CHF exacerbations significantly increases the day after Thanksgiving, undoubtedly as a result of increased salt consumption.
8. **Arrhythmias.** Sudden cardiac death accounts for 30% of deaths in patients with CHF. Patients with ischemic or nonischemic cardiomyopathy, NYHA class II to III heart failure, and an ejection fraction less than or equal to 35% have a significant survival benefit from an implantable cardioverter defibrillator (ICD) for the primary prevention of sudden death. Cardiac resynchronization therapy with biventricular pacing is beneficial in patients with an ejection fraction less than or equal to 35%, a prolonged QRS duration (≥120 msec), and NYHA class III or IV heart failure despite optimal medical therapy. Cardiac resynchronization therapy attempts to correct the dyssynchrony caused by a bundle branch block, which may contribute to symptoms of heart failure.

C. Chronic diastolic dysfunction. Digoxin and vasodilators do not play a major role in the treatment of patients with predominantly diastolic dysfunction. Treatment focuses on controlling blood pressure and heart rate, maintaining fluid balance, and minimizing ischemia if present. Some agents, such as β-blockers and centrally acting calcium channel blockers (e.g., diltiazem, verapamil), are thought to improve left ventricular relaxation directly. None of these drugs has been shown to reduce mortality rates, and further studies are needed to determine an optimal medical regimen.

D. Acute pulmonary edema. If a patient experiencing acute pulmonary edema is not treated correctly and promptly, he or she may die. Both systolic and diastolic dysfunction can lead to acute pulmonary edema; however, in the beginning, initiating prompt therapy is more important than determining the exact cause of the patient's rapid decompensation. Reducing preload is the primary goal of therapy in patients with acute pulmonary edema. Some patients may require the addition of intravenous inotropes (e.g., dobutamine, milrinone) to aid with diuresis. It is easy to remember how to treat "wet" patients:

MNEMONIC **Treatment of Acute Pulmonary Edema ("MOIST 'N DAMP")**

Morphine (2–4 mg intravenously as long as the blood pressure is adequate)
Oxygen (as much as necessary to raise the oxygen saturation over 90%)
Intubation, if necessary (pulmonary edema is rapidly reversible, but if the patient is tiring, intubation can be lifesaving)
Sit 'em up (to reduce preload)
Tourniquet (rotating tourniquets to decrease preload were once used)
Nitrates (acutely decrease preload)
Diuretics (20–40 mg furosemide intravenously to first decrease preload and then induce a diuresis)
Albuterol (may help bronchospastic patients)
More morphine, more nitrates, and more diuretics as needed
Phlebotomy (was once used to reduce preload)

REFERENCES

Cesario DA, Dec GW. Implantable cardioverter-defibrillator therapy in clinical practice. J Am Coll Cardiol 2006;47:1507–1517.

Hunt SA, Abraham WT, Chin MH, et al. ACC/AHA 2005 guideline update for the diagnosis and management of chronic heart failure in the adult: a report of the American College of Cardiology/American Heart Association Task Force on Practice Guidelines. J Am Coll Cardiol 2005;46:e1–82.

McMurray JJ, Pfeffer MA. Heart failure. Lancet 2005;365:1877–1889.

Nohria A, Lewis E, Stevenson LW. Medical management of advanced heart failure. JAMA 2002;287:628–640. [Classic article].

Ware LB, Matthay MA. Acute pulmonary edema. N Engl J Med 2005; 353:2788–2796.

■ Shock

I. INTRODUCTION

A. Definition. Shock occurs when the arterial circulation is unable to keep up with the metabolic demands of the body.

B. Clinical manifestations of shock—regardless of etiology—usually include:

1. **Hypotension**
2. **Tachycardia**
3. **Altered mental status**
4. **Decreased urine output**
5. **Cool skin**

II. CAUSES OF SHOCK.

The many causes of shock must be remembered because treatment must address both the manifestations of shock as well as its underlying cause.

MNEMONIC **The Causes of Shock ("SHOCK")**

Sepsis
Hypovolemia
Obstruction to flow
Cardiac
Kooky disorders

A. Sepsis is a common cause of shock. Bacteremia caused by **gram-negative rods** (e.g., *Escherichia coli, Klebsiella, Proteus, Pseudomonas*) or **gram-positive cocci** (e.g., *Staphylococcus, Streptococcus*) is the usual cause of septic shock.

B. Hypovolemia. Any process that causes a significant reduction in intravascular volume (e.g., trauma, gastrointestinal bleeding, hematoma, burns, pancreatitis, hyperosmolar states, vomiting, diarrhea) can lead to hypovolemic shock.

C. Obstruction to flow. Disorders such as cardiac tamponade, pulmonary embolism, tension pneumothorax, and severe aortic or mitral valve stenosis can lead to shock. Tamponade and tension pneumothorax should always be considered promptly because early treatment can save the patient's life.

D. Cardiac causes. Cardiogenic shock is most commonly the result of "pump failure," caused by a myocardial infarction (of either the left or right ventricle) or dilated cardiomyopathy. Other cardiac causes include tachyarrhythmias or bradyarrhythmias, acute valvular regurgitation (mitral or aortic), and rupture of the septum or ventricular wall.

E. "Kooky" disorders. This category includes diseases only a medical school "DEAN" could remember:

MNEMONIC **"Kooky" Disorders Leading to Shock ("DEAN")**

Drug toxicity (primarily vasodilating drugs)
Endocrine disorders (adrenal insufficiency or myxedema)
Anaphylaxis
Neurogenic (especially after spinal cord injury)

III. APPROACH TO THE PATIENT

A. Physical examination. The ABCs (**airway, breathing,** and **circulation**) should be assessed first.

1. **Blood pressure** should be verified with a manual cuff. Hypotension is usually defined as a systolic pressure that is less than 90 mm Hg but can vary across individuals. Pulsus paradoxus (a >10 mm Hg drop in systolic pressure with inspiration) suggests tamponade.
2. **Temperature.** If the patient is febrile or hypothermic, septic shock is likely.
3. **Oxygen saturation** should be obtained during the initial assessment.
4. **Neck vein assessment.** Elevated neck veins in a hypotensive patient are usually indicative of:
    a. Tamponade
    b. Tension pneumothorax
    c. Pulmonary embolism (with right ventricular failure)
    d. Right ventricular infarct (typically associated with an inferior wall myocardial infarction)
    e. Biventricular dysfunction (the only entity on this list that will also cause rales)
5. **Lung sounds**
    a. **Rales** usually indicate a cardiac cause.
    b. **Wheezing** should increase suspicion of anaphylaxis.
    c. **Asymmetric breath sounds** may represent pneumothorax.
6. **Cardiac auscultation.** Important findings include an abnormal rate or rhythm, distant heart sounds, a third heart sound (S_3), or new murmurs.
7. **Abdominal palpation** is helpful in evaluating whether pancreatitis, a perforated viscus, or an infected hepatobiliary source is the cause of shock.

8. **Rectal examination** is important, especially if gastrointestinal bleeding is likely.
9. **Skin inspection.** A **scarlatiniform rash** may be indicative of toxic shock syndrome, whereas **urticaria** can be a sign of anaphylaxis.
10. **Neurologic examination** is useful to assess mental status and to ensure that the patient does not have spinal cord compression.

B. Laboratory tests. Useful tests include:

1. A **complete blood count (CBC)**
2. A **chemistry panel,** including blood urea nitrogen (BUN) and creatinine levels
3. **Liver function tests**
4. **Urinalysis**
5. **Blood cultures**
6. **Arterial blood gases**

C. A **chest radiograph** and **electrocardiogram (ECG)** are **mandatory.**

D. Other diagnostic modalities [e.g., computed tomography (CT), echocardiography, endoscopy, ventilation-perfusion ($\dot{V}/\dot{Q}$) scan, cardiac biomarkers, or evaluation of thyroid-stimulating hormone (TSH) level or serum cortisol] should be ordered promptly if warranted by clinical suspicion.

E. Occasionally, patients are hypotensive, but the cause is not clear. In these situations, **pulmonary artery (PA) catheterization** can be useful, especially in patients who are both hypotensive and hypoxemic (Table 13-1).

IV. TREATMENT. The goal is to maintain the mean arterial pressure above 60 mm Hg (calculated by adding two thirds of the diastolic pressure to one third of the systolic pressure) while treating the underlying disorder causing the shock. Treatment is usually instituted even before a definitive cause of shock has been determined.

A. Place the patient in the **Trendelenburg position** (head down).

B. Provide **supplemental oxygen.** Intubation may be necessary.

C. Administer **fluids** rapidly through two large-bore intravenous lines, unless the patient clearly has biventricular failure.

D. Insert a **Foley catheter** to monitor urine output.

E. Place an **intra-arterial catheter** (either in the radial or femoral artery) for closer hemodynamic monitoring, especially if manual blood pressure measurements are unreliable.

F. Consider **vasopressor medications.** The decision to use "pressors" is often difficult; usually, they are used if the patient has not responded to a trial of aggressive fluid resuscitation. The choice of which pressor to use depends on the clinical situation and should be guided by hemodynamic monitoring.

TABLE 13-1

PULMONARY ARTERY (PA) CATHETERIZATION FINDINGS IN SPECIFIC DISEASE STATES

Disease	RAP	PCWP	SVR	CO	Comments
Sepsis	↓	↓	↓	Normal to ↑	Few other disorders have a low SVR
Hypovolemia	↓	↓	↑	↓	Source of fluid loss must be identified
Tamponade	↑	Normal to ↓	↑	↓	PCWP = CVP = PADP
Pulmonary embolism	Normal to ↑	Normal	↑	↓	PADP is often 5 mm Hg > PCWP
Biventricular failure	↑	↑	↑	↓	Diagnosis is usually apparent on physical examination and chest x-ray
Right ventricular infarct	↑	↓	↑	↓	If the patient is hypoxemic and the chest x-ray is normal, consider a right-to-left shunt
Neurogenic shock	↓	↓	↓	Normal to ↓	Hemodynamics can be similar in adrenal insufficiency

CO = cardiac output; normal: 3.5–7 L/min.
CVP = central venous pressure
PADP = pulmonary artery diastolic pressure; normal: 5–12 mm Hg
PCWP = pulmonary capillary wedge pressure; normal: 5–12 mm Hg
RAP = right atrial pressure (equivalent to central venous pressure); normal: 0–8 mm Hg
SVR = systemic vascular resistance; normal: 900–1300 dyne/sec/cm^{-5}
↑ = increased; ↓ = decreased

1. **Mechanism of action.** Vasopressors act on the **autonomic nervous system.** Once you understand what each receptor does (Table 13-2), it is easy to remember the actions of each pressor.
2. **Agents.** Table 13-3 contains the most commonly used vasopressors, in order from α_1-adrenergic agents to β_2-adrenergic agents. Get used to remembering the drugs in this order. [If you need a mnemonic to help you, you can think of the following scenario: A patient, Edward, who has severe congestive heart failure (CHF), calls himself "Eddie." Unfortunately, he is a poor speller, so he spells his name "Edi." Every time you see him, you inquire whether he has paroxysmal nocturnal dyspnea (PND). You ask, "PND EDI?"]

MNEMONIC

Vasopressors ("PND EDI?")

Phenylephrine
Norepinephrine
Dopamine
Epinephrine
Dobutamine
Isoproterenol

TABLE 13-2

REVIEW OF AUTONOMIC NERVOUS SYSTEM

Receptor	Major Location	Action
α_1	Peripheral vascular and coronary smooth muscle	Constricts
β_1	Myocardium	Increases heart rate and contractility
β_2	Bronchial, peripheral vascular, and coronary smooth muscle	Dilates
Dopamine	Vascular smooth muscle (renal, gastrointestinal)	Dilates

TABLE 13-3

VASOPRESSORS

Drug	Action	Dose	Indications
Phenylephrine	α_1-Adrenergic	10–200 μg/min	Sepsis
Norepinephrine	α_1-Adrenergic, β_1-Adrenergic	2–64 μg/min	Sepsis
Dopamine*	Dopaminergic	1–2 μg/kg/min	Sepsis, hypotensive cardiogenic shock
	β_1-Adrenergic	2–10 μg/kg/min	
	α_1-Adrenergic	10–20 μg/kg/min	
Epinephrine	α_1-Adrenergic, β_1-Adrenergic, β_2-Adrenergic	1–4 μg/min	Pulseless arrest, sepsis
Dobutamine	β_1-Adrenergic, β_2-Adrenergic	1–20 μg/kg/min	Cardiogenic shock (but not by itself if patient is hypotensive), congestive heart failure
Isoproterenol	β_1, β_2	1–4 μg/min	Bradycardia

*Action depends on the dose.

3. **Vasopressin.** Vasopressin, a hormone typically responsible for osmotic control in the renal collecting ducts, recently has been shown to have significant vasopressor effects through direct constriction of vascular wall smooth muscle cells. Its effect may be seen even when high doses of other agents fail.

REFERENCES

Abraham E, Matthay MA, Dinarello CA, et al. Consensus conference definitions for sepsis, septic shock, acute lung injury, and acute respiratory distress syndrome: time for a reevaluation. Crit Care Med 2000;28(1):232–235. [Classic article].

Annane D, Bellissant E, Cavaillon JM. Septic shock. Lancet 2005;365:63–78.

Cardiovascular drugs in the ICU. Treat Guidel Med Lett. 2002;1:19–24. [Classic article].

Landry DW, Oliver JA. Pathogenesis of vasodilatory shock. N Engl J Med 2001;345:588–595. [Classic article].

Reynolds HR, Hochman JS. Cardiogenic shock: current concepts and improving outcomes. Circulation 2008;117:686–697.

PART III
PULMONARY AND CRITICAL CARE

14

Acute Dyspnea

I. INTRODUCTION. Dyspnea is defined as an uncomfortable sensation of breathing. Acute dyspnea is a common cause of emergency department visits, hospital admissions, and decompensation among hospitalized patients.

II. CAUSES OF ACUTE DYSPNEA. Dyspnea is the cardinal symptom in a variety of disorders, many of which can be immediately life threatening (Table 14-1).

A. Pulmonary

1. **Pneumothorax** is a sudden event that is often accompanied by acute dyspnea and pleuritic chest pain. This diagnosis should be considered carefully in a patient with significant bullous lung disease, with recent chest wall trauma, or on a ventilator.
2. **Pulmonary embolism** is a difficult diagnosis to make because of the poor sensitivity and specificity of the history and physical examination. Consider the diagnosis early, as specialized diagnostic testing is often required.
3. **Airflow limitation** should be suspected in patients with known obstructive lung disease, such as chronic obstructive pulmonary disease (COPD) or asthma. Airflow limitation leads to hyperinflation and air trapping in the lungs. Increased activation of pulmonary stretch receptors is perceived as dyspnea. Wheezing is the hallmark physical finding of airflow limitation.
4. **Aspiration** should be suspected in patients with swallowing dysfunction, alcohol abuse, seizure disorder, or a diminished level of consciousness. Always ask family members or nurses about witnessed aspiration. However, aspiration events are often not witnessed.
5. **Pneumonia.** Patients will usually have other symptoms of infection, including fever or hypothermia, chills, or a productive cough.
6. **Upper airway obstruction.** An acute onset of symptoms with inspiratory stridor should prompt consideration of this diagnosis.
7. **Acute respiratory distress syndrome (ARDS).** ARDS is a clinically defined entity encountered most commonly in

TABLE 14-1

COMMON CAUSES OF ACUTE DYSPNEA

Pulmonary	Cardiac	Other
Pneumothorax	Myocardial ischemia or infarction	Sepsis
Pulmonary embolism	Congestive heart failure	Metabolic acidosis
Airflow limitation	Arrhythmias	Anemia
Aspiration	Pericardial tamponade	Anxiety
Pneumonia		
Upper airway obstruction		
Acute respiratory distress syndrome		

patients with sepsis, trauma, massive blood transfusion, or pancreatitis.

B. Cardiac

1. **Myocardial ischemia** or **infarction.** Dyspnea may occur in the absence of chest pain and thus may represent an anginal equivalent.
2. **Congestive heart failure (CHF).** In hospitalized patients with CHF, acute dyspnea is often precipitated by fluid administration or myocardial ischemia. A significant elevation in brain natriuretic peptide (BNP) may suggest increased ventricular wall stress and a cardiogenic cause of dyspnea. Pulmonary embolism will also elevate BNP due to increased right ventricular wall stress, though to a lesser degree.
3. **Arrhythmias.** Patients may have a history of palpitations. Specific etiologies cannot be reliably diagnosed on physical examination; a 12-lead electrocardiogram (ECG) or a rhythm strip is required.
4. **Pericardial tamponade** is rare but should always be considered in patients with breast and lung cancer, renal failure, recent myocardial infarction, or blunt trauma to the chest.

C. Metabolic

1. **Sepsis.** Tachypnea and acute respiratory alkalosis may be the earliest findings in sepsis.
2. **Metabolic acidosis.** Dyspnea is common as patients hyperventilate to compensate for their acidosis. Kussmaul respiration with large tidal volumes is the most common pattern.

D. Hematologic. Acute anemia (from hemorrhage or hemolysis) can cause acute dyspnea due to the decreased oxygen carrying capacity of blood. Anemia can easily be missed on history and physical examination.

E. Psychiatric. Anxiety can be a primary cause of acute dyspnea; however, a diagnosis of primary anxiety should be considered only after ruling out the more serious possibilities.

III. APPROACH TO THE PATIENT. The key to evaluating a patient with acute dyspnea is to focus on recognizing the most serious disorders.

A. Patient history. There are four key areas of inquiry:

1. What was the **speed of onset** of the dyspnea?
2. Are there any **associated symptoms** (e.g., chest pain, cough, chills)?
3. **What happened immediately before** the onset of the dyspnea? What medications or fluids was the patient receiving?
4. What are the patient's **other medical problems**? If already hospitalized, what is the admission diagnosis?

B. Physical examination. Focus on five key areas:

1. **Vital signs.** Significantly abnormal vital signs in an acutely dyspneic patient may signify impending respiratory failure. An oxygen saturation should be obtained.

Remember, a normal oxygen saturation does not exclude the possibility of a serious disorder!

2. **Chest.** Pay particular attention to the symmetry of breath sounds and the presence of wheezing or rales. Look for tracheal deviation (toward a pneumothorax or collapsed lung, away from an effusion). Look for use of accessory muscles or paradoxical breathing (abdomen retracts with inspiration) to signify increased work of breathing and impending respiratory failure.
3. **Heart.** A complete examination should be performed, focusing on the findings of right-sided and left-sided heart failure. Also note the heart rate (too fast? too slow?).
4. **Extremities.** Look for edema (unilateral versus bilateral) and cyanosis. Cool extremities may suggest poor perfusion and a cardiac etiology.
5. **Mental status.** Evaluating the patient's mental status is crucial for two reasons:
   a. A significantly depressed level of consciousness may necessitate intubation for airway protection.

b. The finding of altered mental status as a result of the dyspnea suggests a significant homeostatic insult.

C. Diagnostic studies. Four studies should routinely be performed when the patient is acutely dyspneic.

1. 12-Lead ECG
2. Arterial blood gas analysis
3. Chest radiograph
4. Complete blood count (CBC)

IV. TREATMENT. Treatment should be aimed at the underlying cause. The following are a few general principles:

A. Supplemental oxygen. Hypoxemic patients with acute dyspnea should be given supplemental oxygen, with the goal of normalizing oxygen saturation (>90%) and partial pressure of oxygen ($PaO_2 \geq 60$ mm Hg). A history of COPD or carbon dioxide retention should not prevent oxygen therapy for hypoxemic patients; however, patients at risk for carbon dioxide retention should be monitored closely. Approximately 35% oxygen can be delivered by standard nasal cannula, with close to 100% oxygen available with a nonrebreather face mask.

B. Diuretics. Cardiogenic pulmonary edema should respond rapidly to diuretic therapy. Other processes associated with excess lung water (e.g., ARDS) may also improve with diuresis.

C. β-Agonists. Regardless of the cause, wheezing will likely improve somewhat with nebulized β-agonist therapy. Albuterol can be given continuously if indicated, but may cause undesired tachycardia. Ipratropium (an anticholinergic agent) may be used in conjunction with albuterol but should be given every 4 hours.

D. Mechanical ventilation (see Chapter 26). The need for mechanical ventilation (either invasive endotracheal intubation or noninvasive face mask) should be assessed. Indications for mechanical ventilation include:

1. **Refractory hypoxemia** (PaO_2 <60 mm Hg despite maximal oxygen therapy)
2. **Hypercapnea** (generally manifested by an increasing $PaCO_2$ despite therapy)
3. **Inability to protect the airway**
4. **Impending upper airway obstruction**
5. **Excessive work of breathing (this may signify impending respiratory failure and may happen before abnormalities appear on the arterial blood gas)**

Hypoxemic or hypercapneic respiratory failure may respond to noninvasive positive-pressure ventilation (NIPPV) in patients who are alert and who are able to tolerate the pressurized mask. Inability to protect the airway demands immediate endotracheal intubation. Impending upper airway obstruction should be approached cautiously, with immediate percutaneous tracheostomy available should endotracheal intubation prove impossible.

REFERENCES

Dyspnea. Mechanisms, assessment, and management: a consensus statement. American Thoracic Society. Am J Respir Crit Care Med 1999;159(1):321–340. [Classic article].

Mahler DA, Baird JC. Are you fluent in the language of dyspnea? Chest 2008;134(3):476–477.

Manning HL, Schwartzstein RM. Pathophysiology of dyspnea. N Engl J Med 1995;333:1547–1553. [Classic article].

15 Massive Hemoptysis

I. INTRODUCTION. Hemoptysis, defined as the expectoration of blood, can be an insignificant symptom of a benign illness, a first manifestation of serious malignancy, or a fatal process in and of itself. Hemoptysis is usually classified as either **massive** or **nonmassive**.

A. Massive hemoptysis, variably defined as expectorating >200–600 ml of blood in a 24-hour period, requires immediate evaluation; it is the focus of this chapter.

B. Nonmassive hemoptysis, usually defined as expectorating <200–600 ml of blood in a 24-hour period, accounts for more than 90% of cases. Patients with nonmassive hemoptysis warrant close attention, because they may develop massive hemoptysis in an unpredictable fashion. However, many can be managed effectively as outpatients.

While the precise volume of expectorated blood is usually difficult to ascertain, if a patient says he or she has coughed up about one cup or more of blood in the last 24 hours, consider this "massive" hemoptysis.

II. CAUSES OF HEMOPTYSIS. The list of differential diagnoses is long. The following mnemonic can help you to remember the many causes of hemoptysis—think of soldiers in a "BATTLE CAMP" coughing up blood.

MNEMONIC **Causes of Hemoptysis ("BATTLE CAMP")**

Bronchiectasis* or **B**ronchitis
Aspergillosis*
Tumor*
Tuberculosis*
Lung abscess*
Emboli
Coagulopathy
Arteriovenous malformation, **A**lveolar hemorrhage
Mitral stenosis
Pneumonia

*Most common causes of **massive** hemoptysis.

A. **Bronchitis** is the most common cause of trivial hemoptysis but rarely causes massive bleeding unless coexisting bronchiectasis is present.

B. **Bronchiectasis** is defined as permanent dilatation of the bronchi or bronchioles. Incidence has declined in the past few decades in the United States due to better recognition and treatment for tuberculosis and pneumonia. Alternatively, patients with cystic fibrosis, a disease defined by bronchiectasis, are now living well into adulthood with a 5%–7% lifetime incidence of massive hemoptysis. Massive hemoptysis can occur from arteriovenous shunts that develop in areas of bronchiectatic lung.

C. **Aspergillosis.** Any fungal pneumonia can cause hemoptysis, but infection with angioinvasive *Aspergillus fumigatus* is the most common cause. This usually occurs in immunocompromised patients and can cause massive hemoptysis.

D. **Tumor** should be suspected in a smoker over the age of 40, especially if there is radiographic evidence of a mass lesion.

E. **Tuberculosis.** Massive hemoptysis in patients with active tuberculosis is often caused by cavitary or noncavitary lung necrosis or the rupture of dilated pulmonary arteries that traverse the tuberculous cavities (so-called Rasmussen's aneurysms). Inactive tuberculosis leaves behind residual bronchiectatic airways and parenchymal cavities where mycetomas (fungal occupation of cavity) cause erosion into blood vessels.

F. **Emboli.** Pulmonary embolism can cause lung infarction, which can bleed (usually after initiation of anticoagulation as it necroses). Septic emboli from right-sided endocarditis also occasionally result in massive bleeding.

G. **Coagulopathy.** Anticoagulation is often associated with hemoptysis but is generally not the sole cause. An underlying lesion should be sought. Rarely, anticoagulation can cause alveolar hemorrhage (see II I).

H. **Arteriovenous malformation** is usually congenital and is often associated with hereditary hemorrhagic telangiectasia (Osler-Weber-Rendu syndrome).

I. **Alveolar hemorrhage** is a syndrome where the alveoli fill with blood. It results from rupture or damage to the alveolar capillaries and is most commonly due to an autoimmune-mediated attack on the alveolar capillaries (e.g., Churg-Strauss syndrome, granulomatous vasculitis, microscopic polyangiitis). Some of these conditions may also involve the kidneys [e.g., Goodpasture's syndrome, granulomatous vasculitis, systemic lupus erythematosus (SLE)] causing hematuria and a cellular ("active") urinary sediment. Other nonimmune causes include idiopathic pulmonary hemosiderosis and acute interstitial pneumonitis.

J. Mitral stenosis causing pulmonary venous hypertension can lead to hemoptysis.

K. Pneumonia associated with hemoptysis is often abscess forming and/or necrotizing (e.g., *Staphylococcus aureus*, *Streptococcus spp.*, and certain gram negatives).

III. APPROACH TO THE PATIENT

A. Maintain airway patency and oxygenation. Arterial blood gas analysis and chest radiographs should be performed immediately to assess oxygenation and determine the extent of blood retained in the lung. Because death from massive hemoptysis usually results from alveolar flooding and hypoxemia, ensuring adequate oxygenation is the most important first step.

To prevent aspiration of blood into the unaffected lung in a patient with massive hemoptysis, have the patient lie in the lateral decubitus position with the bleeding side down. How do you know which lung is bleeding? Ask the patient; he or she may know (clues: known cancer, recent procedure or surgery).

1. If emergent intubation is indicated (see Chapter 14), a large-bore endotracheal tube (8.0 or larger) should be used to enable adequate suctioning and allow for urgent bronchoscopy.
2. In cases of unilateral hemorrhage, selective right or left mainstem intubation with specialized endotracheal tubes protects against spread of blood to the unaffected lung.

B. Identify the bleeding lesion.

1. **Ensure a bronchopulmonary source.** It is necessary to ensure that the patient truly has bronchopulmonary bleeding; gastrointestinal and nasopharyngeal bleeding commonly masquerade as hemoptysis. If the source of the bleeding is not obvious, helpful techniques include the following:
   a. **Evaluation of the pH of the expectorated substance** can provide clues—gastrointestinal contents are usually acidic, whereas pulmonary expectorations are usually alkaline.
   b. **Examination of the pharynx** and **larynx** may reveal the cause of the bleeding to be epistaxis.
2. **Lung auscultation** and **chest radiographs** can help to localize the bleeding but may not be helpful if the bleeding is diffuse or if blood has been aspirated from one lung into the other. A chest radiograph may show a mass lesion or cavity.

3. **Urinalysis** and **assessment of renal function** may show proteinuria, dysmorphic red cells, or red cell casts, suggesting a vasculitis or pulmonary-renal syndrome.
4. **Computed tomography (CT)** may reveal a space-occupying lesion (e.g., lung cancer or abscess).
5. **Early bronchoscopy** is indicated for most patients for both therapeutic and diagnostic purposes.
6. **Arteriography** is useful for actively bleeding patients for purposes of localization of the bleeding lesion and therapy. Massive hemoptysis most commonly comes from the bronchial artery circulation and can sometimes be localized and embolized by interventional radiology.

C. Control the hemorrhage.

1. General measures indicated for all patients with massive hemoptysis include bed rest, cough suppressants, sedatives, and stool softeners or laxatives, which help prevent sudden increases in intrathoracic pressure, thereby minimizing intravascular pressure. Upon presentation, the aforementioned measures may inhibit the ability of the patient to expectorate blood, leading to worsening hypoxemia and clinical status. Await clinical stability and/or intubation before initiating.
2. Coagulopathies should be corrected if present.
3. Bronchoscopic maneuvers such as topical application of epinephrine or thrombin or balloon tamponade may be useful in selected patients.
4. External radiation therapy may be effective for reducing bleeding from tumors.
5. Definitive therapy for massive hemoptysis often requires angiographic arterial embolization or surgical lung resection.

Consult a pulmonologist immediately if the patient presents with massive hemoptysis.

REFERENCES

Jean-Baptiste E. Clinical assessment and management of massive hemoptysis.. Crit Care Med 2000;28(5):1642–1647. [Classic article].

Sareli AE, Janssen WJ, Sterman D, et al. Clinical problem-solving. What's the connection? N Engl J Med 2008;358(6):626–632.

Approach to the Chest Radiograph

16

I. **INTRODUCTION.** It is often necessary to rely on your own interpretation of a chest radiograph pending a formal reading. This chapter provides a consistent, easy-to-use approach to the evaluation of a chest radiograph.

II. **PRELIMINARY CONSIDERATIONS**

A. **What kind of radiograph should I order?**

1. A **posterior-anterior (PA) view** is always preferable to an anterior-posterior (AP) view because the latter exaggerates the size of the heart and other mediastinal structures. However, in an emergency situation, an AP view is often the only option.
2. A **lateral view** should also be obtained to provide supplemental information and to confirm findings on the PA view.

B. **Is it a good film?** Assessing the quality of the radiograph may help avoid common misinterpretations.

1. **Inspiration.** Count the number of ribs; a good inspiration will reveal 10 posterior ribs. A poor inspiration may result in the false appearance of an interstitial process, leading to a misdiagnosis of pulmonary edema or atypical pneumonia.
2. **Rotation.** Look at the clavicles and see if they are symmetric with respect to the vertebrae (asymmetry is an indication of rotation). Rotation often leads to erroneous estimates of cardiac, pulmonary artery, aortic, and mediastinal dimensions.
3. **Penetration.** You should be able to see individual vertebrae in a film that is appropriately penetrated. Decreased penetration will make the lungs seem denser (i.e., white). Mild pulmonary edema or a small infiltrate will appear to be significant pulmonary edema or a large infiltrate, and even normal interstitial markings may appear abnormal.

C. **Is there an old film available for comparison?** There is no substitute for comparison with prior films. A new subtle area of consolidation may be found in a patient with suspected pneumonia, a nodule may be unchanged for 10 years and therefore presumed to be benign, or the mediastinum may be wider in a patient with suspected aortic dissection. In all cases, you need to make sure the view was the same (i.e., AP versus PA). In addition, you must "mentally adjust" for variations in technique (i.e., inspiration, rotation, and penetration).

III. THE OUTSIDE-IN APPROACH. The structures visible on a chest radiograph can be evaluated in any order, but you should be consistent every time you read a film. The outside-in approach is frequently used and ensures that commonly overlooked structures (e.g., bones) are not forgotten.

A. Bones and soft tissues. Look for lytic or blastic lesions that may signal a metastatic malignancy. Evidence of osteoporosis or compression fractures may also be found. Look for subcutaneous air to suggest pneumothorax or pneumomediastinum. Soft tissue masses may also be apparent.

B. Pleura. Follow the pleural border of each lung, looking for evidence of focal thickening suggesting scarring or mass, blunting of the costophrenic angle suggesting effusion, or calcifications suggesting old pleural inflammation from empyema or asbestos exposure.

C. Lungs. Look at both lung fields in an orderly fashion. Pay special attention to the diaphragms, the cardiac borders, and the apices. Although symmetric abnormalities may occur (e.g., with pulmonary edema or bilateral pneumonia), asymmetric findings are particularly suspicious. Infiltrates are generally described as "alveolar" or "interstitial." Alveolar infiltrates are generally fluffy, confluent, poorly demarcated opacities. There may be air-bronchograms (lucent airways surrounded by opaque consolidated lung) visible within them. An alveolar infiltrate may be blood, pus, water, or cells; commonly, hemorrhage, pneumonia, cardiogenic pulmonary edema, and acute respiratory distress syndrome (ARDS) are all considerations. Interstitial infiltrates are generally linear, well-defined, reticular (latticelike), occasionally nodular opacities. Interstitial infiltrates suggest atypical pneumonia, interstitial lung disease, and lymphatic congestion (seen in heart failure and malignancy).

1. **Diaphragms**
   a. If one of the hemidiaphragms is obscured, either an infiltrate is present in the respective lower lobe or there is a pleural effusion.
   b. The retrocardiac area is a common place for abnormalities to be overlooked. The left hemidiaphragm should be visible behind the heart. An obscured left hemidiaphragm

suggests atelectasis or an infiltrate. The presence of air bronchograms favors consolidation.

c. Flattened diaphragms are often found in chronic obstructive pulmonary disease (COPD).

d. An elevated hemidiaphragm suggests diaphragmatic paralysis, a subpulmonic pleural effusion, or a subdiaphragmatic process.

e. Air under the diaphragm on an upright chest radiograph in a patient presenting with abdominal pain suggests visceral perforation and is usually a surgical emergency.

f. A depressed lateral hemidiaphragm with a poorly visible costophrenic angle and surrounding hyperlucency ("deep sulcus sign") suggests a pneumothorax.

2. **Cardiac borders**

   a. A **lingular infiltrate** (lower portion of the left upper lobe) is suggested if the left cardiac border is obscured.

   b. A **right middle lobe infiltrate** is suggested if the right cardiac border is obscured.

3. **Apices**

   a. **Apical pneumothoraces** are easy to miss; always look carefully for these in patients with chest pain or shortness of breath. Follow the interstitial markings to the chest wall to ensure that no pneumothorax is present.

   b. **Congestive heart failure (CHF): Pulmonary venous congestion** is characterized by **cephalization** (redistribution of blood flow toward the apices). Other common findings with CHF include cardiomegaly, pleural effusions, blurring of the usually sharp and well-demarcated blood vessels, prominent pulmonary arteries, Kerley B lines (horizontal lines extending from the pleura toward the heart), and alveolar infiltrates due to pulmonary edema.

   c. **Tuberculosis:** Reactivation disease often presents with apical cavitary infiltration. A **lordotic view** may be ordered if the apex is not well visualized.

D. Heart

1. **Increased cardiac silhouette.** The cardiac silhouette should be less than one half of the thoracic diameter on a PA film; anything larger suggests cardiomegaly or pericardial effusion.

2. **Chamber enlargement**

   a. The left side of the cardiac silhouette represents the left ventricle, whereas the right side represents the right atrium. Prominence in either location may represent enlargement of the respective chamber.

b. Left atrial enlargement may be signified by:
   (1) The loss of the normal concavity on the left side of the heart
   (2) An elevated left mainstem bronchus
   (3) The "**double-density" sign,** which is seen as two parallel lines on the right side of the heart representing the right atrium and the enlarged left atrial borders

c. Right ventricular enlargement is not visible on PA or AP films, but can be seen on a lateral film as filling of the retrosternal space.

3. **Pulmonary hypertension.** The diameter of the pulmonary artery should generally not exceed that of a dime; prominent pulmonary arteries may signify pulmonary hypertension.

E. Mediastinum

1. **Aortic dissection.** Mediastinal widening may signify aortic dissection, but the sensitivity and specificity of this finding are suboptimal.
2. **Lymphadenopathy.** A widened paratracheal stripe (normally a narrow opaque stripe along the right side of the trachea) and fullness of the aortic-pulmonary window (a triangular space on the left side of the mediastinum below the aortic arch) often signify mediastinal lymphadenopathy.

REFERENCES

Dixon AK. Evidence-based diagnostic radiology. Lancet 1997;350(9076): 509–512. [Classic article].

McAdams HP, Samei E, Dobbins J 3rd, et al. Recent advances in chest radiography. Radiology 2006;241(3):663–683.

Hypoxemia

17

I. INTRODUCTION

A. Hypoxemia is not a diagnosis; it is a manifestation of an underlying disease.

B. Hypoxemia is common in hospitalized patients.

C. Patients with hypoxemia should always be evaluated promptly.

II. CLINICAL VALUES

A. Arterial oxygen tension (PaO_2). In strictest terms, one needs to obtain an arterial blood gas report to confirm the presence of hypoxemia. A **normal** PaO_2 at sea level is **80–100 mm Hg.**

B. Oxygen (O_2) saturation. The arterial O_2 saturation is the percentage of oxyhemoglobin in arterial blood. It can be measured by pulse oximetry (indirect) or arterial blood gas analysis (direct).

Pulse oximetry has a variability of at least 4%. Thus, when in doubt, check an arterial blood gas.

C. Alveolar-to-arterial (A-a) gradient. The A-a gradient helps determine the cause of hypoxemia and provides a rough estimate of how ill a patient is.

1. A **normal A-a gradient** is **less than the patient's age divided by 4 plus 4.** For example, a 24-year-old patient should have an A-a gradient less than 10.
2. Calculating the A-a gradient is easy using the alveolar gas equation and values from the arterial blood gas report.
   a. First, the alveolar oxygen tension (PAO_2) is calculated using the **alveolar gas equation:**

$$PAO_2 = (P_{barometric} - P_{water})\, FIO_2 - PaCO_2 / 0.8$$

where

$P_{barometric}$ = the barometric pressure (760 mm Hg at sea level)

P_{water} = the vapor pressure of water at body temperature (47 mm Hg)
FIO_2 = the fraction of oxygen in the inspired gas (0.21 on room air)

Remember, for the simplified equation to work, the patient must be breathing room air.

$PaCO_2$ = the arterial carbon dioxide tension

Thus, at sea level, the equation simplifies to:

$$P_{AO_2} = 150 - P_{aCO_2} / 0.8$$

The value for $PaCO_2$ is obtained from the arterial blood gas report.

b. To calculate the A-a gradient, subtract the PaO_2 (obtained from the arterial blood gas report) from the PAO_2 (obtained from the alveolar gas equation):

$$\text{A-a gradient} = P_{AO_2} - P_{aO_2}$$

III. MECHANISMS OF HYPOXEMIA. There are five pathophysiologic mechanisms that cause hypoxemia (Table 17-1).

A. Ventilation-perfusion (**$\dot{V}/\dot{Q}$**) mismatch accounts for more than 95% of cases of hypoxemia. **$\dot{V}/\dot{Q}$** mismatch occurs when ventilation in a part of the lung is decreased in comparison to perfusion.

B. Right-to-left shunting occurs when systemic venous blood (PVO_2 = 40 mm Hg) enters the left side of the heart without coming in contact with oxygen-rich alveolar air.

1. Right-to-left shunting may result from cardiac abnormalities (e.g., patent foramen ovale, atrial septal defect) or pulmonary abnormalities (e.g., arteriovenous malformations; hepatopulmonary syndrome; completely consolidated area of lung with blood, pus, or water; or because of atelectasis).
2. A shunt exists whenever ventilation equals zero but perfusion continues.

C. Diffusion defects leading to hypoxemia most often manifest when red blood cell (RBC) transit time through the pulmonary vascular bed decreases (e.g., during exercise). The causes include interstitial lung diseases (e.g., idiopathic pulmonary fibrosis), environmental lung disease, *Pneumocystis*

TABLE 17-1

CAUSES OF HYPOXEMIA

Pathophysiologic Mechanism	Clinical Examples
Ventilation-perfusion ($\dot{V}/\dot{Q}$) mismatch	Pneumonia, CHF, ARDS, atelectasis, tumor-filled alveoli
Right-to-left shunting	Any of the causes of $\dot{V}/\dot{Q}$ mismatch if $\dot{V}/\dot{Q} = 0$, congenital cardiac abnormalities, pulmonary arteriovenous malformation
Diffusion defects	Interstitial lung disease, *Pneumocystis* pneumonia, emphysema
Hypoventilation	**Cannot breathe:** impairment of respiratory mechanics with airway obstruction (e.g., COPD, asthma), neuromuscular dysfunction (poliomyelitis, Guillain-Barré syndrome, myasthenia gravis, ALS, myotonic dystrophy) or restriction of the chest wall or lungs (kyphoscoliosis, pulmonary fibrosis) **Will not breathe:** CNS damage, drugs (e.g., opiates and acute alcohol intoxication), obesity hypoventilation syndrome, hypothyroidism
Low inspired O_2 tension	High altitude

ALS = amyotrophic lateral sclerosis; *ARDS* = acute respiratory distress syndrome; *CHF* = congestive heart failure; *CNS* = central nervous system; *COPD* = chronic obstructive pulmonary disease.

pneumonia, and emphysema. In emphysema, loss of alveoli reduces the available surface area for diffusion.

D. **Hypoventilation** is defined by an elevated $PaCO_2$ and a normal A-a gradient. There are many causes of this abnormality; to find the cause, a systematic approach, starting at the head and working to the lungs, is best.

E. **Low inspired oxygen tension.** Unless the patient is at a high altitude, this cause can be ruled out.

REFERENCES

Henig NR, Pierson DJ. Mechanisms of hypoxemia. Respir Care Clin North Am 2000;6(4):501–521. [Classic article].

Rodriguez-Roisin R, Roca J. Mechanisms of hypoxemia. Intensive Care Med 2005;31:1017–1019.

Tierney LM Jr, Whooley MA, Saint S. Oxygen saturation: a fifth vital sign? Western J Med 1997;166(4):285–286.

18 Pulmonary Function Tests

I. INTRODUCTION

A. Uses. Pulmonary function tests can be used to:

1. Differentiate obstructive lung disease from restrictive lung disease
2. Assess the severity of lung disease
3. Evaluate response to therapy

B. Types of information assessed. Pulmonary function tests allow assessment of three types of information:

1. **Lung volumes**
   a. The **total lung capacity (TLC)** is the volume of air in the lungs after a maximal inspiratory effort.
   b. The **functional residual capacity (FRC)** is the volume of air at the end of tidal expiration with the glottis open.
   c. The **residual volume (RV)** is the volume of air remaining in the lungs after a maximal expiratory effort.
   d. The **vital capacity (VC)** is the maximal volume of air that can be expelled from the lungs following a maximal inspiration.
2. **Expiratory flow rate.** The **forced expiratory volume in 1 second (FEV_1)** is the most commonly used screening test for airway disease. FEV_1 represents the volume of air expired during the first second of expiration.
3. **Diffusion capacity.** Evaluation of the diffusing capacity for carbon monoxide (DLCO) indicates the adequacy of alveolar–capillary gas exchange. Common causes of a decreased DLCO are emphysema, interstitial lung disease, and pulmonary vascular disease.

C. Interpretation. An organized and systematic approach to interpretation is required. When interpreting the results of pulmonary function testing, it is important to note both the observed values and the percent predicted. The range of normal for all values will vary slightly depending on the pulmonary function testing laboratory.

II. OBSTRUCTIVE VERSUS RESTRICTIVE LUNG DISEASE

A. The **relationship between flow rate, lung volume, resistance,** and **compliance** is as follows: **Flow rate = Lung volume / (Airway resistance)(Compliance).** Therefore, the flow rate (as measured by

FEV_1) will decrease if the lung volume decreases (as seen in restrictive disorders), airway resistance increases (as seen in asthma or chronic bronchitis), or compliance increases (as seen in emphysema).

B. **Obstructive disorders cannot be distinguished from restrictive disorders on the basis of FEV_1 alone.** To distinguish between obstructive and restrictive lung disorders, the lung volume must be eliminated from the equation; dividing by the forced vital capacity (FVC) will accomplish this goal **(FEV_1/FVC ratio).** The FEV_1/FVC ratio is the percent of the forced vital capacity expelled in 1 second.
   1. If the **FEV_1/FVC ratio** is **decreased (<70%)**, then the patient has **airflow limitation,** suggesting obstructive disease.
   2. If the **FEV_1/FVC ratio** is **normal** or **increased (>80%)** in the setting of a low FEV_1, then the patient may have **restrictive disease.**

III. APPROACH TO THE INTERPRETATION OF PULMONARY FUNCTION TESTS

A. **Look at the FEV_1 first.**
   1. If the patient has a normal FEV_1, TLC, and DLCO, the patient is unlikely to have significant pulmonary disease.
   2. If the FEV_1 is low, look at the FEV_1(%) to document airflow limitation (obstructive disease) or to suggest restrictive disease.
      a. If the FEV_1/FVC ratio is normal or high, the patient may have restrictive disease (which will be confirmed by a low TLC).
      b. If the FEV_1 is less than 80% predicted and the **FEV_1/FVC ratio is less than 70**, the patient has airflow limitation, suggesting obstructive disease.
         (1) If the patient has airflow limitation, then determine if it is reversible.
            (a) If the FEV_1 improves by 12% or more and at least 200 ml after bronchodilator administration, reversible airflow limitation is present.

B. **Now look at the lung volumes.**
   1. Increased TLC, RV: This suggests hyperinflation and gas trapping, consistent with obstructive lung disease.
   2. Decreased TLC, RV: This suggests restriction and is diagnostic of restrictive lung disease.

C. **Finally, look at the DLCO.**
   1. DLCO values should always be corrected for hemoglobin (DLCO-C)
   2. If the patient has obstructive disease, a low DLCO-C suggests the presence of emphysema.

3. If the patient has normal spirometry and lung volumes with a low DLCO-C, pulmonary vascular disease or early interstitial lung disease should be suspected.

REFERENCES

Crapo RO. Pulmonary-function testing. N Engl J Med 1994;7;331(1):25–30. [Classic article].

Pellegrino R. Interpretative strategies for lung function tests. Eur Respir J 2005;26:948.

19 Obstructive Lung Disease

I. INTRODUCTION

A. Disorders. There are four major obstructive lung diseases:

1. **Asthma**
2. **Chronic obstructive pulmonary disease (COPD)**
3. **Bronchiectasis**
4. **Cystic fibrosis**

B. Definitions. Asthma and COPD are by far the most common obstructive lung diseases; therefore, these two disorders are the focus of this chapter. All obstructive diseases are marked by **airflow limitation,** characterized by a **low forced expiratory volume in 1 second (FEV_1)** and a **low FEV_1/forced vital capacity (FVC) ratio.**

1. **Asthma** is characterized by reversible narrowing of the distal airways as a result of chronic inflammation and airways hyperreactivity. Pathologic changes include smooth muscle hypertrophy, mucosal edema, mucus hypersecretion and mucus plugging. The airflow limitation is **usually reversible** with bronchodilators. Because of reversibility, the FVC and FEV_1may be normal between exacerbations. A methacholine bronchoprovocation test showing a drop in FEV_1 of 20% or more supports the clinical diagnosis.
2. **COPD.** The airflow limitation in COPD is **not reversible.** There are two types of COPD:
   a. **Chronic bronchitis,** defined clinically as a productive cough lasting for at least 3 months over 2 consecutive years, results from chronic airway inflammation and hyperproduction of mucus.
   b. **Emphysema** is defined pathologically as permanent enlargement of the airspaces distal to the terminal bronchioles with parenchymal destruction. This is also the result of chronic airway inflammation.

II. CLINICAL MANIFESTATIONS OF ASTHMA AND COPD

A. Asthma is usually seen in children and young adults. Clinical manifestations may include:

1. Episodic wheezing, chest tightness, and dyspnea
2. Chronic cough

3. Tachypnea, reliance on the accessory muscles, and intercostal retraction
4. A prolonged expiration phase and hyperresonance
5. Pulsus paradoxus

B. COPD usually presents in the fifth or sixth decade of life. Most patients have components of both chronic bronchitis and emphysema.

1. **Chronic bronchitis ("blue bloaters")**
   a. Stocky build
   b. Prominent, productive cough
   c. Mild dyspnea
   d. Early hypoxemia and hypercarbia
   e. Wheezes and rhonchi
2. **Emphysema ("pink puffers")**
   a. Barrel-chested with a thin build
   b. Mild cough with severe dyspnea
   c. Hypoxemia and hypercarbia only in end-stage disease
   d. Diminished breath sounds on examination
   e. Hyperresonance with percussion

III. DIAGNOSIS OF ASTHMA AND COPD. These disorders are diagnosed on the basis of the patient's history, physical examination findings, and abnormal pulmonary function test results.

A. Asthma. Patients with asthma are usually diagnosed based on history, pulmonary function testing, and responsiveness to therapy. When the diagnosis is in question, specialized testing can be performed (e.g., methacholine provocation, exercise spirometry) to aid in the diagnosis. Remember, **not all that wheezes is asthma.**

B. COPD. Patients with COPD often have a history of chronic cough, sputum production, and dyspnea that may have been present for many years. The etiology is almost always prolonged cigarette smoking; however, α_1-antitrypsin deficiency should be suspected in patients who are younger than 40 years of age, especially if they have predominantly basilar emphysema.

IV. TREATMENT. The treatment of acute exacerbations of asthma and COPD is very similar.

A. Albuterol and **ipratropium** are first-line agents and have similar efficacy. Ipratropium may be more effective in COPD. β-Agonists appear to have a more rapid onset of action and should be nebulized if patients are too distressed to use metered dose inhalers effectively.

B. Steroids are critical in asthma exacerbations and have been shown to benefit hospitalized patients with COPD flares, also called acute exacerbation of chronic bronchitis (AECB).

Steroids improve symptoms after 4–6 hours and should be used for at least 5–10 days in patients with severe exacerbations. Oral therapy is generally as efficacious as parenteral, if patients are tolerating feeds.

C. **Theophylline** is cautiously used because of concerns regarding toxicity and proven efficacy of other agents. If used, levels should be checked carefully and dosage modified accordingly.

D. **Humidified oxygen** should be used in all patients who are hypoxemic. Caution is needed in patients susceptible to carbon dioxide retention, since high blood levels of oxygen can both blunt the respiratory drive and take away the normal physiologic hypoxemic vasoconstrictive response, leading to worsening $\dot{V}/\dot{Q}$ matching (predominant mechanism). In these patients, oxygen therapy remains vital, but it should be titrated to maintain an oxygen saturation near 90%.

E. **Heliox,** a mixture of oxygen and helium (instead of nitrogen), improves laminar flow, which results in decreased airway resistance. In rare asthmatics with airflow limitation, it may be beneficial, although its efficacy is debated.

F. **Intravenous magnesium,** although controversial, may be beneficial in patients with severe asthma.

G. **Antibiotics** provide a benefit in patients with AECB who have dyspnea and a change in sputum production or color, even in the absence of fevers and radiographic infiltrates. Asthmatic patients should be treated only if a bacterial infection is suspected.

H. **Bi-level noninvasive ventilation** decreases work of breathing and allows for better ventilation and oxygenation, resulting in improved outcomes for patients with COPD exacerbation.

REFERENCES

National Asthma Education and Prevention Program. Expert panel report III: guidelines for the diagnosis and management of asthma. NHLBI 2007. Available at: www.nhlbi.nih.gov/guidelines/asthma/asthgdln.htm

Qaseem A, Snow V, Shekelle P, et al. Diagnosis and management of stable chronic obstructive pulmonary disease: a clinical practice guideline from the American College of Physicians. Ann Intern Med 2007; 147:633.

Rabe KF. Global strategy for the diagnosis, management, and prevention of chronic obstructive pulmonary disease: GOLD Executive Summary. Am J Respir Crit Care Med 2007;176:532–555.

Sutherland ER. Management of chronic obstructive pulmonary disease. N Engl J Med 2004;350:2689.

Restrictive Lung Disease

I. INTRODUCTION. Restrictive lung disease is an uncommon but important group of disorders that is often diagnosed by pulmonary function testing to evaluate dyspnea or by an abnormal chest radiograph. There are more than 100 causes of restrictive lung disease, and distinguishing among them is of critical importance to prognosis and treatment.

A. Definition. The **sine qua non** of restrictive lung disease is a **reduction in lung volumes [total lung capacity (TLC), vital capacity (VC), residual volume (RV)].** The forced expiratory volume in 1 second (FEV_1)/forced vital capacity (FVC) ratio may be increased due to increased elastic recoil of the lung, but this finding is not necessary to make the diagnosis.

B. Etiology. Interstitial lung disease is the focus of this chapter because it is perhaps the most important cause of restrictive lung disease. Remember that diseases of the pleura, chest wall, and nervous system can also cause restriction. Use the following mnemonic to "PAINT" a mental picture of the causes of restrictive lung disease.

MNEMONIC **Causes of Restrictive Lung Disease ("PAINT")**

Pleural (scarring, effusions, pneumothorax)
Alveolar (edema, hemorrhage, inflammation)
Interstitial lung disease
Neuromuscular (myasthenia, phrenic nerve dysfunction, myopathy)
Thoracic or extrathoracic (kyphoscoliosis, obesity, ascites, pregnancy)

II. CAUSES OF INTERSTITIAL LUNG DISEASE (ILD)

A. Interstitial processes can be remembered using the mnemonic "HITS FACED." (For some, the mnemonic may be easier to remember if the "S" is placed before the "H.")

MNEMONIC **Causes of Interstitial Lung Disease ("HITS FACED")**

Histiocytosis X or **H**ypersensitivity pneumonitis
Idiopathic interstitial pneumonia
Tuberculosis or **T**umor
Sarcoidosis
Fungal infection
Alveolar proteinosis
Collagen vascular disease
Environmental or **E**osinophilia associated
Drugs

1. **Pulmonary histiocytosis X (eosinophilic granuloma)** is an idiopathic disorder that may progress to fibrosis.
   a. **Diagnosis.** The typical patient is a 30- to 40-year-old smoker. The upper lung zones are most frequently involved. Birbeck granules (X bodies) are seen within mononuclear cells on biopsy under electron microscopy.
   b. **Treatment** involves smoking cessation and often requires high-dose steroids.
2. **Hypersensitivity pneumonitis** is an immune-mediated inflammatory process that results from repeated inhalation of organic dusts (e.g., mold, grain, bird droppings). The disease can be acute, subacute, or chronic; unrecognized disease can progress to fibrosis.
   a. **Diagnosis** is usually made by history and characteristic radiographic findings. Occasionally, lung biopsy is required.
   b. **Treatment.** The source of the antigen should be avoided; this may involve moving or changing jobs. High-dose steroids may be necessary as well.
3. **Idiopathic interstitial pneumonia (IIP)** is the most common diagnosis for patients presenting with ILD. It has several subtypes, defined by their radiographic and pathologic appearance. The most common of these is idiopathic pulmonary fibrosis (IPF), which presents in the sixth to seventh decade of life with the insidious onset of dyspnea and cough.
   a. **Diagnosis.** A careful history must be taken to exclude other causes of ILD. The chest radiograph generally shows interstitial abnormalities, but a high-resolution computed tomography scan is more sensitive and can be helpful in identifying subtypes [e.g., IPF, desquamative interstitial pneumonia (DIP), nonspecific interstitial pneumonia (NSIP), respiratory bronchiolitis interstitial lung disease (RBILD), cryptogenic organizing pneumonia

(COP), acute interstitial pneumonia (AIP)]. Lung biopsy is generally required for definitive subclassification.

b. **Treatment.** Most subtypes of IIP respond well to steroids. IPF does not, and newer therapies aimed at stopping fibroproliferation are under investigation. An antioxidant, *N*-acetylcysteine, may slow physiologic decline. Lung transplantation should be considered in appropriate patients.

4. **Tuberculosis.** Diffuse micronodular infiltrates can occur with tuberculosis if the infection is disseminated (i.e., miliary tuberculosis). Diffuse parenchymal infiltration can occur during reactivation of disease, usually in immunocompromised hosts.
   a. **Diagnosis** requires the identification of acid-fast organisms on sputum or tissue stain, and culture or polymerase chain reaction (PCR) should be obtained to confirm it is *Mycobacterium tuberculosis.*
   b. **Treatment** entails combination antibiotic therapy for tuberculosis.
5. **Tumor.** ILD due to malignancy is usually due to lymphangitic spread. The most common etiologies are lung and breast cancer.
   a. **Diagnosis** is suggested by diffuse reticular abnormalities on chest radiograph with Kerley B lines. Lung biopsy is often required.
   b. **Treatment** depends on the malignancy and previous radiation and chemotherapy received.
6. **Sarcoidosis** is an idiopathic systemic granulomatous disease usually presenting in the third to fourth decade of life; there is lung involvement in 90% of cases. The incidence is higher in African Americans and in women.
   a. **Diagnosis** is suggested by lymphadenopathy (characteristically bilateral hilar involvement), rash, erythema nodosum, and hepatosplenomegaly. There may be an elevated angiotensin-converting enzyme (ACE) level; however, this finding is neither sensitive nor specific.
   b. **Treatment.** Many patients with mild disease improve without therapy. Glucocorticoids may be appropriate for some patients.
7. **Fungal infections**
   a. **Histoplasmosis** is found in the central and eastern United States and presents as diffuse ILD, often in a miliary pattern, during reactivation in immunocompromised hosts. **Coccidioidomycosis** is endemic in the southwestern United States. Rarely, diffuse involvement occurs during primary infection; it is more common during reactivation in immunocompromised hosts.

b. **Diagnosis.** A history of travel to endemic areas and typical radiography are often diagnostic. Serologic tests may be helpful to confirm exposure. Lung biopsy can confirm the diagnosis.
c. **Treatment.** Active disease is most commonly treated with amphotericin B.

8. **Alveolar proteinosis** is a rare disorder resulting from accumulation of lipoproteinacious material in the alveolar space due to an acquired inability of the alveolar macrophage to digest and clear surfactant. This defect is thought to be due to an antibody-mediated depletion of granulocyte-macrophage colony-stimulating factor (GM-CSF). Diagnosis can be made by high-resolution computed tomography scanning (which shows a characteristic pattern of "crazy paving") and bronchoscopic lavage. Inhaled GM-CSF has replaced whole lung lavage as the primary therapy.
9. **Collagen vascular diseases.** ILD is only one manifestation of pulmonary involvement in these disorders. Rheumatoid arthritis and scleroderma are the two diseases most commonly associated with ILD that ultimately leads to fibrosis. These diseases are often histopathologically indistinguishable from the idiopathic interstitial pneumonias. Diagnosis often requires lung biopsy, although empiric therapy with glucocorticoids is often prescribed.
10. **Environmental exposures** can include organic dusts (leading to hypersensitivity pneumonitis) or inorganic dusts (e.g., asbestos, silica, beryllium) leading to pneumoconioses. Particle deposition leads to inflammation, which can progress to fibrosis. There are dozens of known pneumoconioses, and a careful occupational and environmental history is critical in identifying an agent. Diagnosis is usually made by history and chest radiography. Lung biopsy is occasionally performed. Treatment entails removal from the source of exposure, and steroids are occasionally helpful.
11. **Eosinophil-associated lung diseases** are generally characterized by pulmonary infiltrates, eosinophilic bronchoalveolar lavage fluid, and in many cases, peripheral eosinophilia. Figure 20-1 shows an easy way to remember the major diseases that cause pulmonary infiltrates with eosinophilia (PIE). These diseases are often diagnosed by history, chest radiograph, and bronchoalveolar lavage. Occasionally, lung biopsy is required. Most of these conditions are exquisitely steroid responsive, although prolonged steroid therapy is sometimes required. Relapses are common.
12. **Drugs.** The most common drugs to cause ILD are antineoplastic drugs; antibiotics (sulfa drugs, penicillins,

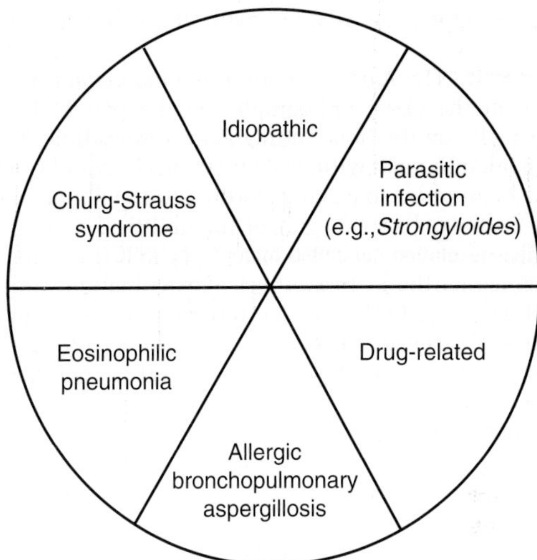

Figure 20-1 Major diseases that cause pulmonary infiltrates with eosinophilia. Just think of six pieces of PIE!

nitrofurantoin); sulfonylureas; gold; phenytoin; penicillamine; and amiodarone. The diagnosis is made by history. Removal of the offending agent is critical. If continued, progressive fibrosis can occur.

III. APPROACH TO THE PATIENT

A. Patient history and physical examination. Although the symptoms of cough and dyspnea are of foremost concern to the patient, they are almost universal and do not distinguish one disease from another. The history should focus on exposures to environmental agents and drugs. The review of systems should be comprehensive; look for symptoms of infection or evidence of collagen vascular disease (e.g., history of rash, arthralgias, photosensitivity, ulcers).

B. Chest radiograph. A chest radiograph is helpful. It will usually reveal bilateral interstitial (reticular) abnormalities. However, it can be diagnostic in other ways:

1. Pleural thickening or effusions in the absence of parenchymal disease will reveal the pleura as the cause of the restrictive physiology. Pleural plaques suggest asbestosis.
2. A normal chest radiograph with evidence of restriction (low TLC) and an elevated RV on pulmonary function testing suggests the possibility of a neuromuscular disorder.
3. A chest radiograph may be diagnostic if normal parenchyma is seen in combination with spinal pathology

(e.g., kyphoscoliosis) or small lung volumes (e.g., ascites, obesity).

C. Other tests. The most common dilemma occurs when ILD is seen on the chest radiograph and the patient history and physical examination findings are unrevealing. Many tests are available, each with its own sensitivities and specificities. Tests should be selected according to the patient's situation and the list of likely diagnostic possibilities.

1. **High-resolution computed tomography (HRCT)** is a logical next step after the history, physical examination, and chest radiograph. HRCT has been reported to have high specificities for the diagnosis of idiopathic pulmonary fibrosis, sarcoidosis, asbestosis, silicosis, and many other forms of ILD.
2. **Bronchoscopy.** Bronchoalveolar lavage can be diagnostic by revealing infectious organisms or malignant cells. Cell count and differential analysis of lavage fluid is sometimes helpful, particularly when looking for eosinophilic lung disease, alveolar hemorrhage, pulmonary alveolar proteinosis, hypersensitivity pneumonitis, and sarcoidosis.
3. **Transbronchial biopsy** increases the risk of pneumothorax and hemorrhage but enables diagnosis of diseases not identified on lavage, particularly sarcoidosis and histiocytosis X. Although it cannot reliably diagnose many forms of ILD, transbronchial biopsy may be beneficial in patients who are too ill to tolerate surgical lung biopsy.
4. **Surgical lung biopsy** is the diagnostic gold standard. It may be performed by open thoracotomy or thoracoscopically. **Video-assisted thoracoscopic surgery (VATS)** involves the insertion of a rigid thoracoscope into the pleural cavity to biopsy the lung. It appears to have a similar yield to open thoracotomy but decreased morbidity.

If the diagnosis is unclear, repeating the history and physical examination (i.e., "the basics") will often lead to the diagnosis more quickly than ordering a battery of invasive and expensive tests.

REFERENCES

Collard HR. Demystifying idiopathic interstitial pneumonia. Arch Intern Med 2003;163:17.

Gross TJ, Hunninghake GW. Idiopathic pulmonary fibrosis. N Engl J Med 2001;345(7):517–525. [Classic article].

King TE. Clinical advances in the diagnosis and therapy of the interstitial lung diseases. Am J Respir Crit Care 2005;172:268–279.

Community-Acquired Pneumonia

21

I. INTRODUCTION

A. Epidemiology. Community-acquired pneumonia is a leading cause of death and the number one cause of infectious disease-related mortality in the United States. Hospitalized patients with community-acquired pneumonia have an in-hospital mortality rate of up to 25%.

B. Classification. Attempting to classify community-acquired pneumonia as "typical" or "atypical" using clinical information is not very useful for predicting the underlying pathogen.

II. CLINICAL MANIFESTATIONS OF COMMUNITY-ACQUIRED PNEUMONIA

A. Symptoms commonly include subjective fever, cough, sputum production, pleuritic chest pain, and dyspnea.

B. Signs commonly include fever, tachypnea (>20 respirations/min), and signs of lobar consolidation (bronchial breath sounds, egophony, dullness to percussion, crackles).

III. CAUSES OF COMMUNITY-ACQUIRED PNEUMONIA

A. Organisms

1. ***Streptococcus pneumoniae*** is the most common organism and can be quite virulent.
2. ***Haemophilus influenzae*** is an especially common cause of community-acquired pneumonia in patients with chronic obstructive pulmonary disease (COPD).
3. ***Legionella*** spp. can cause severe pneumonia. Gram staining usually reveals numerous polymorphonuclear neutrophils (PMNs) but no organisms.
4. **Aerobic gram-negative rods**. For example, *Klebsiella* infection is seen in alcoholics (in whom it can present as a "bulging fissure" on a chest radiograph).
5. ***Staphylococcus aureus*** pneumonia is classically seen in patients who are immunocompromised or who have recently had infection with influenza. The prevalence of *S. aureus* infections has increased in recent years.

6. **Other.** This category includes respiratory viruses [e.g., influenza virus, respiratory syncytial virus (RSV)]; *Mycoplasma pneumoniae; Moraxella catarrhalis; Chlamydia pneumoniae; Mycobacterium tuberculosis; Pneumocystis jirovecii;* and fungi.

B. Polymicrobial oropharyngeal aspiration must be considered in patients with altered mental status, a history of seizures, alcohol abuse, swallowing difficulties, or patients transferred from a nursing home.

1. If aspiration occurs in the upright position, the lower lobes are affected (the right side more often than the left). The distribution follows the law of gravity.
2. It is more of a "**PUSL**" to remember which lobes are involved if aspiration occurs during **recumbency:** the **P**osterior segment of the **U**pper lobe and the **S**uperior segment of the **L**ower lobe.

IV. APPROACH TO THE PATIENT

A. Diagnostic tests

1. Complete blood count (CBC) with differential
2. Electrolytes, blood urea nitrogen (BUN), and creatinine
3. Peripheral blood cultures on samples drawn from two separate sites should usually be performed.
4. Arterial blood gas
5. Urinary antigen test for *Legionella* should be ordered in alcoholics and patients with severe community-acquired pneumonia.
6. Chest radiograph [posterior-anterior (PA) and lateral views]
7. Sputum analysis
   a. Gram staining and culture of even a properly expectorated sputum sample may not be the best way to detect or identify the responsible organism (it has a high sensitivity, low specificity); therefore, this test is not routinely recommended by some experts.
   b. If there is concern that *M. tuberculosis* or *P. jirovecii* is the cause of the pneumonia, sputum analysis using special stains should always be done.
8. Thoracentesis. If a pleural effusion is seen on chest radiography, the pleural fluid should be sampled and sent for cell count and differential, Gram stain and culture, total protein, lactate dehydrogenase (LDH), pH, and glucose to further evaluate presence of a complicated pleural effusion requiring chest tube drainage (see Chapter 24).

B. Criteria for hospital admission. There are no absolute criteria for hospital admission, but there are specific risk factors associated with a complicated clinical course, increased mortality, or both. The following mnemonic can help you remember some of the most important criteria for admitting a patient: "ADMIT NOW." However, sometimes the most important criterion is the "eyeball" test (i.e., how sick a person looks to an experienced physician).

MNEMONIC **Criteria for Hospital Admission of Patients with Community-Acquired Pneumonia ("ADMIT NOW")**

Age older than 65 years
Decreased immunity [e.g., cancer, diabetes, acquired immunodeficiency syndrome (AIDS), splenectomy]
Mental status changes
Increased alveolar-to-arterial (A-a) gradient
Two or more lobes involved
No home (i.e., homeless patients)
Organ system failure (increased creatinine, bone marrow suppression, severe hypotension, liver failure)
White blood cell (WBC) count greater than 30,000/mm^3 or less than 4000/mm^3

V. TREATMENT

A. Empiric therapy. There are several guidelines that exist for the management of patients with community-acquired pneumonia. The American Thoracic Society recommends **risk stratifying patients** by place of therapy (outpatient or inpatient) and the presence of significant risk factors (e.g., nursing home residence, cardiopulmonary disease, alcoholism, immunosuppression). Inpatients should be treated empirically until a pathogen is identified by sputum or blood culture (if a pathogen is identified, appropriate specific therapy for the organism should be used). In general, antimicrobial therapy should be given for 10–14 days. By far, **the most important treatment strategy is to administer appropriate empiric antibiotics as soon as possible** (in the emergency department).

1. **Group 1:** Non-critically ill hospitalized patients without risk factors. These patients can be treated with a macrolide or a respiratory fluoroquinolone (not ciprofloxacin as it lacks adequate *S. pneumoniae* coverage).
2. **Group 2:** Inpatients, not in intensive care, with risk factors. These patients should be treated with intravenous β-lactam plus macrolide or intravenous respiratory fluoroquinolone alone.

3. **Group 3:** Inpatients in intensive care, without risk factors for *Pseudomonas* infection (bronchiectasis, immunosuppression, recent antibiotics, or malnourished). These patients can be treated with intravenous β-lactam plus macrolide or plus intravenous respiratory fluoroquinolone (preferred).
4. **Group 4:** Inpatients in intensive care, with risk factors for *Pseudomonas* infection. These patients can be treated with an antipneumococcal, antipseudomonal β-lactam plus an antipseudomonal fluoroquinolone (or an intravenous aminoglycoside).
5. In patients at risk for community-acquired methicillin-resistant *S. aureus* **(MRSA),** initiate empiric intravenous vancomycin or linezolid.

B. Response to therapy. Most patients will have some improvement by 3 days. However, cough and crackles usually take longer to respond (1 week and 3 weeks, respectively). The chest radiograph can take even longer to return to normal (4–12 weeks depending on patient age and if there is underlying lung disease). In patients not responding to therapy consider the following:

1. Bacterial resistance to antimicrobial agent(s) chosen
2. Unusual pathogen (e.g., *M. tuberculosis, P. jirovecii,* viral infection)
3. Complication of the infection (e.g., empyema, lung abscess)
4. Underlying malignancy leading to postobstructive pneumonia
5. Additional noninfectious causes (e.g., congestive heart failure, Churg-Strauss syndrome, bronchioalveolar cell carcinoma)

C. In patients failing to respond to what appears to be appropriate therapy, consider obtaining a pulmonary consultation (for possible bronchoscopy) and further imaging (e.g., chest computed tomography).

REFERENCES

Mandell LA. Infectious Diseases Society of America/American Thoracic Society consensus guidelines on the management of community-acquired pneumonia in adults. Clin Infect Dis 2007;44:S27–S72.

Metlay JP, Kapoor WN, Fine MJ. Does this patient have community-acquired pneumonia? Diagnosing pneumonia by history and physical examination. JAMA 1997;278(17):1440–1445. [Classic article].

Shefet D, Robenshtok E, Paul M, et al. Empirical atypical coverage for inpatients with community-acquired pneumonia: systematic review of randomized controlled trials. Arch Intern Med 2005;165:1992–2000.

■ Pulmonary Hypertension

22

I. INTRODUCTION

A. Pulmonary hypertension is **defined as a mean pulmonary artery pressure greater than 25 mm Hg at rest or greater than 30 mm Hg with exercise**. It is diagnosed by pulmonary arterial catheterization. It can be suspected by physical examination and confirmed by echocardiography, but the sensitivity and specificity of these methods are too low for definitive diagnosis and initiation of treatment.

B. Untreated pulmonary hypertension historically carried a high mortality, but new treatment options have emerged that have significantly improved outcomes.

II. CLINICAL MANIFESTATIONS OF PULMONARY HYPERTENSION

A. Symptoms include:

1. Progressive dyspnea
2. Chest pain (partially as a result of right ventricular ischemia)
3. Fatigue
4. Syncope or near syncope
5. Peripheral edema (from right ventricular failure)

B. Signs. Pulmonary hypertension often presents with physical examination findings that reflect right ventricular failure.

Evidence of right ventricular failure almost always indicates pulmonary hypertension.

The following findings are **typical:**

1. Increased jugular venous pressure
2. A right-sided third or fourth heart sound (S_3 or S_4)
3. A right ventricular lift
4. Pulmonic component of the second heart sound (P_2) louder than the aortic component of the second heart sound (A_2)
5. Murmurs of tricuspid and pulmonic regurgitation (Graham Steell murmur)

6. Right upper quadrant fullness, abdominal distention, and peripheral edema (signs of right heart failure)

III. CAUSES OF PULMONARY HYPERTENSION.

III. CAUSES OF PULMONARY HYPERTENSION. Pulmonary hypertension has been reclassified **(Venice classification)** into five groups based on histopathologic features, natural history, and response to treatment.

A. Pulmonary arterial hypertension (PAH) is characterized by an imbalance between pulmonary vasoconstrictors and vasodilators, abnormal endothelial cell and smooth muscle proliferation, and in situ thrombosis. In patients with PAH, the aforementioned changes occur regardless of the etiology; the classic arteriolar plexogenic lesion is observed histologically. PAH is divided into two subgroups based on etiology.

1. **Idiopathic and familial PAH:** Most commonly seen in **young women** and represents a subgroup with a historical survival of only 2–3 years from diagnosis. This population has benefitted tremendously from **new pharmacologic therapies.**
2. **Associated causes of PAH:** Connective tissue disorders (scleroderma, lupus erythematosus, mixed connective tissue disease, rheumatoid arthritis, polymyositis, Sjögren's syndrome); left-to-right shunts (atrial or ventricular septal defect, patent ductus arteriosus); portopulmonary hypertension; infection with human immunodeficiency virus (HIV); and drugs and toxins (e.g., anorexic agents, cocaine, methamphetamine). Outcomes are variable depending on the severity of PAH, underlying comorbidities, and ability to withdraw or treat the etiology.

B. Pulmonary venous hypertension (due to left heart disease): Most commonly systolic or diastolic left heart failure and/or mitral valve disease.

C. Respiratory diseases and/or chronic hypoxemia: Most commonly obstructive and restrictive diseases lung diseases such as chronic obstructive pulmonary disease and interstitial lung disease, respectively. Obstructive sleep apnea and obesity hypoventilation syndrome rarely cause severe pulmonary hypertension but remain a common cause of mild to moderate pulmonary hypertension. Other hypoxemic states (e.g., living at high altitude) may cause pulmonary hypertension.

D. Chronic thrombotic or embolic disease: Most commonly due to acute or chronic pulmonary emboli and/or in situ thrombosis. Rarely tumor, foreign body, and parasitic emboli have been described.

E. Miscellaneous: Histiocytosis X, sarcoidosis, lymphangioleiomyomatosis (LAM), schistosomiasis, compression of pulmonary vessels (e.g., due to adenopathy, tumor, fibrosis).

Sleep apnea is increasingly being recognized as a cause of hypoxemia and secondary pulmonary hypertension.

IV. APPROACH TO THE PATIENT

A. Preliminary evaluation

1. **Physical examination findings**
   a. Carefully compare the components of the second heart sound at the upper sternal border. A P_2 (pulmonic component) that is louder than the A_2 (aortic component) suggests pulmonary hypertension.
   b. Listen carefully for a left-sided S_3 or S_4, which may indicate left ventricular dysfunction. Also listen for diastolic murmurs indicating mitral stenosis and a variable S_1 and intermittent "plop" that may indicate a left atrial myxoma.
   c. Look for elevated jugular venous pressure (JVP), prominent V waves, hepatojugular reflux, and lower extremity edema suggesting right-sided heart failure.
2. **Laboratory findings.** If chronic hypoxemia exists, then polycythemia is often present.
3. **Radiographic findings**
   a. Pulmonary hypertension from all etiologies will usually result in enlarged central pulmonary arteries visible on the chest radiograph. Right ventricular and atrial enlargement may also be seen in severe, chronic cases.
   b. Evidence of the underlying cause may also be visible radiographically. For example:
      (1) In emphysema, there may be apical blebs, "pruning" of distal vessels, or hyperinflation indicated by flat diaphragms.
      (2) In left ventricular dysfunction, there may be left ventricular or atrial enlargement or evidence of pulmonary edema.
4. **Electrocardiographic findings**. The electrocardiogram (ECG) typically shows right axis deviation. Right ventricular hypertrophy and right atrial enlargement are also common findings (see Chapter 5 IV, VI B and D).

B. Confirmation.

There are many invasive and noninvasive diagnostic tests that may be used to further define the nature of the patient's pulmonary hypertension. Obtaining tests in the following order is a reasonable way to approach patients with pulmonary hypertension.

1. **Echocardiography**
   a. **Doppler echocardiography.** Measurement of pulmonary pressures can support or dispute the initial clinical diagnosis.
      (1) Right ventricular hypertrophy or enlargement, paradoxic motion of the interventricular septum, and right atrial enlargement indicate right ventricular pressure and volume overload due to pulmonary hypertension.
      (2) The presence of left ventricular dysfunction, mitral stenosis, or left atrial myxoma confirms a diagnosis of left heart disease and resulting pulmonary venous hypertension; no additional workup is necessary and appropriate treatment can be instituted.
   b. **Bubble study.** A bubble study allows detection of a right-to-left intracardiac shunt.
2. **Labs.** Tests looking for connective tissue diseases are usually obtained [e.g., antinuclear antibody (ANA), SCL-70, anticentromere, erythrocyte sedimentation rate, rheumatoid factor], as are HIV antibody and liver function tests.
3. **Pulmonary function tests with arterial blood gases are recommended**
   a. **Hypercarbia** causes pulmonary vasoconstriction. Elevated CO_2 levels indicate alveolar hypoventilation (see Chapter 17 for potential causes).
   b. **Hypoxemia,** a decreased diffusing capacity for carbon monoxide (DLCO), and a mild restrictive defect are common findings regardless of the cause of pulmonary hypertension.
   c. More profound restrictive or obstructive defects should suggest pulmonary parenchymal or airway disease as an underlying cause.
4. **Sleep studies** are usually indicated in patients with risk factors for sleep apnea (i.e., hypercarbia, obesity, or a history of snoring). However, sleep studies do not correlate well with the degree of pulmonary hypertension.
5. **Ventilation–perfusion ($\dot{V}/\dot{Q}$) lung scanning** can evaluate for perfusion defects in the large and small pulmonary arteries. Computed tomographic angiogram may be used to rule out proximal occlusion, but may miss emboli or thrombosis in the smaller blood vessels. Evaluation for chronic thromboembolic disease is usually necessary when the above studies are unrevealing (see Chapter 23 IV).
6. **Right-heart catheterization** is necessary if PAH is suspected and the aforementioned studies do not reveal a diagnosis. This study is used to confirm the diagnosis, assess severity, and test for a vasodilator response, which helps to

determine which pharmacologic treatment approach should be initiated.

V. TREATMENT

A. General therapeutic principles

1. Avoid further exacerbation of vasoconstrictor/vasodilator imbalance.
   a. Ensure oxygen saturation greater than 90% (hypoxemia causes pulmonary arteriolar vasoconstriction).

Do not forget to check nocturnal oxygen saturation.

   b. Consider vasodilator therapy for PAH
2. Avoid right ventricular failure. Avoid increased wall stress (volume overload, increased pulmonary arterial pressures) and/or drop in diastolic blood pressure (causes right ventricular ischemia and leads to failure, especially if wall stress is increased). Diuretics reduce wall stress and relieve symptoms of congestion. Care should be taken to avoid overdiureses since the right ventricle is dependent on preload.
3. Prevent in situ thrombosis. Chronic anticoagulation is recommended.

Always attempt to reverse the underlying cause of pulmonary hypertension.

B. Pharmacologic therapy. Consultation with an expert in the treatment of pulmonary hypertension should be sought as decisions regarding which therapy to initiate are complex and require close outpatient monitoring and titration. During cardiac catheterization, a vasoreactivity test should be performed to determine vasoresponsiveness. Inhaled nitric oxide is the most common vasodilator used. A positive response is defined by a pulmonary arterial pressure decrease by greater than 10 mm Hg to a level less than 40 mm Hg with stable or increased cardiac output. Ten percent of patients with PAH have a positive vasoreactivity test. These patients are eligible for calcium channel blocker treatment (diltiazem or nifedipine) and have an excellent overall prognosis. Approximately 50% (~5% of all patients with PAH) will have a continued long-term positive response to calcium channel blockers. Other vasodilator and antiproliferative therapies include:

1. Prostacyclins (e.g., intravenous epoprostenol, subcutaneous treprostinil, inhaled iloprost)
2. Endothelin-1 antagonists (e.g., bosentan)
3. Phosphodiesterase-5 (PDE-5) inhibitors (e.g., sildenafil)

C. Patients with class II–V pulmonary hypertension require treatment of the underlying disorder. Vasodilator therapy in patients with respiratory disease is being studied but is unproven and puts patients at risk for gas exchange abnormalities. PDE-5 inhibitors may improve symptoms in patients with chronic thromboembolic disease. The following three causes of pulmonary hypertension are encountered frequently:

1. Chronic obstructive pulmonary disease (COPD) can be treated with smoking cessation, bronchodilators, and oxygen therapy when appropriate.
2. Thromboembolic disease is treated with chronic anticoagulation therapy. Thromboendarterectomy may benefit certain patients who develop pulmonary hypertension as a result of thromboembolism.
3. Sleep apnea can be treated with weight reduction, avoidance of alcohol and sedatives, and nighttime oxygen with or without continuous positive airway pressure (CPAP).

REFERENCES

Farber HW. Pulmonary arterial hypertension: mechanisms of disease. N Engl J Med 2004;351:1655–1665.

McLaughlin V. Pulmonary arterial hypertension. Circulation 2006;114: 1417–1431.

Rubin LJ. Evaluation and management of the patient with pulmonary arterial hypertension. Ann Int Med 2005;143(4):282–292.

Rubin LJ. Pulmonary arterial hypertension. Pro Am Thorac Soc 2006;3: 111–115.

23 Pulmonary Embolism

I. INTRODUCTION. Approximately 600,000 cases of pulmonary embolism cause more than 50,000 deaths in the United States per year. Prompt treatment may significantly reduce the mortality rate.

II. CAUSES OF PULMONARY EMBOLISM

A. Most pulmonary emboli (95%) arise from **deep venous thrombosis** of the lower extremities. The highest risk for pulmonary embolism occurs with proximal deep venous thrombosis (i.e., thrombosis of the popliteal, superficial femoral, or common femoral vein).

B. Pulmonary embolism can also originate from upper extremity or pelvic venous thrombosis and right atrial thrombi.

C. Virchow's triad describes the major risk factors for venous thrombosis (and pulmonary embolism):

1. Venous stasis (e.g., an immobile patient in the hospital)
2. Endothelial damage (e.g., hip or knee surgery)
3. Hypercoagulable state (e.g., malignancy, antiphospholipid antibody syndrome)

D. Rare causes of nonthrombotic pulmonary embolism include fat embolism, amniotic fluid embolism, septic embolism, and tumor embolism.

III. CLINICAL MANIFESTATIONS OF PULMONARY EMBOLISM The symptoms and signs of pulmonary embolism are nonspecific, occurring in many disorders.

A. Symptoms. The presence of chest pain, especially the pleuritic variety, is the most common symptom, followed closely by dyspnea. A feeling of apprehension or impending doom is frequently described.

B. Signs. Tachypnea is present in most patients with pulmonary embolism. Tachycardia, low-grade fever, and evidence of lower extremity swelling or tenderness are other important signs.

IV. APPROACH TO THE PATIENT. Pulmonary embolism can pose a substantial **diagnostic challenge.** The differential diagnosis includes other cardiac and pulmonary disorders that cause dyspnea, chest pain, and hypoxemia. **Common competing diagnoses** are pneumonia, congestive heart failure (CHF), asthma, chronic obstructive pulmonary disease (COPD), pneumothorax, myocardial infarction, and aortic dissection.

A. The **history and physical examination** are essential to the diagnosis. A sudden onset of chest pain and dyspnea is typical. The physical examination may reveal an edematous, erythematous, and tender extremity suggesting deep venous thrombosis.

B. Chest radiograph. The chest radiograph provides valuable information in a patient with dyspnea, chest pain, or hypoxemia.

1. A common misconception is that most patients with pulmonary embolism have a normal chest radiograph. In fact, most patients with pulmonary embolism have an abnormal chest radiograph. **Atelectasis and parenchymal opacities are the most common findings (60%–70% of patients).**
2. There are several classic roentgenographic signs of pulmonary embolism:
   a. **Westermark's sign** is a region of oligemia (decreased vascularity) visible as a focal radiolucent area.
   b. **Hampton's hump** is a peripheral wedge-shaped density that may reflect pulmonary infarction.
   c. Subsegmental atelectasis, a small pleural effusion, an enlarged central pulmonary artery, and an elevated hemidiaphragm are other common signs.
3. **These classic radiographic signs of pulmonary embolism are nonspecific** and cannot definitively establish the diagnosis. Therefore, the main utility of a chest radiograph is in identifying alternative diagnoses (e.g., pneumonia, pneumothorax, pulmonary edema).

C. Electrocardiogram (ECG). Most patients with pulmonary embolism will have an abnormal ECG. The findings, however, are nonspecific.

1. The most common finding is **sinus tachycardia;** other arrhythmias are rare.
2. The classic findings of acute right-sided heart strain are seen in only approximately 25% of patients. These include:
   a. Right bundle branch block
   b. P pulmonale
   c. Right axis deviation
   d. **$S_1Q_3T_3$** (a large S wave in lead I, a large Q wave in lead III, and an inverted T wave in lead III)— remember, these patients are SiQ from Thrombus!
   e. T-wave inversions in V1–V4 (McGinn-White pattern) is seen when pulmonary embolism causes significant right ventricular wall stress.

D. Arterial blood gases. Patients with pulmonary embolism may have alveolar hyperventilation (low $PaCO_2$), hypoxemia (low PaO_2), a widened alveolar-to-arterial (A-a) gradient, or any combination of the three. Although most patients with pulmonary embolism have a widened A-a gradient, up to 6% may be normal. Approximately 20% of patients will have a normal oxygen saturation because hyperventilation increases PaO_2. So even if the A-a gradient is widened, the oxygen saturation can remain in the normal range. Do not rule out pulmonary embolism based on a normal oxygen saturation.

E. D-dimer assay. The use of D-dimer in the diagnostic evaluation of suspected pulmonary embolism has been evaluated in several studies. Unfortunately, the poor specificity of an elevated level prevents one from ruling in pulmonary embolism if the test is positive without conducting further testing. The highly sensitive enzyme-linked immunosorbent assay (ELISA) assay has greater than 99% negative predictive value and can be used to rule out pulmonary embolism in patients with an "unlikely" pretest probability (see later).

F. Biomarkers. Brain natriuretic peptide (BNP) has a poor sensitivity and specificity, but can be used to estimate right ventricular strain. BNP levels greater than 90 pg/ml are associated with much worse outcomes, while levels less than 50 pg/ml are generally associated with a benign course. Similar to BNP, troponin has no diagnostic role in acute pulmonary embolism, but correlates physiologically with right strain and clinically with significantly worse outcomes.

G. Ventilation—perfusion ($\dot{V}/\dot{Q}$) scanning. The $\dot{V}/\dot{Q}$ scan is now used primarily in institutions without radiologic expertise in computed tomographic (CT) angiogram interpretation or in patients who cannot tolerate intravenous contrast (e.g., renal insufficiency, history of severe contrast reaction). The $\dot{V}/\dot{Q}$ scan may have improved sensitivity when evaluating for chronic thromboembolic disease. If perfusion defects are seen in areas of normal ventilation, a pulmonary embolism occluding blood flow is probable. $\dot{V}/\dot{Q}$ scans are interpreted as normal or showing low, intermediate, or high probability of pulmonary embolism based on standardized criteria.

1. Using the $\dot{V}/\dot{Q}$ scan result and the pretest probability, a clinical likelihood of a given patient having a pulmonary embolism can be calculated. Unfortunately, only certain combinations yield acceptable clinical certainty.
   a. A low pretest probability combined with a low-probability $\dot{V}/\dot{Q}$ scan rules out pulmonary embolism in 96% of cases.

b. A combination of a high pretest probability and a high-probability $\dot{V}/\dot{Q}$ scan appropriately diagnoses pulmonary embolism in 95% of cases.

c. A normal scan rules out pulmonary embolism, but all other combinations of pretest probability and $\dot{V}/\dot{Q}$ scan result require further testing.

H. Noninvasive lower extremity testing. Most pulmonary emboli arise from proximal lower extremity deep venous thromboses. Because the treatment of deep venous thrombosis and pulmonary embolism are generally the same, documentation of deep venous thrombosis is adequate reason to stop diagnostic testing and initiate anticoagulation therapy.

1. **Compression Doppler ultrasonography** has excellent sensitivity and specificity in patients with clinically suspected symptomatic deep venous thrombosis (i.e., leg swelling or pain). In asymptomatic patients, the sensitivity of compression ultrasonography is much lower (in the 70% range). This is probably due to an inability to detect thrombus in the iliac and femoral veins.
2. Complete lower extremity ultrasound has been shown to have much better sensitivity since the proximal venous system (iliac and femoral) can be imaged, but it is operator dependent and has not been prospectively studied in patients with suspected pulmonary embolism.

I. Computed tomographic (CT) angiography has recently become the gold standard for diagnosis of pulmonary embolism. It can also aid in diagnosis of other causes of dyspnea when no pulmonary embolism is detected (e.g., pneumothorax, pneumonia, heart failure, rib fractures). The sensitivity depends on the experience of the reader and the quality of the study but approaches 90%. Specificity is excellent. The addition of a CT venogram (scanning through the legs after imaging the chest as the dye moves through the venous circulation) also adds sensitivity to the test.

J. Pulmonary angiography. Pulmonary angiography was the previous gold standard for diagnosing pulmonary embolism; however, the CT angiogram has shown to be equivalent in clinical accuracy, and the associated risks of death, major complications, and minor complications with angiography are approximately 0.5%, 1%, and 5%, respectively. Major complications include contrast-induced renal failure, bleeding, and pulmonary arterial rupture.

K. Pretest probability score. Because pulmonary embolism can be deadly, high sensitivity is required to avoid missing the diagnosis. Adding a pretest clinical probability assessment can improve sensitivity and avoid unneeded tests.

TABLE 23-1

DICHOTOMIZED MODIFIED WELLS CRITERIA

3 points	Pulmonary embolism as likely or more likely than alternate diagnosis
3 points	Clinical signs or symptoms of deep venous thrombosis
1.5 points	Prior history of deep venous thrombosis or pulmonary embolism
1.5 points	Heart rate >100 beats/min
1.5 points	Immobilization $\geq$3 days or surgery in previous 4 weeks
1.0 point	Malignancy; hemoptysis (1 point for each)

"Unlikely" pulmonary embolism = Score less than or equal to 4
"Likely" pulmonary embolism = Score greater than 4

Diagnostic approach for pulmonary embolism:

1. Determine if patient is clinically "likely" or "unlikely" to have pulmonary embolism.
   a. If "unlikely" (modified wells $\leq$4) → order D-dimer.
   b. If "likely" (modified wells >4) → perform CT angiogram (CTA).
2. D-dimer
   a. If negative: stop (no pulmonary embolism).
   b. If positive: perform CTA.
3. CTA
   a. If negative: stop (likely no clinically significant pulmonary embolism).
   b. If positive: treat for pulmonary embolism; duration depends on risk factors.
   c. Uninterpretable: treat and repeat or perform other studies.
4. If CTA is contraindicated, perform other diagnostic studies (e.g., $\dot{V}/\dot{Q}$ scan) or empirically anticoagulate until study can be performed.

V. RISK STRATIFICATION. Predictors of clinical complications requiring close monitoring and potential escalation of care (thrombolysis, vasopressors, or embolectomy) include:

A. Hypotension (~30% mortality; consider thrombolysis)

B. Elevated BNP, troponin (both elevated suggest mortality as high as 30%)

C. Evidence of right ventricular dysfunction on echocardiogram and/or right ventricle–to–left ventricle ratio greater than 0.9 on CTA

VI. TREATMENT. The treatment of pulmonary embolism is anticoagulation with heparin (either unfractionated or low molecular weight), followed by warfarin for several months. Inferior vena cava (IVC) filter is an alternative, short-term management option for patients with absolute contraindications to anticoagulation.

A. Anticoagulation is the standard treatment for both deep venous thrombosis and pulmonary embolism.

1. **Heparin,** either unfractionated or low molecular weight, should be administered immediately. The recurrence of venous thromboembolism increases with delayed or inadequate anticoagulation, so rapid achievement of a partial thromboplastin time (PTT) of 1.5–2.5 times control is desirable. Low-molecular-weight heparin has the advantage of achieving therapeutic levels quicker and more reliably. Heparin is usually continued until adequate oral anticoagulation with warfarin is achieved.
2. **Oral warfarin** should be started when the diagnosis is made. The efficacy and safety of early warfarin initiation have been well documented. The duration of therapy depends on risk factors and patient personal history of pulmonary embolism.
   a. **First pulmonary embolism with a removable risk factor** (i.e., trauma, surgery, immobilization): treat with warfarin at international normalized ratio (INR) 2.0–3.0 for 3–6 months or until risk factor has been removed.
   b. **First pulmonary embolism without risk factors** (idiopathic pulmonary embolism): this area is controversial as the stimulus for pulmonary embolism has not been removed and epidemiologic studies show a high incidence of recurrent pulmonary embolism in this population. Recommendations suggest 12 months to lifetime anticoagulation based on an assessment of bleeding risks on warfarin.
   c. **First pulmonary embolism and irreversible risk factor** (e.g., hypercoagulable disorder) **or patients with recurrent pulmonary embolism** should receive lifetime anticoagulation with warfarin at INR 2.0–3.0.

B. IVC filter. For patients with absolute contraindications to anticoagulation and lower extremity clot, an IVC filter may be placed percutaneously via the femoral vein. For patients with short-term contraindication to anticoagulation (e.g., trauma, recent stroke), temporary filters may be placed and removed once anticoagulation is achieved. Filters are also indicated in patients with massive or submassive pulmonary embolism who have poor cardiopulmonary reserve. If it appears that the patient would likely die from another pulmonary embolus, a temporary filter should be placed to protect the patient during this vulnerable period. IVC filters prevent lower extremity thrombus from traveling to the lungs and may lower the risk of recurrent pulmonary embolism.

C. Thrombolytic agents (e.g., urokinase, tissue plasminogen activator) dissolve clot, resulting in more rapid resolution of perfusion abnormalities than standard heparin therapy. Thrombolytics improve initial hemodynamics in massive pulmonary embolism but do not improve mortality rates. Furthermore, there is a substantial risk of bleeding associated with these agents. For these reasons, thrombolytic agents are not used routinely in the treatment of pulmonary embolism. **In patients with massive pulmonary embolism characterized by hemodynamic instability, thrombolytics may be beneficial.**

REFERENCES

Bates SM. Treatment of deep venous thrombosis. N Engl J Med 2004;351: 268–277.

Christiansen SC. Thrombophilia, clinical factors and recurrent venous thrombotic events. JAMA 2005;293:2352–2361.

Huisman MV. Effectiveness of managing suspected pulmonary embolism using an algorithm combining clinical probability, D-dimer testing, and computed tomography. JAMA 2006;295(2):172–179.

Kucher N. Management of massive pulmonary embolism. Circulation 2005;112:28–32.

Piazza G. Clinical update: acute pulmonary embolism. Circulation 2006; 114:28–32.

24 Pleural Effusion

I. INTRODUCTION

A. Because pleural effusions commonly complicate many medical conditions, health-care providers need a straightforward approach to diagnosis and management.

B. The fluid can consist of anything from simple serous liquid to complicated pleural infections and hemorrhage.

II. CLINICAL MANIFESTATIONS

A. History

1. Patients with pleural effusions typically present with **dyspnea** and **pleuritic chest pain,** although they can be **asymptomatic**.
2. Symptoms may be indolent or rapidly progressive depending on the rate of fluid accumulation.
3. Fevers, chills, and night sweats can occur when effusions become infected.

B. Physical examination

1. The physical examination generally reveals **dullness to percussion, absent or diminished breath sounds, and decreased tactile fremitus**.
2. There is often a **horizontal band of egophony** just above the area of dullness, caused by compressive atelectasis of the overlying lung by the effusion.

III. CAUSES

A. Because there are many causes of pleural effusions, the most clinically useful approach is to categorize the effusion as "transudative" or "exudative" (Table 24-1).

1. **Transudative effusions** are fluid collections usually due to an alteration in Starling forces influencing pleural fluid accumulation (i.e., elevated hydrostatic pressure, decreased oncotic pressure). These usually resolve with treatment of the underlying disorder (e.g., heart failure, ascites).
2. **Exudative effusions** are more concerning as they reflect primary pleural disease. They often require removal (either via thoracentesis or tube thoracostomy) to prevent scarring and infection from developing.

The three most common causes of pleural effusion in the United States are (in order) (1) congestive heart failure, (2) pneumonia, and (3) malignancy.

IV. APPROACH TO THE PATIENT

A. Chest radiograph. The chest radiograph is the first test to order when evaluating a patient with suspected pleural effusion. Effusions of more than 200 ml should be visible on the posterior-anterior (PA) view. Smaller effusions (50–200 ml) will be visible on a lateral radiograph only.

1. Small effusions cause blunting of the costophrenic angle (where the diaphragm meets the chest wall laterally).
2. Larger effusions will opacify the lower lung fields.
3. At times, it is difficult to distinguish a pleural effusion from a consolidative process in the lung. Lateral decubitus radiographs can help distinguish between the two by demonstrating dependent layering of pleural fluid.
4. Occasionally, pleural effusions do not layer clearly, and additional imaging [ultrasound or chest computed tomography (CT) scan] is required.

B. Diagnostic thoracentesis

1. **When to perform a diagnostic thoracentesis.** Once a pleural effusion is identified, diagnostic thoracentesis should generally be performed, especially if the cause is unknown. If a patient has clear evidence of congestive heart failure with bilateral effusions of relatively equal size and no evi-

TABLE 24–1

COMMON CAUSES OF PLEURAL EFFUSIONS

Transudative Effusions	Exudative Effusions
Congestive heart failure	Infections (bacterial pneumonia, tuberculosis, fungal disease, viral disease)
Hepatohydrothorax	Collagen vascular disease
Nephrotic syndrome	Neoplasm (mesothelioma, bronchogenic lung cancer, metastatic disease, lymphoma)
Hypoalbuminemia	Gastrointestinal disease (pancreatitis, esophageal rupture, subdiaphragmatic abscess)
Myxedema	Trauma
Pulmonary embolism	Pulmonary embolism
	Miscellaneous (e.g., following coronary artery bypass surgery, asbestos related, chylothorax)

dence of infection, it is reasonable to attempt diuresis and perform diagnostic thoracentesis if the effusions persist for longer than 48 hours.

2. **Distinguishing between a transudate and exudate.** Pleural fluid should be sent to the laboratory for chemical and microbiologic analysis to determine if it is transudative or exudative and if exudative whether it is complicated or uncomplicated (Table 24-2). If certain specific etiologies are suspected, additional studies should be performed (Table 24-3).
   a. Comparison of pleural and serum levels of total protein and lactate dehydrogenase (LDH) allow for distinction between transudative and exudative effusions (Table 24-2).

TABLE 24-2

BASIC PLEURAL FLUID ANALYSIS

Study	Transudate	Exudate	Comment
Lactate dehydrogenase (LDH)	Less than 60% serum value; less than two thirds of upper limit of normal serum value	Greater than 60% serum value; more than two thirds of upper limit of normal serum value	Draw serum LDH at the time of thoracentesis to compare values
Total protein	Less than 50% of serum value	Greater than 50% of serum value	Draw serum total protein at the time of thoracentesis to compare values
Glucose	Normal	Normal or low (below 60 mg/dl)	Very low in empyema and rheumatoid arthritis
pH	Normal	Normal or low (below 7.20)	Must be drawn into heparinized syringe and kept on ice
Cell count	WBC <1000 (poor accuracy)	WBC >1000 (poor accuracy)	RBC >100,000 suggests trauma, malignancy, or pulmonary embolism
Differential	Neutrophil predominance	Neutrophil, occasionally lymphocyte predominance	Lymphocytic predominance (>50%–80%) suggests malignancy or tuberculosis
Gram stain and culture	No organisms	No organisms unless empyema	

RBC = red blood cell; *WBC* = white blood cell.

TABLE 24-3

ADDITIONAL PLEURAL FLUID STUDIES OFTEN REQUIRED AND ASSOCIATED CONDITION(S)

Study	Associated Conditions
Amylase	Pancreatitis, esophageal rupture, malignancy
Triglyceride	Chylothorax
Creatinine	Urinothorax
Acid-fast stain and culture	Mycobacterial disease
Cytology	Malignancy
Adenosine deaminase	Tuberculosis

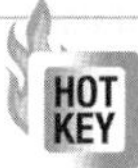

The pleural fluid is considered exudative if any of the following three criteria (i.e., Light's criteria) are met:

1. Fluid LDH–to–serum LDH ratio greater than 0.6
2. Fluid LDH more than two thirds of upper limit of normal serum LDH
3. Fluid protein–to–serum protein ratio greater than 0.5

b. **Pleural fluid glucose, pH, and Gram stain with culture** should be performed on all pleural fluid to determine if the effusion is complicated and/or infected (Table 24-2). A complicated effusion has an unacceptably high likelihood of progressing to cause scarring and lung damage.

An effusion is considered complicated if one of the following criteria is present:

1. Fluid pH less than 7.20
2. Fluid glucose less than 60
3. Gram stain or culture from fluid is positive for organisms

c. **A cell count with differential** should be performed to help determine the etiology of an exudative effusion.

d. Pleural fluid levels of amylase, triglycerides, and creatinine; acid-fast staining and culture; and cytology should be ordered when specific diagnoses are entertained (Table 24-3).

V. TREATMENT. Treatment is based on both etiology and whether there is evidence that the effusion is complicated and/or infected.

A. Transudative effusions rarely require drainage unless they are causing significant discomfort or hypoxemia. Treatment of

Occasionally, some patients who have a transudative effusion will be misclassified as having an exudative effusion based on Light's criteria. If a transudative effusion is clinically probable yet the effusion is misclassified as "exudative" based on Light's criteria (~25%), using more specific tests can confirm or refute your result. A serum albumin level 1.2 g/dl more than the pleural fluid albumin level suggests a transudative effusion. An effusion cholesterol greater than 45 mg/dl coupled with a effusion LDH greater than 200 can confirm an exudative effusion.

transudative effusions should generally be directed at the underlying cause.

B. Complicated effusion or empyema should be surgically drained, either by tube thoracostomy or with a thoracoscope. The diagnosis of empyema is made by positive Gram stain or visibly purulent fluid. Empyema requires antibiotics directed at the causative organism.

C. Exudative effusions that are not obviously complicated may still require surgical drainage if they appear loculated (the fluid is trapped into multiple noncommunicating pockets), an effusion LDH is more than three times the upper limit of normal, or the effusion takes up half the hemithorax on chest radiograph (Table 24-4).

TABLE 24-4

INDICATIONS FOR SURGICAL TREATMENT (TUBE THORACOSTOMY OR THORACOSCOPY)

1. Frank pus on thoracentesis
2. Positive Gram stain or culture
3. pH <7.20
4. Glucose <60 mg/dl
5. Lactate dehydrogenase (LDH) more than three times the upper limit of normal (isolated elevated LDH can be treated with serial thoracentesis in some cases)
6. Evidence of loculation on chest radiograph, ultrasound, or chest computed tomography scan
7. Effusion takes up more than one-half the hemithorax (hepatohydrothorax excluded)

REFERENCES

Light RW. Parapneumonic effusions and empyema. Proc Am Thorac Soc 2006;3:75–80.

Light RW, Macgregor MI, Luchsinger PC, et al. Pleural effusions: the diagnostic separation of transudates and exudates. Ann Intern Med 1972;77(4):507–513. [Classic article].

Porcel JM. Diagnostic approach to pleural effusion in adults. Am Fam Physician 2006;73(7):1211–1220.

25 Respiratory Failure

I. INTRODUCTION. Respiratory failure is a common admitting diagnosis in the intensive care unit (ICU). There are two underlying mechanisms of respiratory failure:

A. Failure to oxygenate. The patient's PaO_2 is less than 60 mm Hg while breathing room air.

B. Failure to ventilate. The patient's $PaCO_2$ is greater than 50 mm Hg.

II. CAUSES OF RESPIRATORY FAILURE

A. Failure to oxygenate (see Chapter 17 III). Of the following five mechanisms of hypoxemia, the last two rarely cause respiratory failure.

1. Ventilation–perfusion ($\dot{V}/\dot{Q}$) mismatch
   a. Diseases of the airways and pulmonary vasculature [e.g., chronic obstructive pulmonary disease (COPD), asthma, pulmonary embolism] may manifest as hypoxemia through a pure $\dot{V}/\dot{Q}$ mismatch mechanism and correct with 100% FIO_2.
   b. Alveolar filling diseases [e.g., acute respiratory distress syndrome (ARDS), pneumonia] usually manifest hypoxemia through mechanisms of both $\dot{V}/\dot{Q}$ mismatch and intrapulmonary shunting. They will not always completely correct with application of 100% FIO_2.
2. Hypoventilation
3. Diffusion defect (rarely a cause of *acute* respiratory failure)
4. Right-to-left intracardiac shunt
5. Low inspired partial pressure of oxygen

B. Failure to ventilate. Hypercapnia is caused by impaired ventilation. Causes can be broken down into two broad categories: "will not breathe" and "cannot breathe." "Will not breathe" suggests a derangement in the respiratory centers of the brain. "Cannot breathe" is defined as an inability to sustain an adequate minute ventilation (V_E) [V_E = respiratory rate (RR) × tidal volume (V_T)] to fully exhale the CO_2 produced in the body. Increased dead space and/or increased production of CO_2 increase minute ventilation requirements.

1. "Will not breathe": Central nervous system (CNS) depression, most commonly from drugs (opiates, benzodiazepines, and alcohol); obesity hypoventilation syndrome (OHS); and rarely brain tumors or strokes.
2. "Cannot breathe":
   a. Processes that reduce or prevent upregulation of V_E and/or increase **CO_2** production while limiting a compensatory increase in V_T and/or RR.
      (1) Upper airway obstruction (e.g., epiglottitis, laryngospasm, obstructive sleep apnea)
      (2) Lower airway obstruction (e.g., asthma, COPD)
      (3) Lung parenchymal abnormalities (e.g., interstitial fibrosis, pneumonia, congestive heart failure, ARDS)
   b. Respiratory muscle weakness: neuromuscular disorders (e.g., botulism, Guillain-Barré syndrome, amyotrophic lateral sclerosis, myxedema), paralyzed or mechanically disadvantaged diaphragm
   c. Chest wall/pleural disorders (e.g., obesity, kyphoscoliosis, pleural effusion)
   d. Dead space ventilation. Pulmonary capillary bed destruction/occlusion (e.g., emphysema, ARDS, pulmonary embolism) can increase dead space ventilation and cause hypercarbia if the patient is unable to mount a compensatory increase in minute ventilation.

III. APPROACH TO THE PATIENT

A. Assess the urgency of the situation.

1. If respiratory failure is acute, evaluate the patient quickly and decide on therapy. The rest of this chapter deals primarily with acute respiratory failure.
2. If respiratory failure is chronic, there is less urgency to treat.

B. Assess the need for intubation.

1. If the patient has any of the following signs, be prepared to intubate:
   a. A significantly elevated respiratory rate (>30 respirations/min)
   b. Fatigue and labored respiration
   c. Use of the accessory muscles to breathe
   d. Stridor (suggests impending upper airway obstruction)
   e. Depressed level of consciousness and inability to protect the airway
2. Indications for intubation are discussed in Chapter 14. **In general, if you think a patient might need to be intubated, he or she probably does!**

C. Attempt to define the cause of the respiratory failure.

1. **Patient history.** Ask about onset, additional symptoms, preceding events, and comorbid conditions.
2. **Physical examination**
   a. Obtain a full set of vitals (including oxygen saturation).
   b. Note the presence or absence of the following:
      (1) Alteration in mental status, gag reflex
      (2) Expiratory wheezes, rales, diminished or absent breath sounds, dullness to percussion
      (3) Third heart sound (S_3) with a sustained point of maximal impulse (PMI), elevated jugular venous pressure, dependent edema
      (4) Abdominal tenderness, bowel sounds
      (5) Peripheral edema and cyanosis
3. **Diagnostic studies.** The following studies should be performed immediately in most patients with acute respiratory failure:
   a. Chest radiograph
   b. 12-Lead electrocardiogram (ECG)
   c. Arterial blood gas analysis [to assess serum pH, oxygenation (PaO_2), and ventilation ($PaCO_2$)]

An arterial blood gas is essential to distinguish failure to oxygenate from failure to ventilate:

Low PaO_2 → failure to oxygenate

High $PaCO_2$ → failure to ventilate

   d. Complete blood count (CBC), serum electrolytes, blood urea nitrogen (BUN), and creatinine

IV. TREATMENT. General therapeutic measures for patients in acute respiratory failure are outlined in Chapter 14. A general approach to mechanical ventilation is described in Chapter 26.

REFERENCES

Penuelas O. Noninvasive positive-pressure ventilation in acute respiratory failure. CMAJ 2007;177(10):1211–1218.

Ware LB, Matthay MA. Acute pulmonary edema. N Engl J Med 2005; 353:2788–2796.

Wheeler AP, Bernard GR. Acute lung injury and the acute respiratory distress syndrome: a clinical review. Lancet 2007;369(9572):1397–1403.

■ Mechanical Ventilation

26

I. INTRODUCTION

A. Definition. A ventilator is simply a pump that delivers a set volume or pressure of mixed gas (usually oxygen and nitrogen).

B. Phases of ventilatory support. The three main phases of ventilatory support can be compared to a plane flight: **initiation** (take-off), **maintenance** (cruising), and **liberation** (landing).

1. **Initiation.** Chapter 14 describes guidelines for making the decision to intubate.
2. **Maintenance.** The goal is to avoid causing or worsening existing lung injury while achieving a balance between making the patient comfortable and allowing enough awareness to make possible assessment of neurologic status and pain. Any of the modes of ventilation detailed in this chapter may be appropriate.
3. **Liberation (also called weaning)** is often the trickiest part (as is landing an airplane). The method should be tailored to the patient, depending on the patient's underlying disease, mental status, and degree of comfort.

II. MODES OF POSITIVE-PRESSURE VENTILATION

A. Volume-cycled modes

1. **Synchronized intermittent mandatory ventilation (SIMV).** The ventilator delivers a set tidal volume at a set rate but delivers no tidal volume for patient-initiated breaths above the set rate. Ventilator breaths are synchronized with patient-initiated breaths, but the ventilator also delivers a breath when the patient does not initiate one. This mode has fallen out of favor because of the disadvantages listed below.
   a. **Advantages.** SIMV offers maximum control of ventilation.
   b. **Disadvantages**
      (1) It is difficult for the patient to overcome resistance of the tubing, which may potentiate respiratory muscle fatigue, when breathing unassisted over the set rate.
      (2) It may prolong liberation from mechanical ventilation when used as a weaning mode.

2. **Assist control (AC).** The ventilator delivers a set tidal volume at a set rate and delivers the same tidal volume for patient-initiated breaths above the set rate. Ventilator breaths are synchronized with patient breaths. Pressures vary.
   a. **Advantages.** The patient receives assistance for every breath.
   b. **Disadvantages**
      (1) The patient may develop respiratory alkalosis because every patient-initiated breath results in a full tidal volume.
      (2) High pressures may result from the delivery of a set tidal volume.
      (3) It may be less comfortable than a pressure-cycled mode.

B. Pressure-cycled modes. In the **pressure control (PC) mode,** the ventilator delivers a constant pressure at a set rate and delivers the same pressure for patient-initiated breaths above the set rate. Tidal volumes vary.

1. **Advantages.** This mode can be used when airway pressures are too high on SIMV or AC.
2. **Disadvantages.** The patient may not receive adequate tidal volumes, especially if the lungs are stiff or the patient has significant airway resistance.

C. Flow-cycled modes

1. **Pressure support (PS).** The ventilator delivers a set pressure only when the patient initiates a breath. Pressure support ceases when flow decreases to 25% of maximum inspiratory flow.
   a. **Advantages**
      (1) Because this method is more physiologic than many of the others, patient comfort is enhanced.
      (2) Since this mode allows the patient to regulate respiratory rate and tidal volume, it is often used in preparation for liberation from mechanical ventilation.
   b. **Disadvantages**
      (1) The patient must trigger every breath.
      (2) The patient may not receive adequate tidal volumes.
2. **Noninvasive positive-pressure ventilation (NPPV).** Ventilation is delivered through a face mask rather than through an endotracheal tube. NPPV is triggered by air flow and delivers a constant pressure throughout inspiration.
   a. **Advantages**
      (1) Patients with hypercapnic ventilatory failure [e.g., an acute exacerbation of chronic obstructive pulmonary disease (COPD)] and hypoxemic respiratory

failure from cardiogenic pulmonary edema may respond well to this mode of ventilation.

(2) NPPV may help delay or avoid endotracheal intubation.

b. **Disadvantages**

(1) The face mask may be uncomfortable for the patient.

(2) It is difficult to deliver high levels of oxygen.

(3) If a patient is unable to control secretions (e.g., sputum, emesis), they can be blown directly into the lungs.

D. Combined modes. Many newer ventilators now have modes that combine both volume-cycled and pressure-cycled ventilation. It is unclear whether these modes offer a clinical advantage over traditional modes. Theoretically they help to ensure adequate ventilation (volume cycled) while attempting to optimize airway pressure and patient comfort (pressure cycled).

E. Liberation modes

1. **Continuous positive airway pressure (CPAP).** The ventilator delivers a continuous pressure, usually 5 cm H_2O, throughout inspiration and expiration.

   a. **Advantages.** The patient does the work of breathing (the low level of support theoretically overcomes the resistance of the ventilator tubing).

   b. **Disadvantages.** It still provides some positive-pressure support and may not completely predict success with unassisted ventilation. Some patients with significant heart failure receive cardiovascular support from positive end-expiratory pressure (PEEP), and therefore, a weaning trial with CPAP may not predict how the patient will perform when liberated from the ventilator.

2. **T-piece.** The endotracheal tube is attached to a T-shaped piece of tubing that delivers only oxygen. The patient is not attached to a ventilator. This method should be used for spontaneous breathing trials (see below) in patients with significant heart failure.

   a. **Advantages.** The patient does the work of breathing without positive pressure support.

   b. **Disadvantages.** Because the patient is not attached to a ventilator, no alarms will sound if the patient becomes tachypneic or apneic.

III. INITIAL VENTILATOR SETTINGS

A. General principles

1. **Hypoxemic respiratory failure.** Patients with respiratory failure and a "white chest radiograph" usually have pulmonary interstitial or alveolar disease. Pneumonia, heart

failure, and acute respiratory distress syndrome (ARDS) make up the majority of cases. If there is no clinical evidence of heart failure, these patients should be placed on a low tidal volume strategy to prevent the development or worsening of ARDS.

a. Tidal volume: 6–8 ml/kg of ideal body weight (IBW)
b. Respiratory rate: 18–35 to ensure adequate ventilation (pH >7.20)
c. PEEP: 5–24 cm H_2O combined with an appropriate fraction of inspired oxygen to maintain PaO_2 greater than 55 mm Hg.
d. In general, tidal volume should be lowered to achieve a plateau pressure less than 30 cm H_2O.

2. **Hypercapnic respiratory failure.** Patients with respiratory failure with a "black chest radiograph" usually have airway disease or a central nervous system (CNS) cause of hypoventilation. Patients with significant airway disease need higher tidal volumes and low respiratory rates to ensure a long expiratory time to empty their lung.
   a. Tidal volume: 8–12 ml/kg IBW
   b. Respiratory rate: 8–12 to achieve adequate ventilation while allowing for a long expiratory time to avoid hyperinflation
   c. PEEP can be set at 5 cm H_2O and titrated as needed to avoid hyperinflation.
3. **Normal lungs.** Intubated for airway protection (e.g., overdose, etc.). Combination of the above strategies is acceptable.
   a. Tidal volume: 6–8 ml/kg IBW
   b. Respiratory rate: 12–16
   c. PEEP: 5 cm H_2O

IV. LIBERATION

A. Methods. Liberation is recommended by the following methods:

1. **Pressure support.** The level of pressure support is turned down gradually.
2. **Spontaneous breathing trial.** The patient is placed on CPAP for 30–120 minutes once a day as a stress test to gauge how the patient will do with very little ventilator support. If the patient passes the stress test and can protect his or her airway and handle secretions, the tube is withdrawn. When coupled with an interruption in sedation, this method has been shown to improve mortality and decrease patient time on the ventilator without increasing the rate of reintubation. A spontaneous breathing trial should be attempted on every day that the following criteria are met.

B. Criteria

1. Reversal or improvement of the condition causing respiratory failure
2. Awake patient able to protect the airway
3. Fraction of inspired oxygen (FIO_2) less than or equal to 0.4 [with an arterial oxygen tension (PaO_2) >60 mm Hg]
4. PEEP less than or equal to 5 cm H_2O
5. Rapid shallow breathing index (RSBI). This is the most predictive measure of successful extubation. The RSBI is the spontaneous respiratory rate/spontaneous tidal volume (V_T) in liters while off positive inspiratory pressure (only PEEP). A ratio of less than 100 is predictive of successful extubation.

MNEMONIC **Most Important Weaning Criteria ("WEANS NOW")**

Wake (patient must be able to protect the airway!)
Electrolytes OK (i.e., no hypomagnesemia or hypophosphatemia)
Acidosis (metabolic) or **A**lkalosis (metabolic) absent
Neuromuscularly intact (beware of prolonged aminoglycoside, steroid, or neuromuscular blockade use)
Suctioning/**S**ecretions controlled
Nutritionally intact
Obstruction of the airways reduced
Weaning parameters
Rapid shallow breathing index less than 100 breaths/L
Negative inspiratory force (NIF) less than –20 cm H_2O (measure if suspect weakness)

V. VENTILATOR EMERGENCIES

Always disconnect the patient from the ventilator and provide support using a bag valve mask and 100% oxygen until the problem is resolved.

A. Low airway pressure alarm. Differential diagnoses include the following:

1. Disconnected tubing
2. Air leak around the cuff (e.g., balloon rupture or tracheal dilatation)
3. Extubation (e.g., tube has slipped into the oropharynx)
4. Tracheoesophageal fistula (rare)

B. High airway pressure alarm. There are two important pressures to understand on the ventilator.

1. **Peak pressure** is the highest pressure needed to inflate the lungs during a tidal volume. It is measured during inspiration and represents both airway resistance and elastic (stretch) resistance of the lung/chest wall complex (plateau pressure).
2. **Plateau pressure** is the elastic (stretch) pressure applied to the lung/chest wall complex. Importantly, airway resistance is not factored in because this pressure is measured during an end-inspiratory static breath hold (no flow state). Chest wall, obesity, and pleural disease can also increase plateau pressure.
   a. **If peak pressure rises without an increase in plateau, there is an increase in airway resistance**. This can occur anywhere from the ventilator to the small airways. Examples:
      (1) Kink in ventilator tubing
      (2) Bronchospasm
      (3) Secretions or aspiration of contents into airways
   b. **If both peak and plateau pressures are elevated, there is an increase in the stiffness of the lung/chest wall complex.** Examples:
      (1) Decreases lung compliance (e.g., pulmonary edema, pneumonia, atelectasis)
      (2) Pneumothorax
      (3) Auto-PEEP (hyperinflation due to stacking breaths)
      (4) Mucous plug (completely occluding airway)
      (5) Asynchronous breathing (patient resistance to ventilator-delivered breath)

C. Apnea alarm. Differential diagnoses include the following:

1. Sedatives
2. (CNS) depression
3. Muscle weakness
4. Neurologic defect

REFERENCES

Fan E. Ventilatory management in patients with acute lung injury and acute respiratory distress syndrome. JAMA 2005;294(22):2889–2896.

Frutos-Vivar F. When to wean from a mechanical ventilator: an evidenced-based strategy. Clev Clin J Med 2003;70(5):389–400.

Tobin MJ. Advances in mechanical ventilation. N Engl J Med 2001;344(26):1986–1996. [Classic article].

27 Abdominal Pain

I. INTRODUCTION

A. The evaluation of a patient with abdominal pain is complicated by the overabundance of potential diagnoses, the frequency of nonspecific signs and symptoms, and the limitations of radiographic studies.

B. Life-threatening conditions can easily "hide" in the abdomen, initially causing few, if any, symptoms. The consequences of wrongly attributing the pain to a benign condition (e.g., gastritis, gastroenteritis) can be catastrophic. Remember, "**Always respect the belly.**"

II. CAUSES OF ABDOMINAL PAIN.

The list of diseases that can cause abdominal pain is almost endless and includes diseases of the liver, gallbladder, pancreas, spleen, kidneys, abdominal aorta, and entire gastrointestinal tract (including the appendix). Pain can also be referred from the thorax (e.g., myocardial infarction or pneumonia) and pelvis [e.g., pelvic inflammatory disease (PID), testicular torsion]. In addition, myofascial, musculoskeletal, and neuropathic pain of the abdominal and flank region can be interpreted as abdominal pain and attributed to the intra-abdominal organs. A thorough approach to abdominal pain consists of the following three steps:

A. Consider the abdominal organs. By remembering that **infection, obstruction,** or **ischemia** may cause abdominal pain in any intra-abdominal organ, you will form a broad differential diagnosis.

B. Rule out referred pain from the thorax and pelvis.

C. Consider metabolic and systemic causes of abdominal pain. These can be remembered using the following mnemonic:

MNEMONIC **Metabolic and Systemic Causes of Abdominal Pain ("Puking My BAD LUNCH")**

Porphyria
Mediterranean fever
Black widow spider bite
Addison's disease or **A**ngioedema
Diabetic ketoacidosis
Lead poisoning

Uremia
Neurogenic (impingement of spinal nerves or roots, diabetes, syphilis)
Calcium (hypercalcemia)
Herpes zoster

III. APPROACH TO THE PATIENT

A. Patient history

1. **Epidemiologic factors** have an important impact on the likelihood of a particular diagnosis (e.g., intravenous drug use can suggest hepatitis; alcohol abuse can suggest pancreatitis or alcoholic hepatitis; hypertension supports the diagnosis of myocardial ischemia or abdominal aneurysm).
2. **Time course.** The progression of certain symptom complexes is critical. For instance, in appendicitis, pain almost always precedes nausea and vomiting.
3. **Symptoms**
   a. **Pain**
      (1) **Quality.** Judgments regarding the quality of pain are often misleading or useless, given the significant variation and overlap among diagnoses. However, acute abdominal pain is often more of a cause for concern than chronic pain, and the chances of finding pathology are significantly higher.
      (2) **Location.** The location of the pain is extremely important and may help order the differential diagnosis (Table 27-1). Because there is a great deal of overlap, you can never be faulted for being too careful (e.g., checking a urinalysis in a patient who has upper quadrant symptoms but lacks the classic costovertebral angle tenderness).
      (3) **Radiation.** The patterns of radiation of the abdominal pain can be useful. As an example, epigastric abdominal pain radiating through to the back is often related to pancreatitis. Evaluation of the pain should include questions regarding radiation.
      (4) **Alleviating and aggravating factors.** Identifying alleviating and aggravating factors for the pain can be helpful in the differential diagnosis. Pain exacerbated by movement and bending may reflect myofascial and musculoskeletal pain. Pain improved with defecation or flatulence is often related to visceral hypersensitivity and increased gas production.
   b. **Other symptoms.** Common symptoms and associated organs or organ systems are summarized in Table 27-2. Remember to ask about cardiac, pulmonary, and pelvic symptoms as well.

TABLE 27-1

DIFFERENTIAL DIAGNOSES FOR ABDOMINAL PAIN AS SUGGESTED BY LOCATION

Location of Pain	Associated Organs	Common Diseases
Right upper quadrant	Liver, gallbladder	Hepatitis, hepatic tumor or abscess, cholecystitis, choledocholithiasis, ascending cholangitis, acquired immunodeficiency syndrome (AIDS) cholangiopathy
Epigastric	Stomach, pancreas, duodenum, abdominal aorta	Gastritis, peptic ulcer disease, pancreatitis, abdominal aortic aneurysm, biliary disease, cardiac disease
Left upper quadrant	Spleen	Splenic enlargement, infarct, or abscess
Left or right lower quadrant	Appendix, intestines, ovary, fallopian tubes, testes, kidney, ureters	Appendicitis,* right- or left-sided diverticulitis, ovarian cyst or torsion, ectopic pregnancy, pelvic inflammatory disease, epididymitis, testicular torsion, nephrolithiasis, pyelonephritis
Periumbilical	Small intestine, appendix, abdominal aorta	Small bowel obstruction, gastroenteritis, appendicitis, abdominal aortic aneurysm, ischemic bowel†
Suprapubic	Bladder, uterus, ovaries, fallopian tubes	Urinary tract infection, pelvic inflammatory disease, endometriosis, ovarian cyst, ectopic pregnancy

*Although the pain of appendicitis eventually localizes to the right lower quadrant, it usually begins in the periumbilical region.
†The location of pain from ischemic bowel is variable.

The pattern of pain migration may help in making the proper diagnosis. For example, pain from appendicitis often begins in the periumbilical region and then shifts and remains in the right lower quadrant.

B. Physical examination

1. **Auscultation** may not provide much information, because the presence or absence of bowel sounds usually does not narrow the differential diagnosis.
2. **Palpation.** Always move gently toward the area of the patient's complaint.
3. **Rectal** and **pelvic examination.** Always perform a rectal examination (with stool guaiac) and a pelvic examination in

TABLE 27-2

SYMPTOMS AND ASSOCIATED ORGAN SYSTEMS

Symptom	Likely Site of Pathology
Dysuria, frequency	Kidney, bladder
Nausea, vomiting, diarrhea	Gastrointestinal tract
Jaundice, pruritus	Liver, gallbladder
Pain that decreases upon sitting up	Pancreas
Abrupt onset of midline pain that is out of proportion to the exam	Mesenteric vessels
Pain exacerbated by flexion of the abdominal musculature	Abdominal wall is possible

patients with abdominal pain. Pain during rectal or pelvic examination may indicate pelvic pathology or a disorder involving a lower intra-abdominal structure (e.g., a retrocolic appendix). Care must be taken in interpreting the guaiac results. The stool guaiac results add no value in patients with frankly bloody or melenic stool. In addition, negative stool guaiacs do not rule out serious intra-abdominal pathology.

C. Diagnostic tests

1. **Basic tests.** The results of the following tests provide a starting point for narrowing the list of possible diagnoses.
   a. **Complete blood count (CBC).** Look for leukocytosis or anemia.
   b. **Renal panel.** Electrolyte disturbances can be the cause or result of the illness. Elevated blood urea nitrogen (BUN) and creatinine levels may suggest volume depletion or renal pathology. Elevated BUN can also suggest reabsorption of blood from above the ligament of Treitz. In the setting of a euvolemic patient with a suggestion of a possible gastrointestinal (GI) bleed, an elevated BUN supports an upper GI source.
   c. **Liver function tests** screen for liver or biliary pathology.
   d. **Amylase.** Evaluating the lipase level in addition to the amylase level may increase the sensitivity and specificity for pancreatitis.
   e. **Urinalysis** is helpful to rule out diabetic ketoacidosis and renal pathology.
   f. **Urine pregnancy test.** If the patient is a woman of childbearing age, a pregnancy test should be performed regardless of how probable pregnancy seems to the patient.
   g. **Coagulation studies.** Prothrombin time (PT) and partial thromboplastin time (PTT). Although these add little

information regarding the etiology of acute abdominal pain, it is worthwhile performing them for anyone who may need an invasive procedure.

2. **Ancillary tests.** Given your initial diagnostic impressions, the following tests may be indicated:
    a. **Serum calcium.** This test can rule out hypercalcemia as a possible diagnosis.
    b. **Serum albumin.** A low value may increase suspicion of an intra-abdominal malignancy.
    c. **Fecal white blood cell (WBC) count.** A fecal WBC count should be performed to screen for bowel inflammation in any patient with diarrhea.
    d. **Radiologic examination of the abdomen.** Flat and upright views are useful for evaluating bowel obstruction, intestinal perforation (free air), or the presence of radio-opaque kidney stones.
    e. **Radiologic examination of the chest.** Posterior-anterior (PA) and lateral views are indicated when the patient is experiencing upper abdominal pain (to rule out a lower lobe pneumonia) or when there is any suspicion of intestinal perforation.
        (1) A lateral radiograph sometimes demonstrates free air not seen on the PA film. The patient should remain upright for at least 5 minutes before PA and lateral radiographs to increase the sensitivity for detecting air beneath the diaphragm. In a patient who cannot sit up (e.g., because of pain or hypotension), a **left lateral decubitus view** can be used to evaluate for free air.
        (2) Enlargement of the aortic or cardiac silhouette may suggest an abdominal aortic aneurysm or a cardiac cause of the pain.
    f. **Abdominal ultrasound** is often the best way of evaluating gallbladder, biliary, and renal pathology; diseases in the liver, spleen, pancreas, abdominal aorta, and some intra-abdominal abscesses can also be detected.
    g. **Abdominal computed tomography (CT) scan.** An abdominal CT scan is better than ultrasound for evaluating most intra-abdominal structures (except for the biliary tree and perhaps the kidney). Triple-contrast studies (intravenous, oral, and rectal) are usually performed, yielding much finer detail. For patients with elevated creatinine levels, intravenous contrast can sometimes be avoided if the bowel is of primary concern; however, abscesses will often be missed unless intravenous contrast is used. [Abdominal magnetic resonance imaging (MRI) is an option for patients in whom radiocontrast dye is contraindicated.]

h. **Paracentesis.** If the patient has ascites, you should always perform a paracentesis to rule out peritonitis. Even if there is a very low likelihood of infected ascites, a paracentesis should be performed within the first few hours of evaluation.

i. **Electrocardiography.** Every patient with a history of cardiac disease or risk factors and abdominal pain (especially upper abdominal pain) should have an electrocardiogram (ECG) to rule out myocardial ischemia. Inferior wall myocardial ischemia is the type of ischemia most likely to cause abdominal pain.

D. General guidelines for the management of a patient with abdominal pain

1. The patient should have nothing by mouth during the initial evaluation because surgery may be necessary.
2. Associated conditions (e.g., severe volume depletion or electrolyte imbalances) should be corrected while the diagnostic workup is proceeding.
3. In the past, it was thought that the use of painkillers (e.g., opiates) during evaluation of the patient would "mask" potential diagnoses. However, it is now generally considered inappropriate to withhold medication in a patient with severe pain. The use of short-acting opiates (e.g., fentanyl) allows careful titration, which helps prevent hypotension.
4. A nasogastric tube is indicated in patients with severe vomiting or bowel obstruction.
5. Early consultation with a surgeon when certain disorders are suspected clinically (e.g., appendicitis, peritonitis, cholecystitis) can prevent long delays and unnecessary tests.
6. When an etiology is not apparent and the patient appears ill (e.g., fever, diaphoresis, resting tachycardia, abdominal tenderness), observation in the hospital is usually necessary. In these situations, there is no substitute for frequent follow-up exams and the tincture of time. In addition, advanced imaging (CT scan with contrast) may be extremely helpful.

REFERENCES

Jacobs DO. Clinical practice. Diverticulitis. N Engl J Med 2007; 357(20):2057–2066.

Suleiman S, Johnston DE. The abdominal wall: an overlooked source of pain. Am Fam Physician 2001;64(3):431–438.

Whitcomb DC. Clinical practice. Acute pancreatitis. N Engl J Med 2006; 354(20):2142–2150.

28

■ Liver Tests

I. INTRODUCTION

A. The liver has been called "the custodian of the milieu interieur." Hepatic disorders therefore have far-reaching effects on homeostasis. Fortunately, there are several tests that can help determine the cause of the injury and allow assessment of the liver's remaining synthetic capacity. The proper interpretation of the liver enzymes and other liver tests is dependent on remembering the core functions of the liver, which are:

1. Synthesis of intravascular proteins
2. Central role in glucose metabolism
3. Production of critical blood clotting factors
4. Detoxification of chemicals that enter the gastrointestinal (GI) tract
5. Metabolism of byproducts of hemoglobin metabolism

B. The blood tests used to assess the liver are commonly called liver function tests (LFTs). Whereas some of these measures reflect the actual function of the liver (e.g., albumin, bilirubin, prothrombin time), many only reflect injury [e.g., aspartate aminotransferase (AST), alanine aminotransferase (ALT), and alkaline phosphatase].

II. GENERAL APPROACH

A. Synthetic function

1. **Albumin.** The liver is an important site of protein synthesis. Assessment of albumin levels can tell us how well the liver is making proteins in general. If dietary intake is constant and the liver fails, it can take several weeks for albumin levels to fall. Therefore, in a patient with acute liver failure, the albumin level may be normal. Conversely, in patients with high levels of metabolic stress (sepsis, shock), albumin levels may drop quickly despite adequate liver function.
2. **Prothrombin time (PT).** The PT is a function of plasma levels and the activity of factors I, II, V, VII, and X. The half-lives of some of these proteins are much shorter than that of albumin; therefore, the PT increases within hours of a significant decrease in the synthetic function of the liver.

3. **Total bilirubin levels** can also be used to assess liver function. Clinical jaundice is usually apparent with bilirubin levels that exceed 3 mg/dl. A complete discussion of bilirubin formation and elimination is beyond the scope of this chapter, but, briefly, bilirubin is formed by the breakdown and cleavage of the heme ring. The bilirubin is then glucuronidated (conjugated) in the liver and excreted in the bile. Elevations can be thought of as being predominantly **unconjugated** or **conjugated.** Most are a mix of both.
   a. **Unconjugated (indirect).** Levels of unconjugated bilirubin increase if production increases (e.g., as a result of hemolysis or hematoma) or hepatic uptake or conjugation decrease (as seen in Gilbert's syndrome and Crigler-Najjar syndrome).

The most common cause of unconjugated hyperbilirubinemia in an otherwise healthy person is Gilbert's syndrome.

   b. **Conjugated (direct).** Levels of conjugated bilirubin increase with decreased secretion of bilirubin into bile canaliculi (as seen in Dubin-Johnson syndrome and Rotor's syndrome). Biliary epithelial damage (as a result of hepatitis, toxins, or cirrhosis) or ductal obstruction (as a result of biliary stones, cholangitis, or pancreatic cancer) can also increase conjugated bilirubin levels.
4. **Glucose levels** may be decreased in patients with severe liver dysfunction secondary to disruptions in glycolysis and gluconeogenesis.

B. **Injury pattern.** The two predominant patterns of liver injury are **cholestatic** and **hepatocellular.**
1. **Cholestatic pattern.** The cholestatic pattern is characterized by elevations in **alkaline phosphatase, bilirubin,** and **γ-glutamyl transpeptidase (GGT).**
   a. **Alkaline phosphatase** is an enzyme that hydrolyzes organic phosphate esters. Alkaline phosphatase is found primarily in liver and bone, but may also be found in the small intestine, kidney, placenta, and leukocytes. In the liver, alkaline phosphatase is found primarily on the surface of the bile canalicular membrane. Disproportionate elevations of alkaline phosphatase occur with any disease that obstructs bile flow (e.g., biliary stones, cholangitis, pancreatic cancer) or diseases that

infiltrate the liver causing micro-obstruction or damage (e.g., tuberculosis, sarcoidosis, metastatic cancer).

b. **GGT** is an enzyme found in many tissues, but notably, not bone. Therefore, it is most useful for evaluating the cause of an elevated alkaline phosphatase level. If both enzymes are elevated, the liver is a likely source, whereas elevation of alkaline phosphatase with a normal GGT suggests a bone source. GGT is also elevated in patients with alcoholic liver disease.

2. **Hepatocellular pattern.** The hepatocellular pattern is associated with elevations in **aspartate aminotransferase [AST,** serum glutamate oxaloacetate transaminase (SGOT)], **alanine aminotransferase [ALT,** serum glutamate pyruvate transaminase (SGPT)], and **lactate dehydrogenase (LDH).**
   a. **AST** is an enzyme found in the cytosol and mitochondria of hepatocytes. It is also found in cardiac and skeletal muscle; renal, brain, pulmonary, and pancreatic tissue; leukocytes; and erythrocytes. AST is a sensitive indicator of hepatic injury but is not specific.
   b. **ALT** is an enzyme found in the cytosol of hepatocytes. Because it is found only in the liver, ALT is a very specific indicator of hepatocellular injury.
   c. **LDH** is an enzyme that is found in many tissues; isoenzyme 5 (LDH-5) is found in the liver. LDH levels increase with any hepatocellular injury.
   d. Bilirubin is typically normal early in a patient with hepatocellular injury. Over the subsequent 2–5 days, however, the bilirubin often becomes elevated in response to the original hepatocellular injury.

MNEMONIC

Causes of Significantly Increased (>1000 U/L) AST and ALT Levels ("Tainted **M**ushrooms **C**an **C**ause **B**ad **H**epatitis, **S**o **W**atch **O**ut!")

Tylenol or **T**etracycline toxicity
Mushrooms (*Amanita phalloides*)
Carbon tetrachloride toxicity (rare)
Congestive hepatopathy
Budd-Chiari syndrome
Hepatitis (viral)
Shock liver (due to hypotension of any cause)
Wilson's disease (subtype associated with fulminant hepatic necrosis)
Other toxins (e.g., halothane, valproic acid, vitamin A)

TABLE 28-1

COMMON LIVER TEST ABNORMALITIES*

Disease	AST	ALT	Alkaline Phosphatase	Bilirubin	Comments
Cholelithiasis	N	N	N	N	Usually asymptomatic; may cause postprandial pain
Choledocholithiasis	N/↑	N/↑	↑↑	↑	Biliary colic; may lead to cholangitis
Cholecystitis	N/↑	N/↑	N/↑	N/↑	Positive Murphy's sign; fever; elevated WBC count
Cholangitis	↑↑	↑↑	↑↑↑	↑↑	Charcot's triad (fever, right upper quadrant pain, jaundice)
Viral hepatitis	↑↑↑↑	↑↑↑↑	↑	↑↑↑↑	ALT > AST
Alcoholic hepatitis	↑↑↑	↑↑↑	↑↑	↑↑↑	AST > ALT; AST usually <300 IU/L unless in combination with another insult
Congestive hepatopathy	↑↑↑	↑↑↑	↑↑	↑↑	PT often rises early
Metastatic disease	↑	↑	↑↑↑	N	Consider this diagnosis with isolated increased alkaline phosphatase

ALT = alanine aminotransferase; *AST* = aspartate aminotransferase; *N* = normal; *PT* = prothrombin time; *WBC* = white blood cell.
*These disorders often present with variable liver function test abnormalities.

III. COMMON LIVER FUNCTION TEST ABNORMALITIES are summarized in Table 28-1.

REFERENCES

Navarro VJ, Senior JR. Drug-related hepatotoxicity. N Engl J Med 2006; 354(7):731–739.

Saini S. Imaging of the hepatobiliary tract. N Engl J Med 1997;336(26):1889–1894. [Classic article].

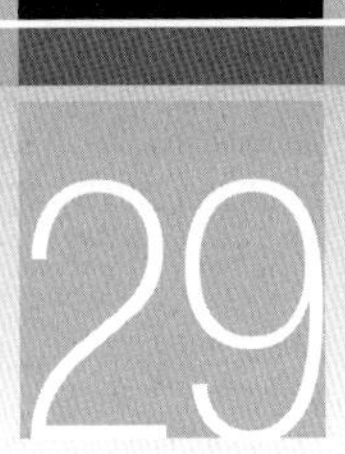

Acute Diarrhea

I. INTRODUCTION. Although we might think of diarrhea as primarily a nuisance, more than 5 million deaths per year worldwide can be attributed to this ailment.

A. Definition. Diarrhea is the excretion of more than 300 g of stool per day. Diarrhea is not a subjective experience of increased frequency or quantity of stool. However, patients often interpret any increase in the number of stools per day or an increase in the liquid nature of the stool as diarrhea. Therefore, quantification of stool is important.

B. Classification. Diarrhea can be classified as acute (<3 weeks in duration) or chronic (>3 weeks in duration). Because acute diarrhea is seen more often in hospitalized patients, it is the focus of this chapter.

II. COMMON CAUSES OF ACUTE DIARRHEA IN HOSPITALIZED PATIENTS

A. Infection. Diarrhea of an infectious etiology is the most common etiology in patients being admitted to the hospital with diarrhea. *Clostridium difficile* colitis warrants special consideration given the potential severity of this illness and the fact that patients can be either admitted with *C. difficile* colitis or develop this complication during hospitalization. *C. difficile* colitis needs to be considered in any patient with diarrhea who has been treated with antibiotics or chemotherapy; however, *C. difficile* colitis can also be seen in patients without an obvious exposure.

B. Inflammation. Diarrhea resulting from an inflammatory process (e.g., inflammatory bowel disease, ischemic bowel disease) often presents with blood and pus in the stool. An infectious etiology must be ruled out to make this diagnosis.

C. Drugs, including laxatives, antacids containing magnesium, antibiotics, and colchicine, are an often overlooked cause of diarrhea.

D. Toxins, including heavy metals, seafood toxins, and mushroom toxins, can cause acute diarrhea.

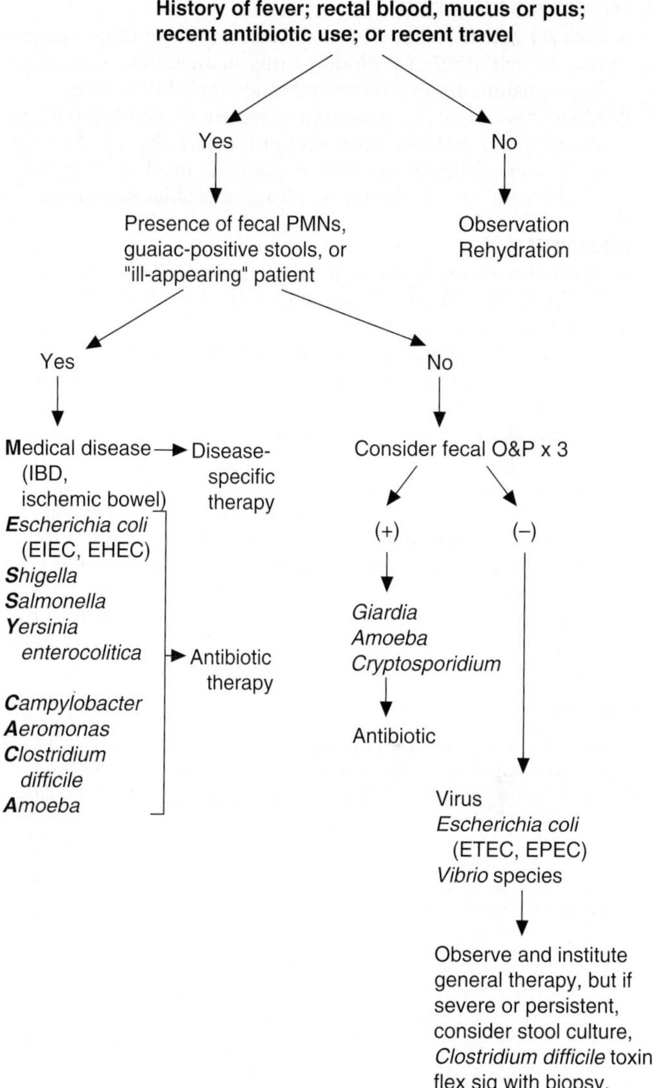

Figure 29–1 Algorithm for evaluating patients with acute diarrhea. *EGD* = esophagogastroduodenoscopy; *EHEC* = enterohemorrhagic *Escherichia coli* (serotype 0157:H7); *EIEC* = enteroinvasive *E. coli; EPEC* = enteropathogenic *E. coli; ETEC* = enterotoxigenic *E. coli; flex sig* = flexible sigmoidoscopy; *IBD* = inflammatory bowel disease; *O&P* = ova and parasites; *PMNs* = polymorphonuclear neutrophils.

III. APPROACH TO THE PATIENT

A. Evaluate volume status. Physical examination findings suggestive of dehydration include resting tachycardia, orthostatic hypotension, dry mucous membranes, and skin tenting.

B. Most cases of acute, infectious diarrhea are self-limited and do not need workup, only supportive care. Figure 29-1 can help you differentiate which patients need a diagnostic workup and which patients need antimicrobial treatment.

IV. TREATMENT

A. Bland diet. Dairy foods, spicy foods, and caffeine should be avoided. The patient should follow the BRAT diet: **b**ananas, **r**ice, **a**pplesauce, and **t**oast.

B. Rehydration. Intravenous fluids may be necessary if the patient is unable to take liquids orally.

C. Pharmacologic therapy

1. **Antimotility agents.** In some patients with infectious diarrhea, antimotility agents pose a theoretical risk of toxic megacolon and prolongation of illness. Infectious etiology should be ruled out before antimotility agents are used.
2. **Bismuth subsalicylate** has antisecretory and antimicrobial properties and can be useful for traveler's diarrhea or viral diarrhea.
3. **Antibiotics,** if necessary, are usually given in 5- to 7-day courses.

REFERENCES

Bartlett JG. Clinical practice. Antibiotic-associated diarrhea. N Engl J Med 2002;346(5):334–339. [Classic article].

Calfee DP. Clostridium difficile: a reemerging pathogen. Geriatrics 2008;63(9):10–21.

Thielman NM, Guerrant RL. Clinical practice. Acute infectious diarrhea. N Engl J Med 2004;350(1):38–47.

Trinh C, Prabhakar K. Diarrheal diseases in the elderly. Clin Geriatr Med 2007;23(4):833–856, vii.

Acute Gastrointestinal Bleeding

I. INTRODUCTION. Gastrointestinal (GI) bleeding is both a common and serious problem in the United States.

A. Classification. GI bleeding is traditionally classified as "**upper**" or "**lower,**" depending on whether the bleed originates above or below the ligament of Treitz.

B. Definitions

1. **Hematemesis** is blood, including "coffee grounds," in the vomitus. Hematemesis clearly represents an upper GI source.
2. **Hematochezia** is red or maroon-colored blood in the stool. Hematochezia can occur with lower GI bleeds and rapidly bleeding upper GI bleeds.

In 10% of patients with hematochezia, the source of bleeding is the upper GI tract.

3. **Melena** is black, tarry stool resulting from digested blood. Melena usually indicates an upper GI bleed because the blood has been digested to hematin, but small bowel and right-sided colonic hemorrhages can also produce melena. Melena has three characteristics that help to distinguish it from other causes of dark stool: (1) it is dark black, (2) it has a characteristic odor (patients say it smells far worse than normal stool), and (3) it has a consistency that is loose and tarry/oily.

Bismuth subsalicylate, iron, spinach, and charcoal can also produce black stools. However, these substances are *not* associated with a positive stool guaiac.

II. CAUSES OF GI BLEEDING

A. Upper GI source. There are many causes of upper GI tract bleeding; the most common can be remembered easily using the mnemonic, "GUM BLEEDING." (The first three causes are the most common.)

MNEMONIC **Gastrointestinal Bleeding—Upper Gastrointestinal Sources ("GUM BLEEDING")**

Gastritis [secondary to nonsteroidal anti-inflammatory drugs (NSAIDs), alcohol, or stress]
Ulcers (often caused by *Helicobacter pylori* or NSAIDs)
Mallory-Weiss tear (often secondary to excessive vomiting)
Biliary (hemobilia, usually secondary to trauma or recent hepatobiliary procedure)
Large varices (seen in patients with portal hypertension)
Esophagitis or **E**sophageal ulcer
Enteroaortic fistula (usually seen in patients with aortic grafts)
Duodenitis or **D**ieulafoy's lesion (an ectatic artery in the stomach)
Inflammatory bowel disease (upper tract Crohn's disease)
Neovascularization (arteriovenous malformation), usually seen in the elderly; more commonly causes lower GI bleeding
Gastric cancer

B. Lower GI source. Use the following mnemonic to remember the causes of lower GI tract bleeding—you may need a "DRAIN" to collect the blood.

MNEMONIC **Gastrointestinal Bleeding—Lower Gastrointestinal Sources ("DRAIN")**

Diverticulosis
Radiation colitis
Arteriovenous malformation (angiodysplasia)
Ischemia, **I**nflammation, or **I**nfection
Neoplasm

1. **Diverticulosis** is the most common cause of lower GI bleeding. The disorder is painless and is almost never a cause of chronic blood loss. Since bleeding is an unusual finding in

diverticulitis, painful bleeding suggests a nondiverticular source.

2. **Radiation colitis** can occur at any time following radiation therapy. It is most commonly seen after radiation of the prostate (men) or cervix/uterus (women).
3. **Arteriovenous malformations (angiodysplasia)** occur primarily in the elderly and may cause both acute and chronic blood loss.
4. **Ischemia.** In widespread mesenteric ischemia, for example, the patient often experiences pain out of proportion to the examination. However, ischemic colitis in the "watershed" area of the left colon typically presents with left lower quadrant pain and bleeding.
5. **Inflammatory bowel disease** is usually accompanied by diarrhea and rarely causes massive bleeding.
6. **Infectious colitis** is also usually accompanied by diarrhea.
7. **Neoplasms** (benign or malignant) usually cause chronic, rather than acute, blood loss.

III. APPROACH TO THE PATIENT

A. Patient history. The history is helpful for distinguishing between an upper and lower source of bleeding, but poor for determining the exact cause of the bleeding. It is important to inquire about the following:

1. Number of episodes
2. Most recent episode
3. Use of NSAIDs and aspirin or other antiplatelet agents
4. Use of anticoagulants
5. Cirrhosis
6. Alcohol abuse
7. Vomiting before hematemesis
8. Presence and location of abdominal pain
9. Prior aortic surgery
10. Previous history of GI bleeding

B. Physical examination

1. **Vital signs.** Check orthostatics—if your patient "tilts" (i.e., moving from a supine position to an upright position causes his or her pulse to increase by more than 20 beats/min or systolic blood pressure to decrease by more than 10 mm Hg), then intravascular volume is 10%–20% below normal. Patients taking β-blockers might have a "normal" pulse rate, despite a large volume loss.
2. **HEENT.** Check for scleral icterus, which may indicate liver disease with associated varices. Rule out epistaxis and oral lesions as a source of the bleeding.
3. **Lungs and heart.** Check for evidence of left ventricular dysfunction, which can affect fluid administration.

4. **Abdomen.** Given the cathartic nature of blood, the absence of bowel sounds may suggest an intra-abdominal catastrophe. Look carefully for rigidity, involuntary guarding, and rebound tenderness, which may suggest peritonitis. Presence of borborygmi (bowel sounds heard without a stethoscope) is caused by increased motility from blood in the small bowel (typically suggesting an upper GI source). If the amount of blood being passed from above or below is not consistent with the patient's clinical picture, consider intraperitoneal bleeding.
5. **Rectum.** Palpate for rectal masses. A stool guaiac should be performed if the stools are not clearly bloody.
6. **Neurologic examination.** Check for asterixis (evidence of liver disease).
7. **Skin.** Look for signs of liver disease, such as jaundice, spider angiomata, and palmar erythema.

C. Diagnostic tests. Important initial tests to run include:

1. Blood typing and cross-matching
2. Complete blood count (CBC) with platelets
3. Electrolyte panel
4. Blood urea nitrogen (BUN) and creatinine levels
5. Liver tests
6. Prothrombin time (PT) and partial thromboplastin time (PTT)
7. Chest and abdominal radiographs
8. Electrocardiogram (ECG)

D. General guidelines for the management of a patient with GI bleeding. In a patient with GI bleeding, **do not delay management because you have not figured out the cause of the bleeding!** GI bleeding is one situation in internal medicine in which the initial management is usually the same regardless of the exact cause.

1. **Ensure that the ABCs (airway, breathing, circulation) are in place.**
2. **Begin fluid replacement.** Intravenous access should be obtained immediately, preferably with two large-bore (18-gauge or larger) intravenous lines.
3. **Insert a nasogastric tube if there is any possibility of an upper GI bleed.** Remember that some patients with upper GI bleeding will have hematochezia. Bolus with 500 ml of water, then withdraw the fluid; keep a tab of how much water it takes for the aspirate to become almost clear.
   a. The nasogastric tube aspirate may be negative, even in the presence of upper GI bleeding, if:
      (1) The source of the bleeding is below the end of the nasogastric tube (e.g., if the nasogastric tube ends in the stomach, bleeding from a duodenal ulcer may not be apparent in the aspirate)
      (2) The bleeding is transient

(3) Nasogastric lavage that does not contain bile is not adequate to assess duodenal bleeding

b. The tube should be kept in place if there is active bleeding or signs of small bowel obstruction.

4. **Hold antihypertensive or diuretic therapy.** In addition, the patient should receive nothing by mouth.
5. **Decide whether to admit the patient to the intensive care unit (ICU).**

a. If your patient needs to take a trip to the ICU, he or she will need a "VISA." Patients generally require admission if any of the following criteria are met:

MNEMONIC **Criteria for Admittance to ICU with a Gastrointestinal Bleed ("VISA")**

Variceal bleeding (suspected or confirmed)
Instability of vital signs
Serious comorbid conditions [e.g., coronary artery disease, chronic obstructive pulmonary disease (COPD)]
Active GI bleeding

b. All patients admitted to the ICU should be seen by a gastroenterologist immediately. However, remember that resuscitation should not be delayed while awaiting a consult with a gastroenterologist.

6. **Stabilize the patient.**

No diagnostic testing (endoscopic or radiologic imaging) can be performed until the patient is adequately resuscitated.

a. **Transfusion**

(1) Elderly patients or those with coronary artery disease are usually transfused to keep their hematocrit greater than 30%. At least 2 units of typed and cross-matched packed red blood cells (RBCs) should be kept in the blood bank at all times.

(2) In a patient with active bleeding, consider a platelet transfusion if the patient's platelet count is less than 50,000/mm^3. Fresh frozen plasma should be used if the patient's international normalized ratio (INR) is greater than 1.5.

b. **Intravenous** proton pump inhibitors should be given for upper GI bleeding.

c. **Vitamin K** should be administered if the patient's PT is abnormal.

A unit of blood entering or leaving the body should change the patient's hemoglobin level by approximately 1 g/dl.

7. **Ancillary tests**
   a. After resuscitation, patients with evidence of ongoing upper GI bleeding will typically undergo upper endoscopy within a few hours. This "urgent" endoscopy will not only assess the source of bleeding but will also attempt to achieve hemostasis. In patients with no clear ongoing bleeding, endoscopy should typically be performed within 12–24 hours.
   b. In the setting of suspected lower GI bleeding that stops, a colonoscopy is typically indicated. Stable patients can often be prepped for colonoscopy the night of admission after consultation with the gastroenterologist; colonoscopy can be performed the following morning.
   c. In patients with ongoing significant GI bleeding without an obvious source or in patients with presumed lower GI bleeding who are not amenable to endoscope evaluation, a technetium-99 (T^{99})–labeled red blood cell scan can be performed. This can help to identify a small bowel source or identify the location of colonic bleeding.
   d. A visceral angiogram is typically indicated when a source has been identified on a labeled RBC scan and is done for both diagnostic and therapeutic (embolization) purposes.
   e. Capsule endoscopy can be done to assess the small bowel. This is typically performed in the setting of chronic GI bleeding with negative colonoscopy and upper endoscopy. However, it can be done in semiacute bleeding suggestive of a small bowel source. The capsule endoscopy is a diagnostic modality and does not provide therapeutic options.

REFERENCES

Gralnek IM, Barkun AN, Bardou M. Management of acute bleeding from a peptic ulcer. [Review]. N Engl J Med 2008;359(9):928–937.

Marmo R, Koch M, Cipolletta L, et al. Predictive factors of mortality from nonvariceal upper gastrointestinal hemorrhage: a multicenter study. Am J Gastroenterol 2008;103(7):1639–1647; quiz 1648.

Rockey DC. Lower gastrointestinal bleeding. Gastroenterology 2006; 130(1):165–171.

Splenomegaly

31

I. INTRODUCTION

A. Splenomegaly is enlargement of the spleen.

1. A normal spleen is 12 cm × 7 cm and weighs less than 200 g. It is surrounded by a thin capsule. The spleen is usually not palpable unless it is enlarged; therefore, **a palpable spleen is always abnormal.**
2. At times the spleen may be difficult to palpate, but dullness to percussion in the 11th left intercostal space (Traube's space) suggests splenic enlargement.
3. **Massive splenomegaly** occurs when the spleen weighs more than 3000 g.

B. Hypersplenism is the term given to any clinical situation in which the **spleen inappropriately removes excess amounts of leukocytes, platelets,** or **erythrocytes** from the circulation.

1. **Hypersplenism and splenomegaly are not synonymous.** Patients with hypersplenism all have splenomegaly; however, only a small percentage of those with splenomegaly have hypersplenism.
2. **Characteristics** of hypersplenism include the following:
   a. **Splenomegaly**
   b. **Splenic destruction/sequestration of one or more cell lines**
   c. **Normal or hyperplastic bone marrow**
   d. **Reversal of the cytopenia following splenectomy**

II. CLINICAL MANIFESTATIONS OF SPLENOMEGALY

A. Nonacute splenomegaly is most common. Clinical presentations include:

1. **Early satiety** (because of impaired gastric filling); may lead to weight loss
2. **Cytopenia** (as a result of hypersplenism); may lead to infections, bleeding, or fatigue
3. **Symptoms of the underlying disease**
4. Many patients have no symptoms referable to splenomegaly.

B. Acute splenomegaly

1. **Clinical signs** include the sudden onset of left upper quadrant pain and a tender, enlarged spleen.

2. **Differential diagnoses**
   a. Subcapsular hematoma
   b. Splenic rupture due to trauma (even remote) or an infectious process (e.g., malaria, mononucleosis, typhoid fever)
   c. Splenic infarct due to embolism or sickle cell disease
   d. Hemorrhage into a splenic cyst

III. CAUSES OF SPLENOMEGALY

A. Congestive causes. This category includes any disease that leads to disordered splenic blood flow, so that the blood "backs up" in the spleen. Think of causes that anatomically head away from the spleen.

1. **Splenic vein obstruction**
2. **Portal vein obstruction**
3. **Hepatic schistosomiasis**
4. **Cirrhosis**
5. **Hepatic vein obstruction**
6. **Constrictive pericarditis**
7. **Congestive heart failure (CHF)**

B. Reactive causes. This category includes those diseases that lead to splenic hyperplasia. Because the spleen is a lymphoid gland, many diseases that cause a systemic immunologic response can cause splenomegaly. In addition, blood disorders that lead to hemolysis can also cause the spleen to enlarge.

1. **Infections**
   a. **Bacterial** (e.g., endocarditis, tuberculosis, sustained bacteremia)
   b. **Viral** (e.g., mononucleosis, viral hepatitis)
   c. **Parasitic** (e.g., malaria, leishmaniasis, trypanosomiasis)
   d. **Fungal** (e.g., disseminated histoplasmosis)
2. **Collagen vascular diseases**
   a. **Rheumatoid arthritis.** Felty's syndrome is the triad of granulocytopenia, rheumatoid arthritis, and splenomegaly.

Rheumatoid arthritis—like CHF, systemic lupus erythematosus, and endocarditis—usually causes mild splenomegaly.

   b. **Systemic lupus erythematosus (SLE)**
3. **Serum sickness.** This immune complex disorder—usually caused by a drug hypersensitivity reaction—occurs 1–3 weeks following primary exposure (or within 36 hours of re-exposure) to an offending agent.

MNEMONIC **Clinical Manifestations of Serum Sickness ("SALT")**

Skin rash (morbilliform, urticarial, or palpable purpura)
Arthralgias or **A**rthritis
Lymphadenopathy
Temperature increase

4. **Work hypertrophy** can be caused by hemolysis.

C. **Infiltrative causes**
   1. **Benign**
      a. **Sarcoidosis**
      b. **Amyloidosis**
      c. **Gaucher's disease,** an autosomal recessive disorder characterized by an accumulation of sphingolipid within phagocytic cells throughout the body
   2. **Malignant**
      a. **Lymphomas**
      b. **Leukemias**
      c. **Myeloproliferative disorders**
      d. **Primary splenic tumors**
      e. **Metastatic tumors**

MNEMONIC **Causes of Massive Splenomegaly ("Hopefully, My Medical Students Can Learn Gastroenterology")**

Hairy cell leukemia (uncommon, resembles chronic lymphocytic leukemia)
Malaria
Myeloid metaplasia with myelofibrosis (one of four myeloproliferative disorders)
Sarcoidosis
Chronic myelogenous leukemia (another myeloproliferative disorder)
Lymphoma (primarily splenic lymphoma)
Gaucher's disease

IV. APPROACH TO THE PATIENT

A. **Patient history.** When taking the history, focus on searching for an underlying cause. Things to look for include:
   1. **Alcohol use**, **viral hepatitis**, or **cirrhosis**
   2. **CHF**
   3. **Febrile illness (current or recent)**
   4. **Arthralgias, arthritis,** or **joint stiffness**
   5. **Fever, weight loss, diaphoresis,** or **lymph node swelling**
   6. **Family history of anemia** or **splenomegaly**

B. **Physical examination.** Look for evidence of hepatomegaly, lymphadenopathy, skin rash, subcutaneous nodules, CHF, liver disease, or an infectious process.
C. **Laboratory tests** usually include a **complete blood count (CBC) with platelets** and analysis of the peripheral smear and **liver tests**.
D. **Other tests.** Blood cultures may be warranted. An **ultrasound** is useful to confirm the presence of splenomegaly and evaluate liver size. Abdominal computed tomography (CT) scanning may add to information from ultrasound. Bone marrow biopsy, lymph node biopsy, serologies, exploratory laparotomy, and other imaging studies may also be performed.

REFERENCES

Carr JA, Shurafa M, Velanovich V. Surgical indications in idiopathic splenomegaly. Arch Surg 2002;137(1):64–68.

Grover SA, Barkun AN, Sackett DL. Does this patient have splenomegaly? JAMA 1993:270(18):2218–2221. [Classic article].

Harmanci O, Bayraktar Y. Clinical characteristics of idiopathic portal hypertension. World J Gastroenterol 2007;13(13):1906–1911.

Ascites

I. INTRODUCTION. Ascites is the accumulation of excess fluid within the peritoneal cavity.

II. CAUSES OF ASCITES. Ascites may occur as part of anasarca (generalized edema) or as isolated peritoneal fluid.

A. Anasarca. The causes of a generalized edematous state can be remembered as the "**osis group"—nephrosis, cirrhosis, cardiosis, and hypothyroidosis**.

B. Isolated fluid collection. There are three primary mechanisms of ascites production. In addition, there are miscellaneous disorders that cause ascites by various mechanisms.

1. **Increased hydrostatic pressure** in the splanchnic capillaries may result from diseases that produce elevated venous pressure. One way of thinking about the causes of increased hydrostatic pressure is to trace the venous blood from the heart down.
   a. **Cardiac. Right-sided heart failure** and **constrictive pericarditis** lead to elevated venous pressure and can cause ascites.
   b. **Hepatic**
      (1) **Postsinusoidal obstruction** includes inferior vena cava obstruction, hepatic vein obstruction (i.e., **Budd-Chiari syndrome**), or hepatic venule obstruction (i.e., **veno-occlusive disease**).
      (2) **Sinusoidal obstruction** is the most common cause of ascites and usually results from **cirrhosis.**
      (3) **Presinusoidal obstruction** may be caused by **schistosomiasis** or **portal vein thrombosis.** (Portal vein thrombosis may cause variceal bleeding but only rarely produces ascites.)
2. **Decreased oncotic pressure** may result from decreased albumin intake (i.e., **starvation**), decreased albumin production (i.e., **severe liver disease**), or increased loss of albumin (e.g., **nephrotic syndrome, protein-losing enteropathy**).
3. **Increased capillary permeability** may occur with **infection** (e.g., tuberculosis) or **malignancy.**
4. **Miscellaneous causes**
   a. **Hypothyroidism.** Myxedema usually produces anasarca, not isolated ascites.

b. **Pancreatitis** may cause **pancreatic ascites.**
c. **Lymphatic obstruction** from **trauma, tumor,** or **infection** (e.g., filariasis, tuberculosis) may cause **chylous ascites.**

III. APPROACH TO THE PATIENT

A. Patient history and physical examination. A complete history and physical examination (including rectal and pelvic examinations) are necessary. By remembering the underlying mechanisms, you can systematically pursue the diagnosis.

1. **Increased hydrostatic pressure**
   a. **Right-sided heart failure** or **constrictive pericarditis.** Ask about symptoms of left-sided heart failure (the most common cause of right-sided heart failure). Perform a careful cardiac examination and evaluate the jugular venous pressure. Assess the patient for evidence of hepatojugular reflux.
   b. **Budd-Chiari syndrome** may be suggested by right upper quadrant pain and an enlarged liver in a patient with a myeloproliferative disorder, hypercoagulable state, or recent pregnancy.
   c. **Hepatic veno-occlusive** disease should be considered in patients with ascites and a history of chemotherapy or bone marrow transplantation.
   d. **Cirrhosis** is the most common cause of ascites. Inquire about risk factors, including alcohol consumption and hepatitis exposures (e.g., intravenous drug use and family history). Look for signs of chronic liver disease (see Chapter 34).
2. **Low oncotic pressure** in the absence of severe liver disease may be suggested by a history of starvation or by the presence of nephrotic syndrome.
3. **Increased capillary permeability** may be suggested by a history of fevers or weight loss, which could suggest infection or malignancy.
4. **Miscellaneous mechanisms**
   a. **Pancreatic ascites** should be considered whenever pancreatitis or pancreatic ductal disruption is a possibility.
   b. **Lymphatic obstruction** is suspected on the basis of the "milky" appearance of chylous ascites.
   c. **Myxedema.** If myxedema is the etiology, the patient will usually have other symptoms of hypothyroidism (see Chapter 80).

B. Laboratory tests. Routinely performed laboratory tests include a complete blood count (CBC) with differential, an electrolyte panel, blood urea nitrogen (BUN) and creatinine levels, prothrombin time (PT) and partial thromboplastin time (PTT), and liver function tests with serum albumin. A urine dipstick test for protein and thyroid function tests are also frequently performed, especially when anasarca is present.

C. Diagnostic paracentesis is always needed to make a definitive diagnosis. Even when the diagnosis seems apparent, diagnostic paracentesis is still indicated to rule out secondary processes [e.g., spontaneous bacterial peritonitis (SBP)].

1. **Procedure**
   a. Make sure the patient has emptied his or her bladder before the procedure. Alternatively, a Foley catheter may be inserted.
   b. A midline approach (i.e., 1–2 cm directly below the umbilicus) may be preferable because this region is avascular. However, prior midline surgery often necessitates a lateral approach because the bowel may be adherent to the peritoneal wall.
   c. A small needle (19-gauge or smaller) is usually used for a diagnostic paracentesis.
2. **Fluid analysis.** A cell count with differential, bacterial Gram stain and cultures, and an albumin level should be obtained on the fluid sample. Lactate dehydrogenase (LDH) and glucose levels may provide additional information. An amylase or triglyceride level should be ordered if there is a possibility of pancreatic or chylous ascites, respectively. In patients in whom malignancy is a concern, cytology can be performed on the fluid (the larger volume assessed, the higher the yield).

Remember to order a serum albumin level at approximately the same time the ascitic fluid is obtained.

3. **Interpretation.** Table 32-1 contains likely etiologies of ascites and their characteristic fluid findings. Remember that the findings given are only generalizations and will not apply in all cases. Furthermore, the presence of two or more disorders may skew the fluid analysis.
   a. **Cell count.** The cell count can be used to assess the likelihood of SBP, tuberculosis, or malignancy.
      (1) **SBP.** Treatment of SBP is usually indicated when the absolute neutrophil count exceeds **250 cells/μl.** Counts greater than 500 cells/μl are more specific but less sensitive for SBP.
      (2) **Tuberculosis** or **malignancy.** A cell count that exceeds 250 cells/μl and is lymphocyte predominant often implies tuberculous or malignant ascites. (However,

SBP can also occasionally have a lymphocyte-predominant pattern.)

b. **Serum–ascites albumin gradient.** Subtract the ascitic fluid albumin value from the serum albumin value.
   (1) If the result is greater than or equal to 1.1, portal hypertension is implicated (i.e., a hydrostatic etiology is responsible).
   (2) If the value is less than 1.1, capillary permeability is probably abnormal (i.e., infection or malignancy may be implicated).

If portal hypertension is accompanied by another disorder that produces increased capillary permeability, the gradient will usually remain greater than or equal to 1.1. SBP usually occurs in patients with portal hypertension; therefore, the gradient is usually greater than or equal to 1.1 in these patients.

c. **Gram stain** and **culture** of ascitic fluid should be performed if peritonitis is suspected.
d. **LDH** and **glucose levels.** An elevated LDH or low glucose level may indicate tuberculosis or malignancy; however, these lab tests have limited value.
e. **Amylase** and **triglyceride levels.** Elevated amylase or triglyceride levels may indicate pancreatic or chylous ascites, respectively.

D. Additional testing may be necessary when the ascitic fluid contains an elevated cell count with a lymphocyte predominance, increasing suspicion for tuberculous or malignant ascites.

1. **Purified protein derivative (PPD) test.** A positive PPD test will increase suspicion for tuberculous peritonitis.
2. **Acid-fast bacillus stain** and **culture of ascitic fluid.** These are relatively insensitive tests, but sending a large volume of fluid (e.g., 1 L) may increase the yield.
3. **Abdominal computed tomography** may reveal an intra-abdominal malignancy.
4. **Laparoscopy** with **peritoneal biopsy** is often performed to make an expedient diagnosis.

IV. TREATMENT. The general management of ascites is discussed in Chapter 35; other specific therapies are tailored to the underlying etiology and will not be discussed here.

TABLE 32-1

CHARACTERISTIC FLUID FINDINGS

Disorder	Serum–Ascites Albumin Gradient	Cell Count (Cells/μl)	Total Protein*	Other Findings
Cirrhosis	≥1.1	<250 (mesothelial)	Moderate	Abnormal liver function tests
Spontaneous bacterial peritonitis (SPB)	≥1.1	>250 (PMNs)	Moderate	Culture may be positive, but typically is negative
Congestive heart failure	≥1.1	<1000 (mesothelial)	High	Elevated neck veins, gallops, abnormal ECG
Hypothyroidism	≥1.1	<250 (variable)	Variable	Decreased free T_4, increased TSH
Liver malignancy (primary or secondary)	≥1.1	Variable	Moderate	Elevated serum AFP with primary malignancy
Nephrotic syndrome	<1.1	<250 (mesothelial)	Low	Positive urine dipstick and 24-hour collection for protein
Tuberculous ascites	<1.1	>1000 (variable)	High	Ascitic acid-fast bacillus stain occasionally positive
Secondary peritonitis	<1.1	>250 (PMNs)	Moderate	Very low ascitic glucose, polymicrobial
Pancreatic ascites	<1.1	>1000 (PMNs)	Moderate	Increased serum and fluid amylase
Peritoneal malignancy	<1.1	>1000 (variable)	High	Cytology, CT scan, peritoneal biopsy may be useful

AFP = α-fetoprotein; *CT* = computed tomography; *ECG* = electrocardiogram; *PMNs* = polymorphonuclear neutrophils; T_4 = thyroxine; *TSH* = thyroid-stimulating hormone.
*Total protein is considered low if it is <1 g/dl, moderate if it is 1–3 g/dl, and high if it is >3 g/dl.

REFERENCES

Gines P, Cardenaw A, Arroyo V, et al. Management of cirrhosis and ascites. N Engl J Med 2004;350(16):1646–1654.

Runyon BA. Management of adult patients with ascites caused by cirrhosis. Hepatology 1998;27(1):264–272. [Classic article].

Sheer TA, Runyon BA. Spontaneous bacterial peritonitis. Dig Dis 2005; 23(1):39–46.

Videos in clinical medicine. Paracentesis. N Engl J Med 2006;355(19):e21.

33 Acute Pancreatitis

I. INTRODUCTION. Pancreatitis implies inflammation of the pancreas.

A. Acute pancreatitis results from the leakage of pancreatic enzymes into pancreatic tissue, leading to autodigestion. Because acute pancreatitis is more common than chronic pancreatitis, acute pancreatitis is the focus of this chapter.

B. Chronic pancreatitis. Causes are varied and ultimately lead to destruction of the pancreatic tissue. The process usually starts with multiple episodes of acute pancreatitis, which subsequently leave the patient with a damaged pancreas.

II. CLINICAL MANIFESTATIONS OF ACUTE PANCREATITIS

A. Symptoms usually include the abrupt onset of epigastric pain that lasts for hours to days and radiates to the back, nausea and vomiting, sweating, weakness, and anxiety. The patient often feels better when sitting up and leaning forward.

B. Physical examination findings

1. The patient may be febrile, tachycardic, tachypneic, and hypotensive.
2. The skin of the periumbilical area may be discolored **(Cullen's sign),** or flank ecchymoses **(Turner's sign)** may be present.
3. The abdomen is hypoactive with mild distention (because of ileus). Upper abdominal tenderness (usually without rebound or rigidity) is present.

C. Laboratory findings

1. **Elevated serum amylase** and **lipase** are the hallmarks of acute pancreatitis.
2. Other findings may include leukocytosis (12,000–15,000/mm^3), hypoalbuminemia, hyperglycemia, and elevated aspartate aminotransferase [AST, serum glutamate oxaloacetate transaminase (SGOT)], alkaline phosphatase, and bilirubin.

III. CAUSES OF ACUTE PANCREATITIS. There are numerous causes of pancreatitis. The simplest way to remember the most important of these causes is with the mnemonic, "BAD HITS." (HINT: If you move the "S" in front of the "H," the mnemonic will be easier to remember but more difficult to utter in public.)

MNEMONIC **Common Causes of Acute Pancreatitis ("BAD HITS")**

Biliary stones
Alcohol abuse
Drugs
Hyperlipidemia or **H**ypercalcemia
Idiopathic or **I**nfectious
Trauma
Surgery [post–endoscopic retrograde cholangiopancreatography (ERCP) or intra-abdominal surgery] or **S**corpion sting

A. **Biliary stones** are the most common cause of acute pancreatitis in suburban hospitals.
B. **Alcohol abuse** is the most common cause in urban hospitals.
C. **Drugs.** Many drugs can cause acute pancreatitis, including thiazide diuretics, sulfa antibiotics, pentamidine, and some antiretroviral agents.
D. **Hyperlipidemia (types I, IV, V).** Pancreatitis usually does not occur in hyperlipidemic patients until their serum triglyceride level exceeds 1000 mg/dl.
E. **Idiopathic causes.** In 15% of patients, no obvious cause of pancreatitis is identified; however, many authors implicate pancreas divisum (a congenital defect) or autoimmune pancreatitis as the cause.
F. **Infectious etiologies** include mumps, cytomegalovirus (CMV), human immunodeficiency virus (HIV), and infections caused by *Escherichia coli.*
G. **Trauma.** Blunt, rather than penetrating, trauma is most often responsible.
H. **Surgical.** Postsurgical pancreatitis occurs in 3% of patients undergoing ERCP.
I. **Scorpion stings.** This cause is really only important to know for residents' report or on attending rounds.

IV. **APPROACH TO THE PATIENT.** The diagnosis is based on finding elevated serum amylase or lipase levels in the context of an appropriate clinical setting. Imaging studies that may be helpful include abdominal ultrasound and computed tomography (CT). When a patient presents with pancreatitis, you should:

A. **Determine the cause** of the pancreatitis.
B. **Assess the severity** and **estimate the prognosis.** Because the serum amylase and lipase levels do not correlate with severity, **Ranson's criteria** are used to assess severity and prognosis.

1. Ranson's criteria are assessed at admission and during the initial 48 hours.

MNEMONIC **Ranson's Criteria at Admission ("WAGLS")**

White blood cell (WBC) count > 16,000/mm^3
Age > 55 years
Glucose > 200 mg/dl
Lactate dehydrogenase (LDH) > 350 U/L
SGOT > 250 U/L

MNEMONIC **Ranson's Criteria During the Initial 48 Hours ("BaCH** wasn't an **SOB**")

Base deficit greater than 4 mEq/L
Calcium less than 8 mg/dl
Hematocrit decrease of more than 10%
Sequestration of fluid greater than 6 L
Oxygen less than 60 mm Hg
Blood urea nitrogen (BUN) increase of greater than 5 mg/dl

2. In general, as the number of criteria increases, so does the mortality rate.

V. TREATMENT is primarily supportive and includes bowel rest, volume resuscitation, pain control, and management of respiratory distress and renal failure. Nasogastric tubes are used for gastric decompression in patients with persistent vomiting. If gallstones are thought to be the cause, ERCP may be indicated. Cholecystectomy should only be considered once the patient recovers from the acute episode.

VI. COMPLICATIONS

A. Pancreatic abscess should be suspected when patients worsen after initial improvement. Radiology-guided drainage or surgical intervention is often necessary in this group of patients.

B. Pancreatic pseudocyst occurs in 10%–20% of patients and usually does not require specific treatment unless it has been present for longer than 6 weeks, is greater than 5 cm in diameter, or is accompanied by significant symptoms.

C. Renal failure and **respiratory failure** are the two most common systemic complications.

REFERENCES

Frossard JL, Steer ML, Pastor CM. Acute pancreatitis. Lancet 2008; 371(9607):143–152.

Skipworth JR, Pereira SP. Acute pancreatitis. Curr Opin Crit Care 2008; 14(2):172–178.

Alcoholic Liver Disease

34

I. INTRODUCTION

A. The amount of alcohol required to produce liver disease in a given patient is variable. Women in general are more susceptible than men, but men are more often affected because of higher alcohol consumption rates.

B. Most authorities believe that a susceptible person must drink 60–80 g of alcohol per day for at least 10 years before developing cirrhosis. Many women, however, develop cirrhosis with much lower alcohol intake. Patients with intercurrent liver disease (e.g., viral hepatitis, nonalcoholic liver disease) are more susceptible to alcoholic liver injury.

C. Alcohol contents of common beverages: (1) beer: 11.5 g in 12 oz (1 can), (2) wine: 11.5 g in 4 oz (1 glass), and (3) hard liquor: 10.3 g in 1 oz (1 shot).

D. There are three commonly discussed degrees of alcoholic liver disease. These three syndromes often overlap in a given patient:

1. **Fatty liver**
2. **Alcoholic hepatitis**
3. **Micronodular (Laënnec's) cirrhosis**

Approximately all heavy drinkers (i.e., those who consume at least 60 g of alcohol per day) develop fatty liver, whereas less than one third develop alcoholic hepatitis and cirrhosis.

II. CLINICAL MANIFESTATIONS OF ALCOHOLIC LIVER DISEASE.

Table 34-1 summarizes the clinical findings that accompany the various degrees of alcoholic liver disease.

III. APPROACH TO THE PATIENT

A. Fatty liver is usually diagnosed in patients with a history of alcohol consumption accompanied by mildly abnormal liver enzymes, hepatomegaly, or both. A definitive diagnosis may be made by biopsy but is rarely necessary. Other possible causes of fatty liver include obesity, diabetes, hyperlipidemia,

TABLE 34-1

CLINICAL FINDINGS IN ALCOHOLIC LIVER DISEASE

Syndrome	Symptoms	Signs	Laboratory Findings
Fatty liver	None	None, or possibly hepatomegaly with or without tenderness	AST mildly elevated
Alcoholic hepatitis	Subjective fever, right upper quadrant pain, nausea, vomiting	Fever, tender hepatomegaly, jaundice (common), splenomegaly, ascites, peripheral edema, encephalopathy (in severe cases)	AST:ALT ratio >2:1, with AST <300 IU/L; elevated PT, alkaline phosphatase,* and bilirubin levels; low hematocrit, platelet count, and albumin
Cirrhosis	Anorexia, weight changes, jaundice, variceal bleeding, encephalopathy	Jaundice, liver size is variable (but usually small), ascites, splenomegaly, palmar erythema, spider angiomas, testicular atrophy, gynecomastia, Dupuytren's contractures, asterixis, altered mental status	Same as for alcoholic hepatitis; prerenal azotemia may also be seen

ALT = alanine aminotransferase; *AST* = aspartate aminotransferase; *PT* = prothrombin time.
*But usually less than three times normal.

steroids (endogenous or exogenous), starvation, parenteral nutrition, and toxins (e.g., carbon tetrachloride).

B. Alcoholic hepatitis can be very mild or life-threatening. The patient often presents with the signs and symptoms summarized in Table 34-1 after a prolonged "drinking binge"; often the onset of symptoms coincides with the cessation of drinking (patients quit drinking because they feel so poorly). Although alcoholic hepatitis is a common disease in alcoholics, other diseases (e.g., cholecystitis and cholelithiasis) may mimic alcoholic hepatitis quite closely. To avoid missing other pathologies, have a low threshold for getting an abdominal ultrasound in an alcoholic patient with right upper quadrant pain. In addition, alcoholic patients who come in with significantly elevated transaminase levels have something in addition to alcohol-related disease (e.g., acetaminophen toxicity, viral infection).

Alcoholic hepatitis does not cause transaminase elevations greater than 300 without an additional cause.

C. Cirrhosis. Alcoholism is one of the most common causes of cirrhosis in the United States. The diagnosis is usually obvious clinically once the patient develops decompensated liver disease (see Table 34-1). It is important to evaluate the alcoholic patient for other common causes of liver disease. Many patients who develop chronic alcoholic liver disease also have other disease affecting the liver (e.g., hepatitis C).

IV. TREATMENT

A. Fatty liver. Abstinence is the mainstay of therapy. Most patients who achieve successful long-term sobriety undergo formal rehabilitation. **Exercise** and **nutritional counseling** are advisable for patients with obesity, diabetes, or hyperlipidemia.

B. Alcoholic hepatitis. The long-term prognosis depends on liver function and the patient's ability to abstain from consuming alcohol.

1. **Supportive therapy** includes correction of fluid and electrolyte status and observation for alcohol withdrawal, seizures, and delirium tremens. Patients with alcoholic hepatitis are often significantly malnourished and need aggressive vitamin, mineral, and calorie supplementation.
2. **Steroid therapy** may benefit some patients with extensive liver dysfunction. However, the risk of infection outweighs the benefit of steroids in most patients.

C. Cirrhosis. Abstinence is critical to prevent worsening of liver function. Management of decompensated cirrhosis is addressed in Chapter 35.

Many patients with alcohol-related liver disease have the potential for dramatic improvement in liver function with abstinence from alcohol and supportive care. It is not uncommon for patients with alcoholic hepatitis and ascites (or even encephalopathy) to have complete clinical resolution with long-term abstinence.

REFERENCES

Cargiulo T. Understanding the health impact of alcohol dependence. Am J Health Syst Pharm 2007;64 (5 suppl 3):S5–11.

Reuben A. Alcohol and the liver. Curr Opin Gastroenterol 2008;24(3): 328–338.

Tilg H, Day CP. Management strategies in alcoholic liver disease. Nat Clin Pract Gastroenterol Hepatol 2007;4(1):24–34.

35 ■ Liver Failure

I. INTRODUCTION

A. Acute liver failure is defined by the presence of **encephalopathy** and **coagulopathy associated with acute hepatic disease.** It is often classified as fulminant or subfulminant, depending on whether it develops within 2 months of, or as many as 6 months after, the onset of illness.

B. Chronic liver failure occurs over a longer period. It is characterized by hepatic fibrosis, evidence of hepatic synthetic dysfunction, and clinical signs such as ascites, encephalopathy, and muscle wasting.

II. CLINICAL MANIFESTATIONS OF LIVER FAILURE

A. Acute liver failure is characterized by the rapid development of coagulopathy, jaundice, altered mental status, and often nonspecific symptoms (e.g., nausea, malaise), usually in a previously healthy patient.

1. **Central nervous system (CNS) signs**
   a. **Altered mental status. Encephalopathy** produces an alteration in mental status that ranges from mild confusion (grade I or II encephalopathy) to stupor or coma (grade III or IV encephalopathy). Patients may also present with agitation and delusions, which are uncommon in chronic liver failure. Unlike chronic liver disease, acute liver failure may not be clinically obvious; it is therefore important to consider hepatic failure in all patients with altered mental status.
   b. **Asterixis** is frequently noted on examination.
   c. **Cerebral edema** accompanies hepatic encephalopathy in the majority of acute liver failure patients with grade IV encephalopathy (coma). Significant cerebral edema can lead to brain herniation and is a common cause of death in patients with acute liver failure. **Cushing's reflex (hypertension and bradycardia), abnormal pupillary reflexes,** and **increased muscle tone progressing to decerebrate posturing** are signs of increasing **cerebral edema.** Cerebral edema occurs more commonly with fulminant liver failure, whereas renal failure and ascites are more often associated with a subfulminant course.

2. **Hematologic signs.** Elevation of the prothrombin time (PT) is universally present and may be accompanied by an elevated partial thromboplastin time (PTT). Thrombocytopenia may also occur.
3. **Cardiovascular signs** may include hypovolemia, a decrease in systemic vascular resistance associated with hypotension, and an increase in cardiac output. Because these findings may also indicate sepsis, infection should be considered and ruled out.
4. **Metabolic changes**
   a. **Hypoglycemia** may aggravate the alteration in mental status. Patients with profound liver injury can develop refractory hypoglycemia. Blood glucose levels should be monitored frequently.
   b. **Hypokalemia** can result from respiratory alkalosis induced by liver failure.
   c. **Hyponatremia** and **hypophosphatemia** may also occur.
5. **Complications**
   a. **Hemorrhage.** Thrombocytopenia is a strong risk factor for gastrointestinal or other bleeding.
   b. **Infections.** Defects in neutrophil function as well as humoral and cell-mediated immunity may result in bacterial or fungal infections. Early use of broad-spectrum antibiotics is encouraged in patients with acute liver failure, evidence of infection, or clinical decompensation.
   c. **Renal failure** is an ominous complication.
      (1) **Hepatorenal syndrome** should be considered in patients with severe liver disease, declining renal function, and prerenal physiology (i.e., a low urinary sodium level). Hepatorenal syndrome is distinguished from hypovolemia by the patient's failure to respond to a fluid challenge. Hepatorenal syndrome must also be distinguished (on the basis of clinical criteria) from other causes of kidney failure that result in prerenal physiology (see Chapter 37).
      (2) **Acute tubular necrosis** may also occur.
   d. **Hepatopulmonary syndrome.** Intrapulmonary shunting of blood leads to hypoxia. Typically, patients are more symptomatic when they are sitting up, as opposed to lying down (i.e., they are platypneic), because sitting up increases blood flow to the lower lobes where more shunting is known to occur. This complication is most commonly seen in chronic liver failure.

B. Chronic liver failure. Clinical manifestations of chronic liver failure are summarized in Table 34-1.

III. CAUSES OF LIVER FAILURE

A. Acute liver failure

1. **Infection**
   a. **Viral hepatitis** is one of the most common causes of acute liver failure (along with acetaminophen toxicity).
      (1) **Hepatitis A** is a rare cause of fulminant hepatitis and never produces chronic disease.
      (2) **Hepatitis B** causes fulminant liver failure in approximately 1% of infected patients.
      (3) **Hepatitis C** usually causes only chronic disease but at a high rate (>70%).
      (4) **Hepatitis D** causes coinfection or superinfection only in the presence of hepatitis B surface antigen (HBsAg) and may account for more than 50% of cases of fulminant disease caused by hepatitis B.
      (5) **Hepatitis E** is endemic in Mexico and parts of Asia; the mortality rate is high among pregnant women.
      (6) **Epstein-Barr virus, cytomegalovirus (CMV),** and **herpesvirus** occasionally cause acute liver failure. Liver failure from these infections is more common in immunocompromised patients.
2. **Drugs and toxins**
   a. **Drugs**
      (1) **Direct hepatotoxicity**
         (a) **Acetaminophen overdose.** Alcoholics and malnourished patients have a higher risk of hepatotoxicity as a result of acetaminophen overdose. At least 50% of cases with acetaminophen hepatotoxicity are not related to overdose attempts but are therapeutic misadventures.

Remember the "**rule of 140s**" when confronted with the possibility of acetaminophen overdose: the approximate toxic dose is 140 mg/kg, a blood level that exceeds 140 μg/ml 4 hours after ingestion may be toxic, and the first dose of acetylcysteine (the antidote) is 140 mg/kg orally or by nasogastric tube (often followed by 70 mg/kg every 4 hours for 17 doses).

         (b) **Heavy metals, phosphorus, vitamin A, valproic acid,** and **tetracyclines** may also be directly hepatotoxic.
      (2) **Idiosyncratic reactions** may also result in acute liver failure. **Isoniazid, halothane, phenytoin,** and **sulfonamides** are some examples of drugs that can cause idiosyncratic hepatotoxicity.

b. **Toxins**. *Amanita phalloides* (the death-cap mushroom) and **carbon tetrachloride** (found in industrial cleaning solvents) can both produce acute liver failure.

3. **Vascular abnormalities**
   a. **Inadequate arterial supply,** as a result of cardiac pathology (e.g., cardiac arrest, myocardial infarction, cardiomyopathy), infiltrating malignancies, or sepsis, may cause liver failure.
   b. **Venous obstruction**
      (1) **Veno-occlusive disease.** Intrahepatic obstruction of the hepatic venules may be associated with bone marrow transplantation, chemotherapy, or oral contraceptive use.
      (2) **Inferior vena cava obstruction** or **hepatic vein obstruction** (i.e., **Budd-Chiari syndrome**) often results from thrombosis associated with a myeloproliferative disorder or hypercoagulable state or from direct tumor invasion.
4. **Inherited metabolic disorders. Wilson's disease** usually presents in younger patients (20–40 years of age) and may result in acute or chronic liver failure.
5. **Miscellaneous causes**
   a. **Pregnancy.** Both acute **fatty liver** and the **HELLP** (**H**emolysis, **E**levated **L**iver enzymes, **L**ow **P**latelets) **syndrome** may complicate pregnancy.
   b. **Reye's syndrome.** Children younger than 15 years may develop Reye's syndrome, which is usually associated with viral illness and concomitant salicylate use.

B. Chronic liver failure

1. **Infections,** including **viral hepatitis** (primarily hepatitis B and C), **schistosomiasis,** and **toxoplasmosis**
2. **Drugs** and **toxins. Alcoholism** accounts for almost 50% of all cases of chronic liver failure.
3. **Vascular abnormalities** (e.g., as a result of cardiac failure, tumors, or venous obstruction)
4. **Inherited metabolic disorders,** including Wilson's disease, hemochromatosis, α_1-antitrypsin deficiency, and glycogen storage disease
5. **Miscellaneous causes**
   a. **Primary biliary cirrhosis.** Women between the ages of 40 and 60 years are most often affected. Pruritus, significantly elevated serum alkaline phosphatase, and the presence of antimitochondrial antibody are typical features (antimitochondrial antibody is noted in 95% of cases).
   b. **Secondary biliary cirrhosis** may result from stones or strictures causing chronic biliary tract obstruction.

c. **Autoimmune hepatitis** is most common in young women. Patients may have other manifestations of autoimmunity; antinuclear and anti–smooth muscle antibodies are found in 20%–40% and 60%–80% of patients, respectively.

IV. APPROACH TO THE PATIENT

A. Patient history. A thorough history is critical if a drug or toxin exposure is thought to be the cause of the liver failure. Vascular disorders may also be suggested by the history (e.g., right upper quadrant pain may imply Budd-Chiari syndrome; weight loss may suggest an intra-abdominal malignancy). Patients need to be specifically asked about over-the-counter and alternative medications.

B. Laboratory tests

1. **General tests.** The following tests are usually performed to evaluate liver function and screen for associated metabolic or hematologic derangements and complications (e.g., bleeding, infection, or renal failure):
   a. Complete blood count (CBC) with differential and platelets
   b. Electrolyte panel with blood urea nitrogen (BUN), creatinine, and glucose levels
   c. Evaluation of PT and PTT
   d. Liver tests [i.e., aspartate aminotransferase (AST), alanine aminotransferase (ALT), alkaline phosphatase, total bilirubin]
2. **Specific tests** can be used to help determine the etiology.
   a. **Hepatitis serologies,** including hepatitis A and C antibodies, HBsAg, and hepatitis B surface and core antibodies are often ordered.
   b. **Acetaminophen level.** An acetaminophen level should be obtained in all patients with signs of acute liver failure. A **salicylate level** and **toxicology screen** are also commonly performed.
   c. **Serum ceruloplasmin.** Wilson's disease should be considered in patients younger than 50 years who have acute or chronic liver failure. A low serum ceruloplasmin level is a sign of Wilson's disease; other findings include a high urinary copper level or the presence of Kayser-Fleischer rings on slit-lamp examination.
   d. **Transferrin saturation** and **ferritin levels** are high in patients with hemochromatosis, a cause of chronic liver failure. These levels may be artificially elevated in acute liver injury; they respond as acute-phase reactants.
   e. **α_1-Antitrypsin level.** Deficiency may result in chronic liver failure.

f. **Antibody tests.** Antinuclear, anti–smooth muscle, and antimitochondrial antibodies may be studied to evaluate the possibility of autoimmune hepatitis or primary biliary cirrhosis.

C. Liver biopsy or **imaging studies** may be performed when the diagnosis is still in question.

V. TREATMENT

A. Identify and treat any treatable causes

1. **Acute liver failure**
   a. **Acetaminophen overdose** can be treated with N-acetylcysteine. Early treatment is desirable, and empiric therapy may be indicated when a toxic dose is suspected. Patients may benefit even when the ingestion occurred as many as 36 hours before therapy.
   b. **Mushroom poisoning** may be treated with penicillin, silybin, or both.
   c. **Pregnancy-related liver failure** is often resolved by delivering the baby.
   d. Patients with **acute hepatitis B** can be treated with antiviral therapy.
2. **Chronic liver failure.** Chronic liver failure is usually not reversible. If administered early in the course of the disease, however, specific treatments may prevent the progression to chronic liver failure. For example:
   a. **Hemochromatosis** may be treated with phlebotomy or deferoxamine chelation therapy.
   b. **Wilson's disease** may be treated with penicillamine chelation therapy.
   c. **Autoimmune hepatitis** is extremely sensitive to steroid therapy.
   d. **Chronic hepatitis B** or **C** may be treated with antiviral therapy.

B. **Prevent** or **treat complications.**

1. **Infections,** such as **spontaneous bacterial peritonitis (SBP),** must be treated aggressively. **A third-generation cephalosporin** is often the initial therapy and is administered for at least 5 days. Following therapy, **norfloxacin** may be used to decrease the rate of recurrent spontaneous bacterial peritonitis. Every attempt should be made to avoid potentially nephrotoxic drugs such as gentamicin in patients with liver disease.
2. **Hemorrhage**
   a. Patients who are not actively bleeding are usually administered **vitamin K** subcutaneously in case vitamin deficiency is partially responsible for the coagulopathy.
   b. **Fresh frozen plasma** and blood products may be required for patients with active bleeding (see Chapter 66).

3. **Bleeding esophageal varices**
   a. **Treatment**
      (1) **Pharmacologic treatment** involves the intravenous administration of **octreotide.**
      (2) **Band ligation** and **injection sclerotherapy via upper endoscopy** are effective procedures but may not be technically feasible in all patients.
      (3) **Transjugular intrahepatic portosystemic shunting (TIPS)** or **surgical shunting** may be used for refractory bleeding.
   b. **Prophylaxis. Propranolol** (20–80 mg orally twice daily) is often given to patients who are stable after a variceal bleed (usually days later) and to those with very large varices.
4. **Ascites** and **edema** are often treated with a **sodium-restricted diet** and **diuretics.**
   a. The primary method of treating ascites in patients with chronic liver disease is sodium restriction. Patients should ingest less than 2 g of sodium per day. Fluid does not need to be limited except in patients with significant hyponatremia. (Up to 80% of patients with ascites can be completely controlled with sodium restriction alone.)
   b. **Spironolactone.** The initial dose is often 100 mg orally once daily; this amount is increased by 100 mg/day every few days while following the serum and urine electrolytes. Spironolactone will take several days before maximal benefit occurs.
   c. **Furosemide** may also be added to the regimen to increase diuresis. Careful monitoring of volume status and electrolytes is always required.
   d. **Large-volume paracentesis** is often necessary for patients with massive ascites whose conditions are refractory to medical therapy or who are symptomatic (80% of patients with ascites can be controlled with sodium restriction and diuretics alone). Intravenous albumin is often given just before large-volume paracentesis is performed to maintain the intravascular volume (especially in patients without peripheral edema).
   e. **TIPS** is being increasingly used for patients with refractory ascites.
5. **Hepatic encephalopathy** may be precipitated by infections, overly aggressive diuresis, electrolyte abnormalities, gastrointestinal bleeding, or drugs (e.g., sedative-hypnotics, narcotics). The reason for increased symptoms must always be sought. Management usually involves identifying and treating precipitating factors and adminis-

tering **lactulose** (often 30 ml orally three times daily or by nasogastric tube, titrated to maintain three loose stools per day). In patients with acute liver failure, cerebral edema may occur and can be treated with **mannitol** (usually 0.3–0.4 g/kg body weight) or hyperventilation. Lactulose is typically not given in acute liver failure.

Intracerebral hemorrhage is always a possibility in patients with coagulopathy and altered mental status and may require further evaluation [e.g., with computed tomography (CT)].

6. **Hepatorenal syndrome.** Midodrine, low-dose dopamine, and calcium channel blockers are still sometimes tried. Patients should be urgently evaluated for liver transplantation.
7. **Metabolic derangements**
   a. **Hypoglycemia** may require intravenous administration of a 10% glucose solution.
   b. **Hypokalemia** and **hypophosphatemia** may require electrolyte replacement.
   c. **Hyponatremia** may require free water restriction.

C. Consider the appropriateness of liver transplantation. Liver transplantation may be performed in patients with acute or chronic liver failure.

1. In the acute setting, liver transplantation is usually indicated when a variety of prognostic factors (e.g., PT, grade of encephalopathy, etiology) suggest a poor chance of survival without it. Because safe transport to a specialized facility is easier when patients have low-grade encephalopathy, a liver transplant should be considered as soon as possible following a diagnosis of acute liver failure.
2. Patients with chronic liver disease should be evaluated for liver transplantation when they first develop evidence of decompensated cirrhosis or hepatocellular carcinoma.
3. The 5-year survival rate after liver transplantation for cirrhosis is greater than 75%.

REFERENCES

Fontana RJ. Acute liver failure including acetaminophen overdose. Med Clin North Am 2008;92(4)761–794, viii.

Parikh S, Hyman D. Hepatocellular cancer: a guide for the internist. Am J Med 2007;120(3):194–202.

Schuppan D, Afdhal NH. Liver cirrhosis. Lancet 2008;371(9615):838–851.

PART V
RENAL/ACID-BASE

Overview of Nephrology

36

I. INTRODUCTION

A. In nephrology, there are many syndromes, each with a set of causative diseases. Specific diseases are often capable of causing more than one syndrome.

In medicine, a "syndrome" refers to a set of clinical manifestations occurring together.

TABLE 36-1

OVERVIEW OF RENAL SYNDROMES

Syndrome	Key to the Diagnosis	Examples of Causes
Acute kidney injury	Classify the cause as prerenal, postrenal, or intrarenal	Dehydration, shock, toxins, interstitial nephritis, obstruction due to enlarged prostate, RPGN, HUS/TTP
Nephrotic syndrome	Classify the cause as renal or systemic	Primary renal diseases (e.g., membranous, focal segmental glomerulosclerosis, minimal change disease); systemic diseases (e.g., diabetes, amyloid, SLE)
Nephritic syndrome	Classify the cause as pauci-immune (ANCA), anti-GBM, or immune complex related	Wegener's disease, Goodpasture syndrome's, various infections (e.g., poststreptococcal and hepatitis C), SLE, IgA, MPGN
Renal tubular acidosis	Classify the acidosis as type 1, 2, or 4	Amyloid, multiple myeloma, drugs (e.g., amphotericin), diabetes, Addison's disease

ANCA = antineutrophil cytoplasmic antibodies; *GBM* = glomerular basement membrane; *HUS/TTP* = hemolytic-uremic syndrome/thrombotic thrombocytopenic purpura; *IgA* = immunoglobulin A; *MPGN* = membranoproliferative glomerulonephritis; *RPGN* = rapidly progressive glomerulonephritis; *SLE* = systemic lupus erythematosus.

B. Know the clinical manifestations and lab data that correspond to each renal syndrome and then think of the diseases that could cause that syndrome. The differential diagnoses for most of the renal syndromes are easy to remember; just match the diagnosis with the patient's complaints and data, and you will be off to the right start.

II. RENAL SYNDROMES. The renal syndromes are discussed in more detail in Chapters 37–40. Table 36-1 provides an overview.

37 Acute Kidney Injury

I. INTRODUCTION

A. Definition. Acute kidney injury is defined as a rapid decrease in glomerular filtration that results in abnormal fluid and electrolyte balance and inappropriate nitrogen waste accumulation (azotemia). Because nitrogen accumulation is initially asymptomatic, the diagnosis is commonly made when the serum creatinine level rises abruptly (e.g., by 0.5 mg/dl or more) during a 24- to 48-hour period.

Although serum creatinine (SCr) is almost solely filtered by the glomerulus and therefore provides a good estimate of the glomerular filtration rate (GFR), it is slightly secreted by the tubules. Some drugs (e.g., cimetidine) can block this secretion, raise the SCr, and cause an underestimation of the actual GFR and, therefore, renal function.

B. Epidemiology. Approximately 5% of all hospitalized patients are diagnosed with acute kidney injury; the incidence can be as high as 30% in the intensive care unit (ICU).

C. Clinical manifestations. Symptoms of acute kidney injury are usually present when the **blood urea nitrogen (BUN) exceeds 100 mg/dl,** but may occur at lesser values. Clinical manifestations include **cardiovascular complications** (e.g., arrhythmias, volume overload, pericarditis); **neurologic abnormalities** (e.g., altered mental status, seizures); or **gastrointestinal complications** (e.g., bleeding, nausea, vomiting).

II. CAUSES OF ACUTE KIDNEY INJURY.

The causes of acute kidney injury can be conveniently classified as **prerenal, intrinsic renal,** or **postrenal** (Figure 37-1).

A. Prerenal causes account for more than half of acute kidney injury cases. Prerenal is actually preglomerular. Any disease state that results in a **decrease in blood flow to the glomerulus** will result in decreased glomerular filtration and, consequently, an elevated serum creatinine level. One way to remember the prerenal causes of acute kidney injury is to begin with the

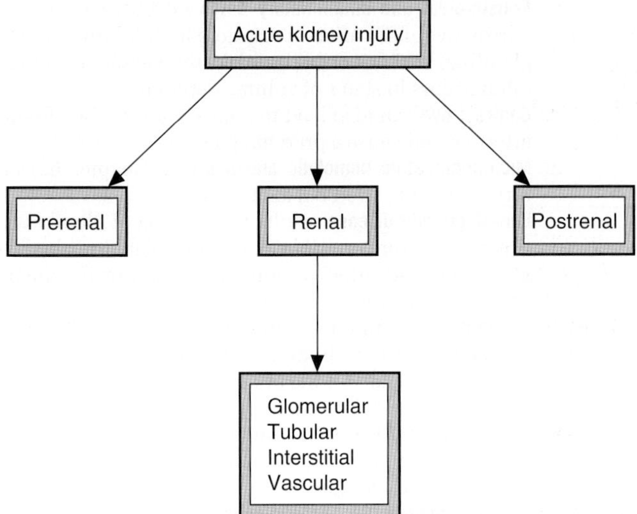

Figure 37-1 The causes of acute kidney injury can be categorized as prerenal, intrinsic renal, or postrenal.

filling of the left ventricle and work your way distally toward the glomerulus.

1. **Decreased filling of the left ventricle** results in decreased cardiac output and, therefore, decreased flow to the glomerulus. **Hypovolemia** is the most common cause, but right ventricular failure and mitral stenosis can also result in poor left ventricular filling and subsequent prerenal azotemia.
2. **Decreased left ventricular function** results in decreased cardiac output even with normal or elevated left ventricular filling.
3. **Aortic stenosis.** Even with normal left ventricular filling and function, critical aortic stenosis can block forward flow to the kidney.
4. **Renal artery stenosis** from atherosclerotic disease or fibromuscular dysplasia decreases flow to the glomerulus. (Fibromuscular dysplasia, most often seen in young women, is much less common than atherosclerotic disease.)
5. **Narrowing of the afferent arteriole** from vasoconstriction, inflammation, or thrombosis can result in prerenal azotemia.
   a. **Sepsis** can lead to constriction of the afferent arteriole via inflammatory mediators.

b. **Nonsteroidal anti-inflammatory drugs (NSAIDs)** can lead to narrowing of the afferent arteriole by inhibiting prostaglandins, which normally dilate the vessel. This most often occurs in states of volume depletion.
c. **Contrast dye** can also lead to constriction of the afferent arteriole and cause a prerenal picture.
d. **Microangiopathic hemolytic anemias** (see Chapter 62) are rare causes of a prerenal azotemia.
e. **End-stage liver disease** results in shunting of blood away from the afferent arteriole (e.g., from splanchnic bed vasodilation and arteriovenous malformations), causing prerenal azotemia.

B. Postrenal causes account for approximately 5%–10% of all cases of acute kidney injury. Because one kidney can adequately compensate for the other, injury will only occur if both kidneys are not functioning properly.

1. **Bladder neck obstruction** is the most common postrenal cause of acute renal failure. Common causes of bladder neck obstruction include:
   a. **Prostatic hypertrophy** or **malignancy**
   b. **Neurologic disorders** (e.g., neuropathy)
   c. **Anticholinergic medications**
2. **Ureteral obstruction**
   a. **Unilateral ureteral obstruction** (e.g., from stones, blood clots, or pus) can result in acute kidney injury in a patient with only one kidney.
   b. **Bilateral ureteral obstruction** may result from retroperitoneal fibrosis, malignancy, or lymphadenopathy.

C. Intrinsic renal causes. Think of the causes as anatomic components of a kidney (i.e., glomeruli, tubules, interstitium, vessels).

1. **Acute glomerulonephritis** affects the glomeruli. The many causes of acute glomerulonephritis are discussed in Chapter 39 II.
2. **Acute tubular necrosis (ATN)** affects the tubules.
   a. **Ischemia** and **shock** from all causes, but particularly septic shock, can lead to ATN.
   b. **Contrast dye agents** used for radiographic studies are toxic to the tubules, but most commonly result in kidney injury in patients with underlying chronic kidney disease (particularly diabetic patients).
   c. **Endogenous pigments** (e.g., **myoglobin, hemoglobin**), **crystals,** and **proteins.** Myoglobinuria (from rhabdomyolysis) or hemoglobinuria (from intravascular hemolysis), uric acid deposition (from tumor lysis), and Bence Jones proteins (from multiple myeloma) can all cause tubule injury and result in ATN.

d. **Medications** (e.g., aminoglycosides) and **toxins** (e.g., heavy metals) can be directly nephrotoxic.
e. **Surgery** or **trauma.** Ischemic injury (as a result of hypotension and inflammatory mediators), tissue destruction (from myoglobin), or a combination of the two can lead to ATN.

The most common causes of ATN are ischemia, contrast dye agents, nephrotoxic drugs, and sepsis.

3. **Acute interstitial nephritis** affects the interstitium. **Medications** (e.g., β-lactam antibiotics, sulfa antibiotics, furosemide, thiazide diuretics, NSAIDs) are the most common causes of acute interstitial nephritis.
4. **Vasculitis** and **microangiopathic hemolytic anemias** affect the blood vessels (see Chapters 62 and 76). Do not be confused by the fact that many of the vasculitides are listed as causes of glomerulonephritis (i.e., inflammation of the glomerulus); because the glomerulus contains a capillary bed, small vessel vasculitis can result in glomerulonephritis.

III. APPROACH TO THE PATIENT. Using data gleaned from the patient history, physical examination, and basic laboratory tests and procedures, the cause is classified as primarily prerenal, postrenal, or renal.

The same disorder may cause more than one type of acute kidney injury.

A. Obtain a patient history.

1. **Prerenal.** A history of congestive heart failure (CHF), dehydration, or new or increased use of diuretics or NSAIDs often signifies a prerenal etiology.
2. **Postrenal.** A history of benign prostatic hypertrophy, kidney stones, nephrectomy, anticholinergic medication use, or a retroperitoneal malignancy may alert you to postrenal causes.
3. **Renal**
   a. **Glomerulonephritis.** The causes of glomerulonephritis can help guide your questions regarding relevant symptoms. For example, a recent sore throat or skin infection may suggest postinfectious glomerulonephritis.

b. **ATN** or **acute interstitial nephritis.** The medication history (including use of over-the-counter NSAIDs) may suggest a tubular or interstitial etiology.

c. **Vasculitis.** Ask about rashes, arthralgias, and fevers (see Chapter 76).

B. Perform a physical examination. Always assess the vital signs, oxygen saturation, and urine output.

1. **Blood pressure. Hypotension** can denote a prerenal cause and sustained hypotension can lead to ATN; **hypertension** may be a sign of glomerulonephritis. Additional evaluation and treatment are aimed at the underlying etiology.
2. **Temperature. High** or **low temperatures** can indicate sepsis (although interstitial nephritis, glomerulonephritis, or vasculitis may also be associated with temperature abnormalities).
3. **Oxygen saturation.** Hypoxemia may signal impending pulmonary edema (e.g., from kidney injury with volume overload).
4. **Urine output measurements** will help you classify the acute kidney injury (AKI) as **oliguric (<400 ml/day)** or **nonoliguric (>400 ml/day).** Nonoliguric AKI is associated with lower mortality and dialysis rates. In patients with oliguric ATN, increased urine output often heralds the return of renal function.
5. **Heart and lung examination.** A complete physical examination is important, with special attention given to the heart and lungs. Heart and lung examination may provide information about the cause of the acute kidney injury (e.g., critical aortic stenosis, severe left ventricular dysfunction) and also permits assessment of some of the consequences (e.g., volume overload, pericarditis).
6. **Abdomen.** Auscultation of renal bruits may indicate renal artery obstruction. Palpation of increased bladder size and tenderness often signify postrenal obstruction.
7. **Skin.** Rashes such as a butterfly facial rash as seen in lupus or palpable purpura as seen in Henoch-Schönlein purpura can be seen in patients with glomerulonephritis. Dry skin with tenting could be a sign of volume depletion.
8. **Neurologic exam.** Asterixis can be a sign of uremia. Coma or seizures can result from advanced uremia.

C. Rule out obstruction.

1. **Postvoid residual (PVR).** A PVR is often performed before laboratory tests because if obstruction is the cause, a diagnosis can be made quickly and an extensive workup is avoided. This procedure is especially useful in older men, in whom obstruction from benign prostatic hypertrophy is not uncommon. The PVR is measured by catheterization

or portable ultrasonographic bladder scan after the patient has "emptied" the bladder.

a. If the PVR is greater than 200–250 ml, obstruction is diagnosed, and a Foley catheter should be left in place.
b. If the patient already has an indwelling catheter, make sure to flush the catheter to evaluate obstruction by encrusted materials or blood clots.

2. **Ultrasound.** The PVR does not help you evaluate the upper urinary tract. In patients with one kidney or suspected bilateral obstruction, renal ultrasound should be performed early in the workup. Occasionally, a non-contrast computed tomography (CT) scan will be performed first depending on the patient's history; CT can also visualize the lower urinary tract.

D. Perform laboratory studies to help determine the diagnosis and the consequences of the kidney injury.

1. **Complete blood count (CBC) with platelets.** The white blood cell (WBC) count helps assess the possibility of infection or interstitial nephritis. Anemia may indicate more chronic kidney disease or bleeding from uremia.
2. **Electrolyte panel** (including Na^+, K^+, Cl^-, HCO_3^-, Ca^{2+}, PO_4^{3-}, Mg^{2+}, and glucose). Common electrolyte or metabolic derangements include hyponatremia, hyperkalemia, hypocalcemia, hyperphosphatemia, and hypermagnesemia as well as a mixed anion and nonanion gap acidosis.
3. **Blood urea nitrogen:creatinine (BUN:Cr) ratio.** A normal BUN:Cr ratio is 10. In prerenal states, urea gets passively reabsorbed along with sodium and water from the proximal tubules while creatinine does not; therefore, a BUN:Cr ratio higher than 10 (and certainly one >20) supports a prerenal diagnosis.
4. **Urinalysis.** A urinalysis is an essential part of the evaluation because an active urinary sediment implies an intraparenchymal cause of kidney disease.
   a. **Red blood cell (RBC) casts** or **dysmorphic red cells** often imply glomerulonephritis.
   b. **WBC casts** are usually a sign of infection (i.e., pyelonephritis) or inflammation (i.e., interstitial nephritis).
   c. **Coarse granular** or **"muddy" brown casts** may signify ATN.
5. **Urine electrolytes** can be a useful diagnostic test in patients with acute kidney injury.
   a. **Urinary sodium** and **chloride** can be used to help delineate a prerenal cause from an intrarenal one. Values less than 20 mEq/L imply a prerenal etiology; values lower than 10 mEq/L are even more specific.

(1) Early obstruction and contrast dye nephropathy can also result in a low urine sodium or chloride level.

(2) With a concomitant metabolic alkalosis, the urinary chloride is a better indicator of a prerenal state because sodium may be excreted with bicarbonate to maintain electroneutrality. In this situation, the urinary sodium may be falsely increased, although prerenal physiology is present.

b. **Fractional excretion of sodium (FENa).** FENa is another way of diagnosing prerenal physiology and can also help evaluate tubulointerstitial dysfunction when a patient is oliguric. To calculate the FENa, remember "UP ... UP" with "sodium over creatinine":

$$\text{FENa} = \frac{\text{Urine Na}^+/\mathbf{P}\text{lasma Na}^+}{\text{Urine Cr}/\mathbf{P}\text{lasma Cr}} \times 100\%$$

(1) A value less than 1% usually signifies prerenal physiology, whereas one greater than 1%–2% usually indicates tubulointerstitial disease (because there is a defect in sodium reabsorption).

Glomerulonephritis without tubular dysfunction will not produce an abnormal FENa, because sodium reabsorption is primarily a renal tubular function.

(2) When a patient is not oliguric, however, the FENa could be high or low in the setting of ATN depending on what intravenous or oral fluid is being administered to the patient. (Oliguria is defined as <30 ml of urine production per hour.) Therefore, the FENa is only useful in an oliguric patient.

Patients receiving diuretics may have an increased FENa despite being prerenal; on the other hand, a patient taking diuretics with a FENa less than 1% usually can be assumed to be severely volume depleted.

c. **Fractional excretion of urea (FEUrea).** When a patient is using diuretics, the urine sodium may not accurately reflect renal tubular function. The FEUrea may be a more accurate tool than FENa in such cases to distinguish between prerenal AKI and ATN.

$$\text{FEUrea} = \frac{\text{Urine Urea}/\mathbf{BUN}}{\text{Urine Cr}/\mathbf{P}\text{lasma Cr}} \times 100\%$$

The FEUrea should not be used alone, but in conjunction with clinical history, exam, and laboratory tests. A FEUrea less than or equal to 35% is consistent with a prerenal state. On the other hand, a FEUrea above this level (typically >50%) is consistent with ATN.

6. **Creatine kinase.** Evaluation of the creatine kinase level is helpful **if the urine dipstick is positive for blood, but no or few RBCs** are noted microscopically. This implies that urinary myoglobin (from **rhabdomyolysis**) or hemoglobin (from **intravascular hemolysis**) is present. **Evaluate the possibility of rhabdomyolysis first;** then consider working up intravascular hemolysis. Creatine kinase levels **greater than 6000 IU** (and often more than 15,000 IU) are usually needed to cause tubular necrosis; however, creatine kinase levels may be normal if the rhabdomyolysis and ATN occurred a few days before the workup.
7. **Ancillary tests.** If glomerulonephritis or vasculitis is suspected or diagnosed, additional tests need to be ordered (see Chapters 39 and 76). Liver function tests are ordered when the hepatorenal syndrome is suspected, but the clinical diagnosis is usually obvious.

E. Perform additional diagnostic studies if the diagnosis remains unclear.

1. **Renal ultrasound.** In addition to ruling out **obstruction,** renal ultrasound helps to **distinguish acute from chronic kidney disease.**
   a. The kidneys are usually normal in size in patients with acute kidney injury.
   b. They are **usually small in patients with chronic kidney disease.** It is easy to remember the chronic diseases that lead to enlarged kidneys because the SHAPE is large:

MNEMONIC

Chronic Diseases That Lead to Enlarged Kidneys ("SHAPE")

Scleroderma
HIV (human immunodeficiency virus)–associated nephropathy
Amyloidosis/infiltrative diseases
Polycystic kidney disease
Endocrinopathy (i.e., diabetes mellitus)

2. **Renal biopsy** is usually unnecessary but is indicated for unresolving acute renal failure of unknown etiology or to define the need for potentially toxic treatment of glomerulonephritis.

IV. TREATMENT

A. Disease specific

1. **Prerenal causes**
   a. **Fluids** are usually indicated because hypovolemia is the predominant prerenal cause of acute kidney injury.

Remember—if the cause of acute kidney injury is cardiac in origin (e.g., CHF, critical aortic stenosis), giving fluids may not be appropriate. Consider these possibilities before giving fluids!

      (1) Administration of **small, defined boluses** (e.g., 250 ml of 0.9% saline) can prevent volume overload.
      (2) **Reevaluate the patient frequently.** The goal urine output is at least 30 ml/hr. Boluses can be continued with that goal in mind as long as the oxygen saturation is maintained and the lungs remain clear (i.e., there is no evidence of pulmonary edema).

   b. **Other treatments** tailored to the specific etiology may also be necessary (e.g., discontinuing medications, administering antibiotics for sepsis).

2. **Postrenal causes**
   a. **Catheterization.** A Foley catheter should be placed, if one has not been placed already.
      (1) **Clamp the catheter** if more than 750 ml drains acutely to prevent the patient from becoming hypotensive. If, after 30 minutes, no hypotension develops, you can allow more drainage while monitoring blood pressure.
      (2) **Observe for postobstructive diuresis.** If the blockage has been present for a few days, a postobstructive diuresis often ensues. This may result from urea accumulation with an osmotic diuresis as well as salt accumulation with a physiologic diuresis. Although this diuresis is partly a physiologic phenomenon, transient tubular dysfunction can contribute to severe volume depletion unless fluids are replaced.

(a) **Fluid replacement.** It is customary to give back approximately half of the urinary losses with half normal saline. Giving normal saline will only exacerbate the problem by adding to the volume overload and leading to a solute diuresis.

(b) **Electrolyte replacement.** Depletion of electrolytes, particularly potassium and magnesium, occurs frequently.

b. **Percutaneous drainage** through a percutaneous nephrostomy tube may be needed in cases of upper tract obstruction.

3. **Renal causes** are treated based on the specific pathology, but there are general treatments that are common to all.

a. **General measures**

(1) **Fluid restriction.** Fluids may need to be restricted to 1–1.5 L/day. Volume status should be monitored using daily weights and input/output measurements.

(2) **Diet.** The diet should be low salt, low potassium, and low phosphorous.

(3) **Adjust medication dosages.** The dosages of medications that are excreted renally should be adjusted. Magnesium- and phosphorous-containing medications should be avoided.

b. **Specific measures**

(1) **Glomerulonephritis.** Treatment is discussed in Chapter 39.

(2) **ATN**

(a) **Fluids** may help prevent further ischemic insults and oliguric states, and may also dilute the effects of certain toxins (i.e., myoglobin, contrast dye).

(b) **Furosemide** in high doses is sometimes successful in converting oliguric to nonoliguric renal failure, but this has not been shown to change patient outcomes. Also, maintaining volume status and appropriate renal blood flow is critical, and the patient should never be "on the dry side."

(c) **Mannitol** is an antioxidant and osmotic diuretic. It can be used for patients with rhabdomyolysis but may precipitate CHF, and should be avoided in susceptible patients.

(3) **Acute interstitial nephritis** is usually treated by discontinuing offending medications and administering fluids as tolerated. A short course of corticosteroids

(1 mg/kg/day for 1–2 weeks with a rapid taper) is occasionally used.

(4) **Vasculitis.** Treatment is discussed in Chapter 76.

MNEMONIC **Indications for Acute Dialysis ("AEIOU")**

Acidosis
Electrolytes (e.g., hyperkalemia, hypercalcemia)
Intoxication
Overload
Uremia

B. Acute dialysis. The following indications are usually applicable regardless of the cause of kidney disease.

1. **Acidosis.** Dialysis is usually necessary when the patient is experiencing complications of a metabolic acidosis (e.g., arrhythmias, left ventricular dysfunction) or if the serum pH starts to fall below 7.2. Sodium bicarbonate is sometimes used as a temporizing measure until dialysis can be initiated.
2. **Severe, refractory hyperkalemia** (usually >6.5–7 mEq/L) or hyperkalemia with persistent electrocardiogram (ECG) changes is an indication for acute dialysis. Temporizing measures include the following: (1) intravenous calcium, which acts as a cardiac membrane stabilizer; and (2) sodium bicarbonate, albuterol nebulizers, and/or insulin and glucose, which cause potassium to move intracellularly. Sodium polystyrene sulfonate is an exchange resin that can be given orally or rectally to decrease potassium levels over several hours. However, as potassium is bound, sodium is released; thus, caution should be used when giving this medication to patients with CHF.
3. **Intoxication.** Dialysis may be necessary when acute kidney injury results from a dialyzable, toxic ingestion (e.g., salicylates, ethylene glycol).
4. **Overload.** Volume overload that is refractory to diuretics is an indication for dialysis. Temporizing measures include nitrates and furosemide (which cause venodilation and may therefore decrease pulmonary edema).
5. **Uremia.** Altered mental status, seizures, pericarditis, intractable nausea and vomiting, and uncontrolled bleeding from platelet dysfunction are all indications for acute dialysis.

REFERENCES

Kellum JA. Acute kidney injury. Crit Care Med 2008;36(4 Suppl):S141–145.
Palevsky PM. Indications and timing of renal replacement therapy in acute kidney injury. Crit Care Med 2008;36(4 Suppl):S224–228.
Pannu N, Nadim MK. An overview of drug-induced acute kidney injury. Crit Care Med 2008;36(4 Suppl):S216–223.
Warnock DG. Towards a definition and classification of acute kidney injury. J Am Soc Nephrol 2005;16(11):3149–3150.
Weisbord SD. Iodinated contrast media and the kidney. Rev Cardiovasc Med 2008;9(Suppl 1):S14–23.

38 Nephrotic Syndrome

I. INTRODUCTION

A. Pathophysiologic mechanism. Nephrotic syndrome results from increased glomerular permeability to serum proteins via changes in either charge-selective or size-selective properties of the glomerular basement membrane.

B. Clinical manifestations of nephrotic syndrome. Onset is insidious, and renal function as measured by glomerular filtration rate (GFR) may be normal. Clinical findings include proteinuria, low serum albumin, hyperlipidemia, and edema. Glomerular hematuria occurs infrequently but is seen with some diseases that traditionally cause nephrotic syndrome (e.g., diabetic nephropathy). (These patients may look "PALE" because they are excreting so much protein—this is not really so, but it makes the following mnemonic easier to remember.)

MNEMONIC **Characteristics of the Nephrotic Syndrome ("PALE")**

Proteinuria (>3.0–3.5 g/24 hours)
Albumin (<3.0 g/dl)
Lipids (often elevated)
Edema

II. CAUSES OF NEPHROTIC SYNDROME

A. Primary glomerular disease. Among patients without diabetes, nephrotic syndrome is caused by primary glomerular disease in the vast majority. Specific etiologies change frequency by age (i.e., the frequency of minimal change disease decreases while that of membranous nephropathy increases with age). Primary glomerular diseases associated with nephrotic syndrome in adults include:

1. **Membranous nephropathy**
2. **Minimal change disease**
3. **Focal segmental glomerulosclerosis (FSGS)**
4. **Membranoproliferative glomerulonephritis**
5. **Rapidly progressive glomerulonephritis**

B. Secondary causes. Commonly, nephrotic syndrome occurs secondary to systemic disease. Although there is a long list of possible secondary causes, most can be remembered easily using the mnemonic, "THIS LAD HAS nephrotic syndrome."

MNEMONIC **Secondary Causes of Nephrotic Syndrome ("THIS LAD HAS nephrotic syndrome")**

Tumors
Heroin, **H**eavy metals, and other toxins/medications [nonsteroidal anti-inflammatory drugs (NSAIDs)]
Infection
  Hepatitis B and C
  AIDS (acquired immunodeficiency syndrome)
  Subacute bacterial endocarditis, **S**yphilis, **S**chistosomiasis
Systemic disorders
  Lupus
  Amyloid
  Diabetes

Among patients with a systemic cause of their nephrotic syndrome, diabetic nephropathy is the most common cause.

1. **Tumors.** Many cancers can cause nephrotic syndrome. In elderly patients with unexplained nephrotic syndrome, an underlying malignancy is a real concern. Both hematologic malignancies (e.g., lymphoma, leukemia, multiple myeloma) and solid tumors (e.g., cancer of the colon, lung, or breast) can cause nephrotic syndrome.
2. **Heroin, heavy metals,** and **toxins/medications.** "Street" heroin, organic gold, mercury, lead, antitoxins, lithium, NSAIDs, and angiotensin-converting enzyme (ACE) inhibitors can cause nephrotic syndrome.
3. **Infections.** There are many infections that can cause nephrotic syndrome; some important ones are **hepatitis B** and **C, AIDS, subacute bacterial endocarditis, syphilis,** and **schistosomiasis.**
4. **Systemic disorders.** Major causes of nephrotic syndrome include **systemic lupus erythematosus (SLE), amyloid,** and **diabetes mellitus.**

The incidence of diabetes mellitus is increasing dramatically in the general U.S. population; thus, diabetic nephropathy is increasing as well (accounts for more than 40% of patients starting hemodialysis).

III. APPROACH TO THE PATIENT. Once it has been determined that a patient has nephrotic syndrome, the search for the underlying cause begins. A thoughtful history and physical examination should be performed, looking for symptoms and signs of diseases listed previously. Depending on the suspected cause, the following laboratory tests and procedures can be useful:

A. **Serum chemistries,** including blood urea nitrogen (BUN), creatinine, glucose, and liver function test measurements
B. **Complete blood count (CBC)**
C. **Antinuclear antibody (ANA) assays**
D. **Hepatitis serologies**
E. **Rapid plasma reagin (RPR)** or **Venereal Disease Research Laboratory (VDRL) test** for syphilis
F. **Human immunodeficiency virus (HIV) test**
G. **Fat pad** or **rectal biopsy** (to look for amyloidosis)
H. **Blood cultures** (to rule out endocarditis)
I. **Chest radiograph**
J. **Serum and urine protein electrophoresis**
K. **Renal biopsy**
L. **Other routine cancer screening appropriate for age and sex (e.g., colorectal cancer screening, Pap smear, mammogram)**

IV. TREATMENT focuses on the underlying disorder. General management strategies include:

A. **ACE inhibitors** to slow progression of renal disease, to decrease proteinuria, and to treat hypertension
B. Specific **therapy for hyperlipidemia** (e.g., HMG CoA reductase inhibitors)
C. A **diet** low in sodium and saturated fat
D. Strict **treatment of hypertension** with a goal blood pressure of less than 125/75 mm Hg.
E. **Fluid restriction** and **diuretics** (if hyponatremia and/or edema are present)
F. **Protein restriction** (0.6–0.8 g/kg/day) to slow the rate of disease progression is controversial.

V. COMPLICATIONS

A. **Infections.** Patients with nephrotic syndrome are prone to infections due to urinary losses of immunoglobulins and complement.
B. **Thrombosis** (both arterial and venous) can occur with loss of antithrombin III, protein C, and protein S in the urine, but is primarily seen in patients with membranous nephropathy as the cause of their nephrotic syndrome.
C. **Hypovolemia** may be a consequence of overdiuresis or intravascular fluid losses if serum albumin is <2.0g/dl.

D. Wasting results from protein depletion, although monitored protein restriction may be beneficial.

E. Atherosclerosis may result from hyperlipidemia.

REFERENCES

Charlesworth JA, Gracey DM, Pussell BA. Adult nephrotic syndrome: non-specific strategies for treatment. [Review]. Nephrology 2008;13(1):45–50.

Hull RP, Goldsmith DJ. Nephrotic syndrome in adults. [Review]. BMJ 2008;336(7654):1185–1189.

Rapidly Progressive Glomerulonephritis

I. CLINICAL MANIFESTATIONS OF RAPIDLY PROGRESSIVE GLOMERULONEPHRITIS (RPGN). Rapidly progressive glomerulonephritis—one type of glomerulonephritis commonly encountered in the inpatient setting—is characterized by the rapid onset of hematuria, proteinuria (usually <3 g/24 hours), rising creatinine levels, and sodium retention with accompanying hypertension over the course of days to weeks. (Compare with the clinical manifestations of nephrotic syndrome, described in Chapter 38 I B.) The diagnosis of RPGN is based on a characteristic renal biopsy. The prognosis is quite poor unless treatment is initiated early and aggressively.

- **A.** The presence of **red blood cell (RBC) casts** or **dysmorphic RBCs** is usually diagnostic of a glomerulonephritis, which can be chronic or acute. White blood cells (WBCs) or WBC casts may also appear in the urine as a sign of inflammation.
- **B. Hematuria** may be microscopic but is often macroscopic, (Patients complain of dark or "smoky" urine.)
- **C. Edema** usually appears initially in areas of low tissue tension (e.g., the periorbital region or scrotum) but may progress to pleural effusions, lower extremity edema, and ascites.
- **D. Hypertension** results from sodium and water retention.

II. CAUSES OF RPGN

- **A. Immune complex diseases.** Activation of the complement system by immune complexes is usually a cause of low complement (C3 and/or C4 and C1q) levels. This accounts for about half of all cases of RPGN.
  1. **Systemic diseases**
     - a. **Postinfectious glomerulonephritis** (most commonly due to streptococcal infection) is the prototype for acute glomerulonephritis. Nephritis usually occurs 1–2 weeks after a pharyngeal or cutaneous infection with a group A (β-hemolytic) streptococcus. Ninety percent of patients recover fully.
     - b. **Systemic lupus erythematosus (SLE).** Complement levels are decreased in 75%–90% of patients with SLE. Other manifestations of lupus are usually present as well.

c. **Subacute/acute bacterial endocarditis.** More than 90% of patients have low complement levels. Blood cultures confirm the diagnosis.

d. **Hepatitis C.** Most patients have low complement levels with over 90% having serum **cryoglobulins** present; hepatitis C antibody is positive.

e. **"Shunt" nephritis** is usually caused by infection of a ventriculoperitoneal shunt used to relieve hydrocephalus. As with bacterial endocarditis, sustained bacteremia is the cause of glomerulonephritis.

f. **Immunoglobulin A (IgA) nephropathy (Berger's disease),** the most common primary glomerular disease in the United States. This is the one immune complex disease with **normocomplementemia**. IgA nephropathy is the renal lesion seen with Henoch-Schönlein purpura.

(1) IgA nephropathy can present as **gross hematuria** (lasting 2–6 days) that occurs a few days after an upper respiratory tract or gastrointestinal infection (termed synpharyngitic), as opposed to the hematuria that occurs with postinfectious glomerulonephritis (after 7–21 days).

(2) Progression to renal failure occurs in up to one third of patients within 20 years. Up to one third of patients will fully recover renal function. Renal function in the last third typically remains stable.

2. **Renal causes**

a. **Membranoproliferative glomerulonephritis (MPGN)** is a disease of children and young adults, and is relatively rare.

(1) It can be classified as **type I** (the most common type, usually with more subendothelial deposits), **type II** (dense deposit disease, which has a higher incidence of hypocomplementemia), or **type III** (prominent subepithelial and subendothelial deposits).

(2) MPGN can also present as nephrotic syndrome and has a generally progressive clinical course with poor outcome.

B. Pauci–immune diseases. These account for approximately 40% of cases of RPGN. These diseases appear as necrotizing glomerulonephritis on renal biopsy but without immune complexes. These patients are **normocomplementemic**.

1. **Small vessel vasculitis syndromes** (see Chapter 76). **Wegener's granulomatosis, Churg-Strauss syndrome,** and **microscopic polyangiitis** can cause acute glomerulonephritis. Over 90% of these patients will have a positive test for an antineutrophilic cytoplasmic antibody (ANCA).

2. **Primary ANCA-associated glomerulonephritis.** While these patients usually present without systemic manifestations, some progress and develop a systemic vasculitis.

C. Anti–glomerular basement membrane (GBM)–associated diseases. These account for about 10%–15% of cases of RPGN; patients are normocomplemententemic.

1. **Systemic diseases. Goodpasture's syndrome** is characterized by the presence of anti-GBM antibodies, pulmonary hemorrhage, and acute glomerulonephritis. It is caused by serum antibodies that react with glomerular and alveolar basement membranes.
2. **Renal disease.** Anti-GBM–associated disease can also be limited to just the kidneys.

III. APPROACH TO THE PATIENT

A. Make the diagnosis. The most important aspect of making the diagnosis of rapidly progressive glomerulonephritis (after taking the history and performing a physical examination) is to personally examine a **freshly voided urine** specimen, preferably before attending rounds! A spot urine protein-to-creatinine ratio is also important. A ratio of 1 is equivalent to 1 g of proteinuria per day.

The best way to increase the chance of finding RBC casts is to obtain an early morning urine specimen after the patient has placed a pillow behind the lumbar spine a few minutes after waking up.

B. Categorize the glomerulonephritis. Once the diagnosis is made, the search for the underlying cause begins.

1. **Laboratory studies.**
   a. The **serum complement (C3 and C4) levels** allow classification of the glomerulonephritis as hypocomplementemic or normocomplemententemic since all RPGNs can be classified in this manner. Immune complex RPGNs (except for IgA nephropathy) are hypocomplementemic. Pauci-immune and anti-GBM–associated RPGNs are normocomplemententemic. One way of remembering this is to use the following mnemonic to recall the causes of RPGN that lead to hypocomplementemia. The causes of RPGN not on the list below are normocomplemententemic.

MNEMONIC **Causes of Hypocomplementemic RPGN ("S**he **S**aw **S**ally **C**ook **P**oisoned **M**acaroni")

SLE
Subacute bacterial endocarditis
Shunt nephritis
Cryoglobulinemia in the setting of hepatitis **C**
Postinfectious glomerulonephritis
MPGN

b. **Additional lab tests**. Other tests that may be useful, depending on the clinical setting, include antistreptolysin O (ASO), antinuclear antibody (ANA), anti-GBM antibody, antineutrophil cytoplasmic antibody (ANCA) titers, serum cryoglobulin, blood cultures, liver function tests, hepatitis serologies (B and C), and erythrocyte sedimentation rate (ESR).

2. **Renal biopsy** is the definitive procedure for diagnosing rapidly progressive glomerulonephritis. Anticoagulation tests and a complete blood count are necessary prior to the biopsy.

IV. TREATMENT

Rapidly progressive glomerulonephritis is a renal emergency!

A. Inflammatory renal disorders should be treated with steroids and cytotoxic agents. If the glomerulonephritis is secondary to a systemic disease, the primary disorder should be treated as well.

B. Indications for **hemodialysis** are given in Chapter 37 IV B.

C. The patient's electrolyte status [including blood urea nitrogen (BUN) and creatinine levels], volume status, and blood pressure should be monitored frequently. Hypertension should be treated.

REFERENCES

Jennette JC. Rapidly progressive crescentic glomerulonephritis. Kidney Int 2003;63:1164.

Morgan MD, Harper L, Williams J, et al. Anti-neutrophil cytoplasm-associated glomerulonephritis. [Review]. J Am Soc Nephrol 2006;17(5):1224–1234.

Renal Tubular Defects

40

I. INTRODUCTION

A. The various diseases, **congenital** and **acquired,** that cause renal tubular defects have one thing in common: they tend to affect the tubules to a greater extent than the glomeruli.

B. Defects may be **anatomic** or **physiologic.**

1. Diseases that cause **anatomic defects** are usually hereditary and include polycystic renal disease, medullary sponge kidney, and medullary cystic disease. Anatomic defects can be diagnosed by intravenous pyelography or ultrasound.
2. Diseases that cause **physiologic** defects in tubular transport usually present as polyuria, electrolyte imbalance, and/or a nongap metabolic acidosis. This chapter focuses on the most confusing aspect of physiologic tubular defects, **renal tubular acidosis.**

II. RENAL TUBULAR ACIDOSIS

A. Definition. Renal tubular acidosis (RTA) results from a net decrease in tubular hydrogen secretion or bicarbonate reabsorption, causing a nongap (or hyperchloremic) metabolic acidosis. Chloride is a marker for acid loss in the urine. If the urinary chloride is low, then the urinary anion gap [Urinary anion gap = $(UNa^{+} + UK^{+}) - UCl^{-}$] is "positive," indicating a kidney problem with acid secretion, and is therefore consistent with an RTA. If the urinary anion gap is "negative," this indicates that the kidney can excrete its acid load, and the source is unlikely to be the kidney (and is usually due to diarrhea).

Nonrenal causes of a nongap metabolic acidosis lead to a **n**egative urinary anion gap.

Just asking the patient whether he or she has diarrhea is usually an efficient and reliable way to distinguish between an RTA and a gastrointestinal (GI) cause of a nongap metabolic acidosis.

B. Classification. Most patients with a nongap metabolic acidosis who do not have diarrhea or an anatomic gastrointestinal abnormality will have one of the three types of renal tubular acidosis (Table 40-1).

1. **Type 1 renal tubular acidosis** occurs as a result of defective hydrogen ion secretion; therefore, urinary pH will be elevated. Hypokalemia results when potassium is excreted instead of H^+ cations. (Usually, Na^+ is reabsorbed, and H^+ is excreted to some degree. H^+ secretion does not occur effectively in type 1 RTA, so K^+ is secreted instead. Thus, electroneutrality is maintained.)
2. **Type 2 renal tubular acidosis** occurs as a result of decreased bicarbonate reabsorption in the proximal tubule. Initially, the urinary pH will be elevated because of

TABLE 40-1

OVERVIEW OF RENAL TUBULAR ACIDOSIS

	Type 1 (Distal)	Type 2 (Proximal)	Type 4
Defect	Decrease in hydrogen secretion	Decrease in bicarbonate reabsorption	Aldosterone deficiency or resistance
Serum [K^+]	Decreased	Decreased	Increased
Urinary pH	>5.3	<5.3 (>5.3 with base load)	<5.3
Major causes	Amphotericin toxicity, hyperparathyroidism, obstructive uropathy, sickle cell anemia, cirrhosis	Fanconi's syndrome, drugs, Wilson's disease, vitamin D deficiency, amyloidosis, multiple myeloma, renal transplant	Diabetes mellitus, nephrosclerosis from hypertension, chronic kidney disease, chronic interstitial nephritis, Addison's, disease, ACE inhibitors, heparin
Treatment	Bicarbonate and K^+	Bicarbonate and K^+*	Mineralocorticoids and potassium restriction

ACE = angiotensin-converting enzyme.
*But not in Fanconi's syndrome.

bicarbonate loss; with continued bicarbonate loss, however, the serum bicarbonate and, thus, the urine bicarbonate concentrations will decrease. Then, all urine bicarbonate can be reabsorbed by the distal tubule, and urinary pH will fall. Hypokalemia occurs as potassium secretion is enhanced to accompany the bicarbonate excreted in the urine. (The body always tries to retain electroneutrality.)

3. **Type 4 renal tubular acidosis** is usually caused by aldosterone deficiency or resistance. Hyperkalemia occurs for the same reason hyperaldosterone states cause hypokalemic metabolic alkalosis. Relative hypoaldosteronism from hyporeninemic states can be seen in diabetic nephropathy, hypertensive nephropathy, tubulointerstitial diseases, and acquired immunodeficiency syndrome (AIDS).

REFERENCES

Batlle D, Moorthi KM, Schlueter W, et al. Distal renal tubular acidosis and the potassium enigma. Semin Nephrol 2006;26(6):471–478.

Laing CM, Unwin RJ. Renal tubular acidosis. J Nephrol 2006;19(Suppl 9):S46–52.

Ring T, Frische S, Nielsen S. Clinical review: renal tubular acidosis–a physicochemical approach. Crit Care (London, England) 2005;9(6):573–580.

41 Urinary Tract Infections

I. INTRODUCTION. Urinary tract infections (UTIs) are extremely common and include cystitis, pyelonephritis, and urosepsis.

A. Etiology. *Escherichia coli* accounts for approximately 80% of all infections. *Staphylococcus saprophyticus, Klebsiella* spp., *Proteus mirabilis, Enterococcus* spp., and other bacteria account for the rest.

B. Epidemiology

1. Women are more susceptible than men to UTIs because the female urethra is shorter, facilitating bacterial access to the bladder.
   a. Sexual intercourse and the use of diaphragms and spermicide are predisposing factors.
   b. In postmenopausal women, estrogen deficiency may predispose patients to acute cystitis (from increased colonization with *E. coli*).
2. Uncircumcised men are at higher risk than circumcised men.

II. CLINICAL MANIFESTATIONS OF UTIs

A. Dysuria (i.e., pain or burning with urination) is usually present and is commonly associated with other irritative symptoms (i.e., urinary frequency, urgency, and nocturia). Although dysuria often indicates acute cystitis, it is important to remember that other disorders may also present with dysuria. There is a FUND of irritative symptoms that may indicate the presence of a UTI:

MNEMONIC **Irritative Symptoms Suggestive of UTI ("FUND")**

Frequency
Urgency
Nocturia
Dysuria

B. Suprapubic or costovertebral angle pain or **tenderness** is usually indicative of cystitis or pyelonephritis, respectively.

C. Fever usually indicates a systemic response, possibly due to pyelonephritis. **Hypotension** and **altered mental status** may indicate urosepsis.

III. DIFFERENTIAL DIAGNOSES OF DYSURIA. Dysuria does not always signal acute cystitis. It is especially important to consider the alternative causes of dysuria in men, because acute cystitis is less common in men than in women. Non-UTI causes of dysuria include the following:

A. Women

1. **Infectious causes**
   a. **Urethritis** (e.g., from *Neisseria gonorrhea, Chlamydia trachomatis,* or herpes simplex virus) may also cause dysuria. Compared with the dysuria of acute cystitis, the dysuria of urethritis usually evolves gradually, is less severe, and is less often accompanied by urinary frequency and urgency. A history of vaginal discharge or a new sexual partner also raises suspicion for urethritis.
   b. **Vaginitis** (e.g., from *Candida* or *Trichomonas*) usually presents with a malodorous vaginal discharge. The patient may also complain of dyspareunia.
2. **Noninfectious causes**
   a. **Interstitial cystitis** presents with dysuria, urinary leukocytes, and a negative urine culture.
   b. **Chemotherapy** and **pelvic irradiation** may cause symptoms that mimic UTI.

B. Men

1. **Bladder pathology** may result in dysuria in both men and women, but the relative paucity of UTIs in men increases the likelihood that some other diagnosis is responsible. Both bladder stones and tumors should be considered.
2. **Prostate syndromes.** With the exception of acute bacterial prostatitis, which usually results in dysuria that is accompanied by significant systemic toxicity, prostate syndromes may be easily confused with cystitis. Laboratory testing is usually needed to differentiate among these disorders (see V F in this chapter).
3. **Urethritis** from gonorrhea or chlamydia is often associated with penile discharge.

IV. LABORATORY STUDIES. Not all of the following tests need to be obtained in every patient. The indications for tests are discussed in part V of this chapter.

A. Urine dipstick testing allows for the determination of urinary pH, leukocyte esterase, nitrite, blood, and protein levels.

1. **Urinary pH.** An alkaline urine may indicate a urease-splitting organism (e.g., *Proteus*).
2. **Leukocyte esterase** usually indicates the presence of inflammatory cells [i.e., white blood cells (WBCs)] and, therefore, infection. The sensitivity may exceed 75%. False-positive results may occur with urinary contamination.
3. **Nitrite** is detected when certain bacteria are present. The sensitivity is relatively low, and false-positive results are noted with bacterial contamination.
4. **Blood** in the urine may indicate myoglobin, hemoglobin, or intact red blood cells (RBCs). Cystitis can cause hematuria, but other causes of bladder pathology should also be considered (e.g., a malignancy anywhere along the urinary tract).
5. **Protein** in the urine may indicate a glomerulopathy, although low levels of proteinuria are seen with bladder irritation. Large numbers of WBCs may lead to a falsely positive protein determination.

B. Urine microscopic analysis. The presence of more than five leukocytes per high-power field denotes pyuria and is indicative of some urinary tract abnormality. Gram staining may also be performed but is not a sensitive test for UTI. **Sterile pyuria** (i.e., pyuria with a negative urine culture) may occur with contained bacterial infections (renal abscesses), systemic bacterial infections (endocarditis), other infections (miliary tuberculosis), inflammatory processes (interstitial nephritis), and partially treated UTI.

C. Urine culture provides the gold standard for diagnosing UTI. Previously, a colony count of 10^5 was considered the cut-off point for diagnosing a UTI, but more than 50% of symptomatic women have a lower colony count. In fact, the presence of as few as 100 colonies may signal infection in a symptomatic woman.

D. Prostatic secretion analysis. Prostatic secretions may be elicited through prostatic massage. In elderly men with possible chronic prostatitis, a urinalysis with culture is often sent before and after prostatic massage.

E. Urine pregnancy test. Because pregnant patients are often treated with different antibiotics and with a longer course of therapy, a urine pregnancy test should be obtained in all patients for whom pregnancy is a possibility.

F. Renal imaging [ultrasound or computed tomography (CT) scan]. In patients who are systemically ill, and especially in those with a history of kidney stones or a presentation compatible with urolithiasis, an ultrasound may be obtained to rule out "pus under pressure" (i.e., an infection behind an obstruction that mimics an abscess).

V. APPROACH TO THE PATIENT

A. Uncomplicated cystitis

1. **Women.** Empiric treatment is one possible approach in healthy, nonpregnant women who present with the classic symptoms of acute UTI without any evidence of pyelonephritis (i.e., no systemic symptoms such as fever, costovertebral angle pain, or nausea) or another cause of dysuria (urethritis, vaginitis). Another option is to obtain a **urinary dipstick,** which is usually the only test that is required. If the urinary dipstick is negative or if the patient has pelvic pain or abnormal vaginal discharge, a **pelvic examination** and a **urine culture** are often indicated as well.
2. **Men.** A **urine dipstick** and a **culture** are generally performed before therapy.

B. Uncomplicated pyelonephritis. Patients usually present with **irritative symptoms** associated with **fever, costovertebral angle pain** or **tenderness,** or both. The **urinary dipstick** is usually positive, and a **urine culture** is usually sent for definitive diagnosis and to ascertain the antimicrobial sensitivities of the causative organism.

C. Recurrent cystitis (e.g., three or more episodes per year) is much more common in women than men. Before diagnosing recurrent cystitis, **rule out relapse.**

1. **Relapses** typically occur early after the completion of therapy. The same species and strain of organism are isolated, and additional urologic evaluation is usually necessary.
2. **Recurrences** typically occur later. A different organism is usually isolated, and additional evaluation is often unnecessary.

D. Complicated UTIs may occur in men or women and are often suspected in patients whose conditions relapse or do not improve with initial therapy. A complicated infection results when a patient has an anatomic or functional abnormality of the urinary tract or a resistant infection. Urinary catheter-related infection (see Chapter 4) is considered to be complicated. A urine culture is always recommended.

E. Asymptomatic bacteriuria. In most patients, screening for asymptomatic bacteriuria is unnecessary. Exceptions include the following:

1. Pregnant women are often screened and treated if the bacteria count is 10,000 or more (to decrease the risk of pyelonephritis).
2. Patients undergoing renal or urologic procedures also benefit from screening.

F. Prostate syndromes. The presence of obstructive symptoms (i.e., hesitancy, difficulty starting and stopping the stream, decreased urinary flow) may favor a diagnosis of chronic prostatitis or prostatodynia. Of note, prostate tenderness on examination is not a sensitive marker for these disorders. If a prostate syndrome is suspected, a urine sample is obtained for urinalysis and culture, and then a second sample is obtained following prostate massage.

1. **Chronic bacterial prostatitis.** An increase in leukocytes usually occurs with massage; culture of prostatic secretions is positive.
2. **Chronic nonbacterial prostatitis** usually demonstrates an increase in leukocytes after massage, but the culture is negative. *Ureaplasma* or *Chlamydia* may be the cause.
3. **Prostatodynia** (a misleading term because the prostate is normal) is a diagnosis of exclusion that is made when the patient has typical symptoms but no increase in leukocytes with massage and a negative culture.

VI. TREATMENT

A. Uncomplicated cystitis. Empiric therapy is generally appropriate when the urine dipstick test is positive. It may also be appropriate for patients with no alternative diagnosis and a high clinical suspicion for UTI.

1. **Trimethoprim (TMP)/sulfamethoxazole (SMX)** (e.g., TMP 160 mg/SMX 800 mg) is often administered orally twice daily for 3 days. A longer course of therapy (e.g., 7 days) may be appropriate in higher-risk patients (e.g., patients with diabetes, elderly patients). Men are usually treated for 7 days.
2. **Fluoroquinolones.** A fluoroquinolone can be substituted if the patient has a sulfa allergy or if resistant strains have emerged in the local area.
3. **Amoxicillin** or **nitrofurantoin** is indicated if the patient is pregnant.

B. Uncomplicated pyelonephritis

1. **Outpatient treatment** is appropriate for many patients. TMP/SMX (TMP 160 mg/SMX 800 mg orally twice daily) may be prescribed for 14–21 days, unless resistant strains of bacteria have emerged in the area (in which case a fluoroquinolone would be an appropriate agent).
2. **Inpatient treatment** may be necessary for diabetic patients, for the elderly, and in patients who appear severely ill or who are unable to maintain hydration secondary to nausea and vomiting. Inpatient treatment is also recommended for pregnant patients. A **third-generation cephalosporin, a fluoroquinolone,** or the **combination of ampicillin and gentamicin** is often used.

C. Recurrent cystitis is often an indication for prophylaxis.

1. **General recommendations.** Postmenopausal women may benefit from topical estrogen to help prevent *E. coli* colonization.

Women who use diaphragms or spermicide should consider alternative methods of birth control. These measures may obviate the need for prophylaxis.

2. **Prophylaxis**
   a. **Postcoital prophylaxis** is often used in patients who relate their UTIs to sexual intercourse. One tablet of TMP/SMX may be taken following intercourse, and patients should be advised to urinate soon after intercourse.
   b. **Daily or three-times-per-week prophylaxis** with TMP/SMX may be used in patients with recurrent UTIs unrelated to sexual intercourse.
   c. **Early therapy** may be preferred in patients who have infrequent recurrences (e.g., two episodes per year). Patients initiate their own 3-day treatment with the onset of symptoms.

D. Complicated UTIs. If a resistant infection is the cause, therapy is generally aimed at the organism and often given for an extended period (e.g., 10–14 days or longer). A fluoroquinolone is often given to outpatients, while broad-spectrum intravenous antibiotics may be required for initial inpatient therapy. If the infection is related to the use of a urinary catheter (see Chapter 4), urine culture and appropriate antimicrobial treatment for 7–14 days is usually required.

If a patient develops a Foley catheter–related infection and still requires an indwelling catheter, the catheter should be replaced before initiating antimicrobial treatment. (Biofilm development along the surface of the catheter harbors microorganisms and may "protect" these organisms from the antimicrobial agent.)

E. Prostate syndromes

1. **Chronic bacterial prostatitis.** Prolonged treatment (often with TMP/SMX for 6 weeks or more) is generally given.
2. **Chronic nonbacterial prostatitis.** Empiric treatment against *Ureaplasma* or *Chlamydia* (e.g., with erythromycin) is often initiated for 2 weeks and should be continued for 3–6 weeks only if symptoms have improved.
3. **α-Blocking** agents may be helpful for bladder neck and urethral spasms.

REFERENCES

Bent S, Nallamothu BK, Simel DL, et al. Does this woman have an acute uncomplicated urinary tract infection? JAMA 2002;287(20):2701–2710.

Leone M, Perrin AS, Granier I, et al. A randomized trial of catheter change and short course of antibiotics for asymptomatic bacteriuria in catheterized ICU patients. Intensive Care Med 2007;33(4):726–729.

Nicolle LE. Uncomplicated urinary tract infection in adults including uncomplicated pyelonephritis. Urol Clin North Am 2008;35(1):1–12.

Stamm WE, Hooton TM. Management of urinary tract infections in adults. N Engl J Med 1993;329(18):1328–1334. [Classic article].

42 Approach to Acid-Base Disorders

I. INTRODUCTION

A. All acid-base disorders can be placed in one of the following categories:

1. **Metabolic acidosis**
    a. **Nonanion gap**
    b. **Anion gap**
2. **Metabolic alkalosis**
    a. **Chloride responsive**
    b. **Chloride unresponsive**
3. **Respiratory acidosis**
4. **Respiratory alkalosis**

B. Often, there is more than one metabolic derangement, which can make interpretation more difficult. However, the approach discussed in this chapter will enable you to diagnose most acid-base disorders.

II. STEPS IN THE EVALUATION OF ACID-BASE DISORDERS.[1] An arterial blood gas and electrolyte panel are needed to fully evaluate all acid-base disorders.

A. Decide whether the patient is acidemic or alkalemic. Although a pH of 7.35–7.45 is considered "normal," mixed disorders or the body's compensatory mechanisms (see IV) may hide significant acid-base derangements within this range. It is therefore useful to decide on acidemia or alkalemia simply on the basis of whether the pH falls below or above 7.40.

1. **Acidemia** is diagnosed when the pH is less than 7.40.
2. **Alkalemia** is diagnosed when the pH is greater than 7.40.

B. Determine whether the acid-base abnormality has a metabolic or respiratory cause. You can make this determination by looking at the arterial carbon dioxide tension ($PaCO_2$). A high $PaCO_2$ and a low pH is a respiratory acidosis, whereas a high $PaCO_2$ and a high pH is a metabolic alkalosis. A low $PaCO_2$ and a

[1]Modified with permission from Haber RJ. A practical approach to acid-base disorders. West J Med 1991;155(2):146–151.

low pH is a metabolic acidosis, and a low $PaCO_2$ and a high pH is a respiratory alkalosis.

1. **Acidemia**
   a. If the patient is acidemic and the $PaCO_2$ is high, you have diagnosed **respiratory acidosis.** An **acute** respiratory acidosis will cause serum bicarbonate to rise about 1 mEq/L per 10 mm Hg rise of $PaCO_2$. After 6–12 hours, the kidney can begin to generate more bicarbonate, and over days a patient can develop **chronic** respiratory acidosis with serum bicarbonate increasing about 3 mEq/L per 10 mm Hg rise in $PaCO_2$.
   b. If the patient is acidemic and the $PaCO_2$ is low, you have diagnosed **metabolic acidosis** (because the $PaCO_2$ does not account for the acidosis). Pure metabolic acidosis results in about a 1.0–1.3 decrease in $PaCO_2$ per 1 mEq/L decrease in serum bicarbonate.
2. **Alkalemia**
   a. If the patient is alkalemic and the $PaCO_2$ is low, you have diagnosed **respiratory alkalosis.** Acute respiratory alkalosis will cause serum bicarbonate to fall about 2 mEq/L per 10 mm Hg fall in $PaCO_2$. **Chronic** respiratory alkalosis will cause serum bicarbonate to fall about 5 mEq/L per 10 mm Hg fall in $PaCO_2$.
   b. If the patient is alkalemic and the $PaCO_2$ is high, you have diagnosed **metabolic alkalosis.** Pure metabolic alkalosis results in about a 0.7 mm Hg increase in $PaCO_2$ for each 1 mEq/L increase in serum bicarbonate.

C. Calculate the anion gap. The anion gap equals **the measured cations minus the measured anions** [i.e., $Na^+ - (Cl^- + HCO_3^-)$]. Because the measured cations are normally more than the measured anions, the unmeasured anions must be greater than the unmeasured cations by exactly the same amount to maintain electroneutrality. Any disorder that increases unmeasured anions will decrease measured anions or increase cations and cause an increased anion gap.

1. Normal is 8–12.
2. If the anion gap is **more than 20, anion gap acidosis** is present. The presence of an anion gap acidosis always represents a primary abnormality (see III A 2).
3. If the anion gap is 12–20, there still might be an underlying anion gap acidosis.

D. Calculate the corrected serum bicarbonate.

1. The purpose of this calculation is to determine what the serum bicarbonate would be if no anion gap existed (i.e., the corrected serum bicarbonate).

a. If correcting the anion gap results in an elevated serum bicarbonate (i.e., >28), the patient has an underlying metabolic alkalosis.
b. If correcting the anion gap results in a reduced serum bicarbonate (i.e., <23), the patient has an underlying nonanion gap acidosis.
c. If correcting the anion gap results in a normal serum bicarbonate, then the decreased serum bicarbonate is completely explained by the anion gap acidosis.

2. The following formula can be used to calculate the corrected serum bicarbonate:

$$CB = \text{Measured AG} - \text{Normal AG} + \text{Measured } HCO_3^-$$

(CB = corrected bicarbonate and AG = anion gap)

By subtracting the normal anion gap from the measured anion gap, you have a measurement of the "extra acid" that is present. Because each extra acid titrates approximately one base, this calculation approximates the amount of bicarbonate consumed in titrating the anion gap acidosis. By adding this value to the measured bicarbonate value, you correct the bicarbonate for the effect of the anion gap acidosis.

Steps for Determining Acid-Base Abnormalities

- Determine whether the pH is greater than or less than 7.4.
- Look at the $PaCO_2$.
- Calculate the anion gap.
- Calculate the corrected serum bicarbonate.

III. DIFFERENTIAL DIAGNOSES. Once you have completed the four steps described in section II, you will have identified most possible acid-base disorders. Three disturbances simultaneously (the "triple ripple") is the maximum because respiratory alkalosis and respiratory acidosis cannot exist simultaneously. The following differentials can help you arrive at a cause for the patient's acid-base disorder or disorders.

A. Metabolic acidosis

1. **Nonanion gap.** The common causes of nonanion gap acidosis include two renal, two gastrointestinal, and two "post" causes.

a. **Renal**

(1) **Acute or chronic kidney disease** usually causes a mixed anion and nonanion gap acidosis.

(2) **Renal tubular acidosis** (see Chapter 40)

b. **Gastrointestinal**

(1) **Diarrhea.** Bicarbonate loss can result in a nonanion gap metabolic acidosis.

(2) **Colovesicular fistula** or **ileostomy** can also cause bicarbonate loss.

c. **"Post" disorders**

(1) **Posthyperventilation.** The kidney compensates for a respiratory alkalosis by "spilling" bicarbonate to generate a nonanion gap metabolic acidosis. If the respiratory alkalosis ceases (e.g., following treatment of heart failure), a nonanion gap acidosis may remain until the kidney can regenerate bicarbonate.

(2) **Postanion gap acidosis.** For the kidney to maintain the body's electroneutrality, the increase in unmeasured anions that accompanies an anion gap acidosis is associated with chloride loss, producing hypochloremic acidosis. If a significant volume loss accompanies the anion gap acidosis (e.g., diabetic ketoacidosis with an osmotic diuresis from hyperglycemia), the kidney will try to correct by reabsorbing salt and water. In doing so, chloride is reabsorbed, and a hyperchloremic (i.e., nonanion gap) acidosis may occur until the kidney can replace the consumed bicarbonate. (This often takes a few days).

2. **Anion gap.** Metabolic anion gap acidoses result from an increase in unmeasured anions. Armed with the following mnemonic, "MUDPLIERS," you can zero in on the cause or causes of an anion gap acidosis.

MNEMONIC **Causes of Anion Gap Acidosis ("MUDPLIERS")**

Methanol intoxication (through conversion into formic acid)
Uremia (urea is an anion)
Diabetic or alcoholic ketoacidosis
Paraldehyde (a medicine no longer in use)
Lactate (usually from anaerobic metabolism during shock or extensive tissue injury)
Isoniazid or **I**ron overdose
Ethylene glycol intoxication (antifreeze ingestion)
Rhabdomyolysis
Salicylate intoxication

a. **Uremia.** Check the blood urea nitrogen (BUN).
b. **Rhabdomyolysis.** Check creatine kinase.
c. **Diabetic ketoacidosis.** Diabetic ketoacidosis can be ruled out on the basis of a negative urine dipstick for ketones.
d. **Salicylate overdose.** A salicylate level should be obtained for all unexplained anion gap acidoses.

e. **Methanol** or **ethylene glycol intoxication. A simultaneous blood sample for osmolarity, serum electrolytes,** and **ethanol level** is especially important in patients with altered consciousness and in alcoholics with an anion gap acidosis because the probability of a methanol or ethylene glycol ingestion is increased.

(1) **Calculate the osmolar gap.** All alcohols (including ethanol, isopropyl alcohol, methanol, and ethylene glycol) can produce an osmolar gap (a difference between measured and calculated osmolarity), but only methanol and ethylene glycol lead to osmolar gaps with significant anion gap acidoses. Calculate the osmolar gap as follows:

$$\text{Calculated osmolarity} = 2 \times \text{Na} + \text{BUN} / 2.8 + \text{glucose} / 18$$

(2) **Correct for ethanol.** The ethanol level divided by 4.6 equals the amount of osmoles that ethanol is contributing to the gap.

(3) **Calculate the remaining osmolar gap.** Subtract the osmoles due to ethanol from the original osmolar gap. The remaining osmolar gap is still unexplained. A value greater than 5 mOsm/kg H_2O is concerning (but not specific) for a toxic ingestion of another alcohol (e.g., methanol or ethylene glycol). Other clinical evidence that may confirm your suspicion includes visual disturbances (with methanol ingestion) and urinary oxalate crystals (with ethylene glycol ingestion).

f. **Lactate.** Often a lactic acidosis is diagnosed on a clinical basis (e.g., obvious sepsis) or by exclusion. An elevated lactate level confirms your clinical suspicion.

g. **Alcoholic ketoacidosis** is probably much more common than we think and deserves to be a diagnosis of exclusion so that other potentially treatable and life-threatening conditions are not missed.

B. Metabolic alkalosis. To determine the cause of metabolic alkalosis, first obtain a urine chloride level. Causes are referred to as **chloride responsive** or **chloride unresponsive.**

1. **Urine chloride less than 20 mEq/L.** Metabolic alkalosis resulting from the following causes **will correct with sodium chloride administration.**

a. **Prerenal states** (e.g., severe heart failure). Most metabolic alkaloses are generated by the kidney reacting to a decrease in renal blood flow. Any of the prerenal states (see Chapter 37 II A) can lead to metabolic alkalosis. **Mechanisms** by which a **prerenal state** produces a metabolic alkalosis include:

(1) **Increased proximal bicarbonate reabsorption.** Avid reabsorption of sodium in the proximal tubule induces increased bicarbonate reabsorption in order to maintain electroneutrality.

(2) **Increased distal acid secretion.** A prerenal state results in higher renin and aldosterone levels, which increases sodium uptake in the distal tubule while leading to potassium and hydrogen ion secretion.

b. **Gastric fluid loss** (from vomiting or a nasogastric tube) can lead to a metabolic alkalosis.

c. **Prior diuretic therapy** leading to volume depletion can result in metabolic alkalosis.

2. **Urine chloride greater than 20 mEq/L.** Metabolic alkalosis resulting from the following causes **will not correct with sodium chloride administration.** The most common causes can be remembered easily if you think of the first four letters of the alphabet:

MNEMONIC

Common Causes of Chloride-Unresponsive Metabolic Alkalosis ("ABCD")

Aldosteronism (primary)
Bartter's syndrome
Cushing's syndrome
Depletion of magnesium

a. **Primary hyperaldosteronism** increases excretion of potassium and hydrogen ion at the distal tubule, resulting in hypokalemia and alkalosis.

b. **Bartter's syndrome** results from defects in salt reabsorption in the thick ascending limb of the renal tubule. Salt and water loss trigger aldosterone production, which causes hypokalemia and alkalosis. (Hypomagnesemia may also be seen.)

c. **Cushing's syndrome** may produce hypokalemia and alkalosis by mechanisms similar to those of primary hyperaldosteronism.

d. **Depletion of magnesium** may result in potassium wasting. Hypokalemia may cause hydrogen ions to shift intracellularly and may also result in increased excretion of hydrogen at the distal tubule; both mechanisms may lead to alkalosis.

Bartter's syndrome and magnesium depletion are generally associated with normal or low blood pressure, whereas primary hyperaldosteronism and Cushing's syndrome are generally associated with hypertension.

Diuretics often produce a confusing picture because although urinary chloride is greater than 20 mEq/L, metabolic alkalosis is usually responsive to sodium chloride administration.

C. Respiratory acidosis (hypoventilation). See Chapter 25 II.

D. Respiratory alkalosis (hyperventilation). There are seven common etiologies:

1. **Primary central nervous system (CNS) disorders**
2. **Pulmonary disease** (including all causes of hypoxemia)
3. **Sepsis**

Respiratory alkalosis can be the first acid-base abnormality seen in patients with sepsis.

4. **Pregnancy**
5. **Drugs** (e.g., salicylates)
6. **Liver disease**
7. **Pain or anxiety**

IV. COMPENSATION

A. Clinicians look at compensatory mechanisms for two reasons:

1. To determine whether compensation is occurring or if there is another primary abnormality
2. To estimate the acuity of an acid-base abnormality

B. Compensation refers to the body's natural mechanisms of counteracting a primary acid-base disorder. For example, the lungs will compensate for the kidneys through hyperventilation during metabolic acidosis and, to a lesser extent, hypoventilation during metabolic alkalosis. The kidneys will compensate for the lungs by excreting or retaining bicarbonate when respiratory alkalosis or acidosis, respectively, is present.

Winter's formula may be used to see if an acid-base disorder is a pure metabolic acidosis.

$$PaCO_2 = 1.5\ [HCO_3^-] + 8 \pm 2$$

(If the patient's actual $PaCO_2$ is in the range predicted by this formula, there is a pure metabolic acidosis with appropriate respiratory compensation.)

For every change of 10 mm Hg in the $PaCO_2$ (up or down) in respiratory acid-base disorders, the pH changes 0.08 if the process is acute and 0.03 if the process is chronic (in the opposite direction of the $PaCO_2$).

REFERENCES

Haber RJ. A practical approach to acid-base disorders. West J Med 1991; 155(2):146–151. [Classic article].

Rastegar A. Use of the DeltaAG/DeltaHCO3- ratio in the diagnosis of mixed acid-base disorders. J Am Soc Nephrol 2007;18(9):2429–2431.

Rose BD, Post TW. Clinical Physiology of Acid-Base and Electrolyte Disorders. [Classic text]. 5th Ed. New York: McGraw-Hill, 2001.

Hyponatremia

I. INTRODUCTION

A. Definition. Hyponatremia refers to a **serum sodium concentration of less than 135 mEq/L.** Hyponatremia is the most common electrolyte disturbance in hospitalized patients.

B. Action of antidiuretic hormone (ADH). Understanding the action of ADH is essential to understanding hyponatremia.

1. Normally, the body regulates serum osmolality very closely by increasing or decreasing ADH secretion. When the effective circulating volume (ECV) decreases, the body senses that there is a lack of intravascular fluid and secretes ADH to help expand intravascular volume at the expense of serum osmolality.
2. Hyponatremia is usually caused by either an:
   a. Appropriate increase in ADH (as seen with hypovolemic or some hypervolemic causes), or
   b. Inappropriate increase in ADH [as seen in the syndrome of inappropriate ADH secretion (SIADH)]

C. Clinical manifestations of hyponatremia depend on the cause, level, and rapidity of hyponatremia; they include confusion, muscle cramps, nausea, and lethargy that may progress to seizures and coma.

D. Approach to the patient

1. The initial step in evaluating patients with hyponatremia is to check the **serum osmolality** to ensure that the patient does not have hypertonic or isotonic hyponatremia.
   a. **Hyperosmolar hyponatremia** is caused by hyperglycemia or hypertonic infusions [e.g., mannitol, total parenteral nutrition (TPN)]. For every 100 mg/dl of glucose above 100 mg/dl, serum sodium will decrease by about 1.6 mEq/L.
   b. **Iso-osmolar hyponatremia** can be caused by hyperlipidemia or hyperproteinemia **(pseudohyponatremia)** and is attributable to laboratory error. Iso-osmolar hyponatremia can also be caused by hyperglycemia and hypertonic infusions, but to a lesser degree than what would cause a hypertonic state.
2. If the serum osmolality is low (<280 mOsm), the next step is to evaluate the patient's **volume status.** With this information,

TABLE 43-1

CAUSES OF HYPO-OSMOLAR HYPOVOLEMIC HYPONATREMIA

Common Causes	Urine Sodium (mEq/L)	Serum Uric Acid
Skin loss	<10	>5 mg/dl
Gastrointestinal loss	<10	>5 mg/dl
Lung loss	<10	>5 mg/dl
Third spacing of fluids	<10	>5 mg/dl
Adrenal insufficiency	>20	>5 mg/dl
Renal loss (diuretics, tubular damage)	>20	>5 mg/dl

it is possible to narrow down the possible causes of the **hypo-osmolar hyponatremia.**

II. HYPO-OSMOLAR HYPONATREMIA

A. Hypovolemic

1. **Physical examination** will reveal signs of **volume depletion** (e.g., orthostasis, resting tachycardia, poor skin turgor, dry mucous membranes, low jugular venous pressure).
2. **Causes** are summarized in Table 43-1.
3. **Treatment** entails **intravascular fluid expansion** (usually with normal saline) and **treatment of the underlying cause.** The initial goal of treatment for any cause of hyponatremia is to increase the sodium only **halfway** during the first 24 hours, and no faster than 0.5 to 1.0 mEq/L/hr. Overly rapid correction increases the risk for central pontine myelinolysis. Demyelination occurs when pontine brain cells undergo rapid shrinkage due to fluid shifts, which can cause neurologic deficits, coma, and death.

B. Hypervolemic

1. **Physical examination** reveals signs of **volume expansion** (e.g., elevated jugular venous pressure, peripheral edema, ascites, pleural effusions, pulmonary edema).
2. **Causes** are summarized in Table 43-2.
3. **Treatment** usually involves a combination of fluid restriction and diuretics.

C. Euvolemic

1. **Physical examination** is notable for the lack of signs indicative of volume depletion or expansion.
2. **Causes** of euvolemic hypo-osmolar hyponatremia are summarized in Table 43-3.
3. **Treatment** involves fluid restriction plus treatment of the underlying cause.

III. SIADH is often a difficult but important diagnosis to make. Because the management of SIADH usually requires fluid

TABLE 43-2

CAUSES OF HYPO-OSMOLAR HYPERVOLEMIC HYPONATREMIA

Common Causes	Urine Sodium (mEq/L)	Serum Uric Acid
Nephrosis (i.e., nephrotic syndrome)	<10	>5 mg/dl
Cirrhosis	<10	>5 mg/dl
Cardiosis (i.e., congestive heart failure)	<10	>5 mg/dl

TABLE 43-3

CAUSES OF HYPO-OSMOLAR EUVOLEMIC HYPONATREMIA

Common Causes	Urine Sodium (mEq/L)	Serum Uric Acid
SIADH	>20	<4 mg/dl
Water intoxication (polydipsia)	Variable	<5 mg/dl
Hypothyroidism, adrenal insufficiency	Variable	>5 mg/dl
Renal dysfunction	>10	>5 mg/dl

SIADH = syndrome of inappropriate antidiuretic hormone excretion.

restriction in a hospitalized patient (who may be NPO, febrile, or both), it is important to be fairly sure of the diagnosis to prevent dehydration. If a hyponatremic patient meets all (or at least most) of the following five criteria, you can feel reasonably confident about treating the patient for SIADH:

A. The patient should have an **underlying reason** to have SIADH. The most common causes are malignancies, central nervous system (CNS) and pulmonary disease, and various drugs.

B. The patient should be clinically **euvolemic** but is actually slightly hypervolemic.

C. The patient should have **normal renal, adrenal,** and **thyroid** function.

D. The patient's **urine osmolality** is inappropriately **increased** and is usually greater than the serum osmolality.

E. The patient may also have a **low serum uric acid level.** Of all the causes of hyponatremia, only two—SIADH and primary polydipsia—are characterized by hypouricemia. In these two disorders, the intravascular volume is actually expanded (even though the disorders are categorized as euvolemic). The kidney handles uric acid the same way it handles sodium; therefore, in states of intravascular expansion, sodium and uric acid elimination are enhanced. Thus, a patient with SIADH should have **a urine sodium greater than 20 mEq/L**, indicating mild volume expansion.

REFERENCES

Adrogue HJ, Madias NE. Hyponatremia. N Engl J Med 2000;342(21):1581–1589. [Classic article].

Liamis G, Milionis H, Elisaf M. A review of drug-induced hyponatremia. Am J Kidney Dis 2008;52(1):144–153.

Lien YH, Shapiro JI. Hyponatremia: clinical diagnosis and management. Am J Med 2007;120(8):653–658.

Hypernatremia

I. INTRODUCTION

A. **Definition.** Hypernatremia refers to **serum sodium concentration greater than 145 mEq/L.**

B. **Severe hypernatremia** is rare if a patient has access to water and has an intact thirst mechanism. Those prone to hypernatremia include the very old, the very young, and the very sick.

C. **Plasma osmolality.** Unlike hyponatremia, hypernatremia is associated with only one state of serum osmolality: hyperosmolality.

D. Hypernatremia is usually due to **water loss out of proportion to electrolyte losses.**

II. CLINICAL MANIFESTATIONS OF HYPERNATREMIA depend on the cause, level, and rapidity of changing serum sodium.

A. **Symptoms** are primarily neurologic in origin due to a contracted intracellular fluid volume, which leads to contracted brain cells, which undergo osmotic adaptation. Symptoms may include altered mental status, hyperthermia, delirium, seizures, and coma.

B. Polyuria and polydipsia may also be prominent.

III. APPROACH TO THE PATIENT.

The initial step in evaluating patients with hypernatremia is to check the patient's **volume status** and **urine osmolality.** A high urine osmolality (>400 mOsm/kg) ensures that renal water conservation is intact. Dilute urine (<250 mOsm/kg) is characteristic of diabetes insipidus (DI).

A. **Hyperosmolar urine**

1. **Nonrenal losses that are hypotonic (e.g., excessive sweating, respiratory tract or gastrointestinal water loss).** Hypernatremia can occur if water intake cannot keep up with hypotonic fluid loss. Urine sodium is typically less than 10 mEq/L due to appropriate attempts to conserve total body volume.
2. **Renal losses (e.g., due to diabetic hyperglycemia, mannitol use).** Progressive volume depletion occurs with the ensuing osmotic diuresis. During these conditions, renal sodium and water conservation is not present, and the urine sodium is typically greater than 20 mEq/L.

3. Rarely, hypernatremia reflects an **increased amount of total body sodium.** Causes include hypertonic fluid administration (e.g., during cardiopulmonary resuscitation with hypertonic fluids), sodium chloride tablet ingestion without adequate water, and mineralocorticoid excess (e.g., primary hyperaldosteronism or Cushing's syndrome). Patients appear volume expanded on physical examination. In these cases, urine sodium is typically greater than 20 mEq/L.

B. Hypo-osmolar urine in the setting of hypernatremia indicates DI. Patients with DI are typically either euvolemic or mildly hypovolemic.

1. **Nephrogenic DI** stems from renal resistance to the action of antidiuretic hormone (ADH). Causes include drugs such as lithium and demeclocycline, chronic kidney disease affecting the collecting ducts (e.g., interstitial nephritis and ureteral obstruction), and electrolyte disorders (hypercalcemia and hypokalemia).
2. **Central DI** is most commonly caused by lack of ADH production in the posterior pituitary [e.g., brain surgery in the area of the pituitary or hypothalamus, head trauma, and idiopathic causes (50%)].

IV. TREATMENT. Extracellular fluid (ECF) status and the speed of development of hypernatremia must be assessed. Before the steps described below are taken, the initial underlying disorder must be corrected. Intranasal desmopressin is used for central DI, and the concentrating defect in nephrogenic DI can be treated with a low-sodium diet and a thiazide diuretic.

A. ECF depletion should be corrected first with isotonic fluids until ECF is restored. Then, water or hypotonic fluids can be administered.

$$\text{Free water deficit} = \text{current TBW} \times ([\text{Na}^+] - 140) / 140$$

(TBW = total body water = 0.5 (for women) or 0.6 (for men) × ideal body weight. TBW may be 10% lower than this calculated value in patients who are significantly volume depleted with hypernatremia. Large urine or stool output also should be considered, in addition to TBW calculations.)

B. ECF expansion can be treated with diuretics. If renal failure is present, dialysis may be necessary.

C. Chronic hypernatremia should be corrected at no faster than 0.5 mEq/L/hr, and no more than 8–12 mEq/day.

REFERENCES

Adrogue HJ, Madias NE. Hypernatremia. N Engl J Med 2000;342(20):1493–1499. [Classic article].

Reynolds R, Padfield P, Seckl J. Disorders of sodium balance. BMJ. 2006; 332(7453):702–705.

45 Hypokalemia

I. INTRODUCTION

A. Definition. Hypokalemia refers to **serum potassium concentration less than 3.5 mEq/L.**

B. Maintenance of plasma potassium

1. Ninety-five percent of potassium is intracellular.
2. Plasma potassium is maintained in a narrow range primarily via two mechanisms:
   a. Intracellular and extracellular shifts of potassium
   b. Renal potassium excretion
3. Increased intracellular shifts and increased renal and gastrointestinal potassium losses lead to hypokalemia.

II. CLINICAL MANIFESTATIONS primarily arise from alterations in membrane polarization.

A. Cardiac. Altered cardiac conduction is the most life-threatening abnormality. An electrocardiogram may display **flat T waves** and **prominent U waves.** Patients are at risk for significant ectopy, which does not always correlate with potassium levels.

Hypokalemia predisposes patients to digoxin toxicity.

B. Neuromuscular. Patients can experience a range of abnormalities from **mild weakness to overt paralysis.** Paralysis is not typically seen with potassium levels greater than 2.0 mEq/L. Muscle cramps, muscle weakness, respiratory failure, and ileus can occur.

Hypokalemia predisposes patients to rhabdomyolysis.

C. Renal. Hypokalemia leads to direct thirst stimulation and a urinary concentrating defect, which causes polydipsia and polyuria. Also, hypokalemia can both initiate and maintain a metabolic alkalosis. Prolonged hypokalemia can lead to renal tubular damage and interstitial fibrosis.

D. **Endocrine.** Aldosterone levels are depressed, and pancreatic insulin release is inhibited.

III. CAUSES OF HYPOKALEMIA

A. Hypokalemia with transcellular redistribution

1. **Alkalosis.** Metabolic alkalosis results in major total body potassium deficits up to 500 mEq; however, respiratory alkalosis typically induces much less of a potassium deficit.
2. **Insulin excess** indirectly stimulates the transcellular Na^+, K^+-ATPase pump, which leads to muscle and liver cellular potassium uptake.
3. **β-Adrenergic agonists** cause direct stimulation of the Na^+, K^+-ATPase pump.
4. **Hypokalemic periodic paralysis** is a rare hereditary disorder leading to rapid recurrent attacks of flaccid paralysis, lasting from 4–24 hours, due to intracellular potassium shifts. Asians and patients with thyroid disease are particularly vulnerable to this entity.
5. **Pseudohypokalemia** occurs in patients with very high white blood cell counts ($>10^5$). Redistribution occurs with leukocyte uptake of potassium.

B. Hypokalemia due to true potassium depletion.

Urinary potassium **excretion** can only be interpreted in a euvolemic patient. Otherwise, volume contraction may reduce urinary potassium excretion and obscure a state of hyperaldosteronism.

1. **Extrarenal potassium loss.** If the kidney is not the source of potassium loss in a hypokalemic patient, the urinary potassium excretion should be less than 25 mEq/day. **Diarrhea, fistula drainage**, and **villous adenomas** are usually easily diagnosed. **Laxative use** may be more difficult to diagnose, however, requiring stool electrolyte measurement. Inadequate potassium intake is a rare cause but can be seen in patients with **eating disorders**.
2. **Renal potassium loss.** Urinary potassium excretion is greater than 20–25 mEq/day. The causes of hypokalemia in this setting can be subdivided based on the patient's blood pressure.
   a. **Patients with elevated blood pressure.** Mineralocorticoid excess leads to potassium loss in these disorders.
      (1) **Hyperreninemic states** include hypertensive emergencies, renovascular hypertension, and rare renin-producing tumors.

(2) **Hyporeninemic states** include primary hyperaldosteronism, Cushing's syndrome, excessive licorice ingestion, and congenital adrenal hyperplasia.

b. **Patients with normal or low blood pressure.** These disorders can be categorized based on serum bicarbonate concentration.

(1) **Low bicarbonate syndromes** include renal tubular acidoses (see Chapter 40).

(2) **High bicarbonate syndromes** include diuretic use, Bartter's syndrome (genetic defects in the thick ascending limb of the loop of Henle), magnesium depletion, and Gitelman's syndrome (genetic defects in the distal cortical tubule). All have urinary chloride excretions greater than 10 mEq/day. Vomiting typically causes volume depletion and metabolic alkalosis, leading to renal potassium wasting and urinary chloride excretion less than 10 mEq/day.

IV. TREATMENT. The underlying disorder, if known, should be treated along with the serum potassium level.

A. Oral repletion is the preferred method. This can be accomplished both with pharmacologic potassium preparations and high-potassium diets.

1. Intravenous (IV) administration can be considered with severe, symptomatic hypokalemia or if patients are unable to tolerate oral medication.
2. Peripheral IV rates should not exceed 10 mEq/hr, with central IV rates not exceeding 20–40 mEq/hr.

High rates of potassium repletion require continuous electrocardiographic monitoring.

B. Hypomagnesemia, and glucose or alkali administration, can worsen hypokalemia and should be corrected before or during potassium administration.

C. Serum potassium levels should be followed very closely. For every 10 mEq of supplemental potassium given, serum potassium rises by 0.1 mEq/L; however, this approximation is less valid when serum potassium levels are less than 3.0 mEq/L.

REFERENCES

Gennari FJ. Hypokalemia. N Engl J Med 1998;338(7):451–458. [Classic article].

Groenveld J, Sipkins Y, Lim S et al. An approach to the patient with severe hypokalemia: the potassium quiz. Q J Med 2005,98:305.

46 Hyperkalemia

I. INTRODUCTION

A. Definition. Hyperkalemia refers to **serum potassium concentration greater than 5.0 mEq/L.**

B. Maintenance of plasma potassium

1. Plasma potassium is **maintained in a narrow range** primarily via two mechanisms:
   a. Intracellular fluid (ICF) and extracellular fluid (ECF) shifts of potassium
   b. Renal potassium excretion
2. **Increased potassium shifting to the extracellular space** and **decreased renal potassium losses** lead to hyperkalemia.
3. **Increased potassium intake** is rarely associated with hyperkalemia unless a patient is oliguric or has significant kidney disease. [Typically, a glomerular filtration rate (GFR) > 20 ml/min is sufficient to maintain potassium balance provided that the diet is not extremely high in potassium.]

II. CLINICAL MANIFESTATIONS.

Symptoms primarily arise from **alterations in membrane polarization.**

A. Cardiac

1. **Altered cardiac conduction** is the most life-threatening abnormality.
2. An electrocardiogram (ECG) may first show **peaking of the T wave;** then **flattening of the P wave** and **prolongation of the PR interval;** then **widening of the QRS complex;** and finally a **deep S wave or sine wave,** heralding ventricular fibrillation and cardiac arrest.

Hyperkalemia with ECG abnormalities is an emergency! Once any ECG abnormality is seen, life-threatening arrhythmias can rapidly occur.

B. Neuromuscular. A range of abnormalities from **mild weakness to tingling and paraesthesias** may occur. Rarely, flaccid paralysis takes place.

C. Renal. Hyperkalemia reduces renal ammoniagenesis and NH_4^+ secretion, leading to less net acid excretion and **metabolic acidosis.** The acidosis then worsens the degree of hyperkalemia.

D. Endocrine. Aldosterone, insulin, and glucagon release are stimulated. Plasma renin levels are suppressed.

III. CAUSES OF HYPERKALEMIA

A. Hyperkalemia with transcellular redistribution

1. **Acidosis-induced hyperkalemia** occurs primarily as a result of **acidosis due to inorganic acids.** Cations move intracellularly in exchange for potassium; potassium levels rise about 0.7 mEq/L for every decrease of 0.1 pH units. Respiratory acidosis causes a small rise in serum potassium levels.

Metabolic acidosis from organic acids (e.g., lactic acid) **does not** typically result in hyperkalemia, because both the cation and organic anion are freely permeable across the cell membrane.

2. **Insulin deficiency and hypertonicity** (e.g., hyperglycemia) promote potassium shift from the ICF to the ECF.
3. **β-Adrenergic antagonists** cause hyperkalemia but do not lead to life-threatening potassium levels.
4. **Hyperkalemic periodic paralysis** is a rare hereditary disorder leading to recurrent weakness or paralysis. Stimuli that lead to mild hyperkalemia (e.g., exercise) can precipitate an episode.
5. **Pseudohyperkalemia** occurs with redistribution of potassium out of cells after blood is drawn (the laboratory will usually report that the blood sample analyzed was a hemolyzed specimen).

B. Decreased potassium excretion

1. **Kidney disease.** A **GFR less than 5 ml/min** is usually accompanied by oliguria and hyperkalemia, whereas a GFR greater than 20 ml/min rarely leads to hyperkalemia.

It is extremely important to educate patients with significant kidney dysfunction about the high potassium content of certain foods, such as citrus fruits and juices, tomatoes, potatoes, and salt substitutes.

2. **Renal secretory defects** associated with interstitial nephritis, sickle cell disease, obstructive uropathy, and renal transplantation all may lead to renal tubular defects and hyperkalemia.

3. **Drugs**
   a. **Heparin,** regardless of molecular weight, suppresses aldosterone excretion.
   b. **Spironolactone, triamterene,** and **trimethoprim** inhibit potassium excretion via sodium channels in the distal nephron.
   c. **Angiotensin-converting enzyme inhibitors** suppress aldosterone production.
   d. **Nonsteroidal anti-inflammatory drugs** cause a reversible form of hyporeninemic hypoaldosteronism.
   e. **Cyclosporine** and **tacrolimus** also cause renal potassium secretory defects.
4. **Mineralocorticoid deficiency** leads to a hyperchloremic metabolic acidosis and hyperkalemia. Causes include Addison's disease and hyporeninemic hypoaldosteronism, as seen in patients with type 4 renal tubular acidosis (see Chapter 40) from diabetes mellitus or acquired immunodeficiency syndrome (AIDS).

IV. TREATMENT. As with hypokalemia, the underlying disorder, if known, should be treated along with the serum potassium level. Always ask if a lab specimen was hemolyzed. The potassium level should be confirmed with a repeat blood draw, particularly in asymptomatic patients, by measuring plasma levels rather than serum. This avoids the leakage of potassium out of cells in the course of clotting.

A. Antagonism of cardiac conduction abnormalities can be accomplished with the administration of **calcium.**
1. Give 10 ml of **10% calcium gluconate** administered intravenously over 2–3 minutes.
2. The onset of action is minutes, and the effect lasts for up to 1 hour. Repeat as needed; continuous calcium infusions are occasionally required.

Intravenous calcium does not lower serum potassium levels, but this therapy should be used whenever there is any ECG evidence of hyperkalemia-induced changes.

B. Intracellular shifting of potassium occurs relatively rapidly.
1. **Bicarbonate** distributes potassium into cells within 15–30 minutes, lasting 1–2 hours.
2. **Insulin** and **albuterol** begin to act over 15–30 minutes, lasting from 4–6 and 2–4 hours, respectively.

C. Potassium removal can be accomplished in several ways.
1. **Loop diuretics** (e.g., 40–160 mg of furosemide, preferably intravenously) is given if the patient is making urine.

2. **Sodium polystyrene sulfonate (Kayexalate)** is an ion-exchange binding resin that administers a sodium load in exchange for binding potassium.
   a. Consider giving 15–60 g by mouth or up to 60 g per rectum.
   b. Its onset is over a few hours. If a patient stools, you know this is working.
3. **Hemodialysis and peritoneal dialysis** result in the extracorporeal removal of potassium. As much as 300 mEq of potassium can be removed during each treatment.

REFERENCES

Evans K, Greenberg A. Hyperkalemia: a review. J Int Care Med 2005;20: 272–290.

Hypertension

47

I. INTRODUCTION

A. Definition. Patients who consistently have **systolic blood pressure greater than 140 mm Hg** or **diastolic blood pressure greater than 90 mm Hg** are considered to be hypertensive. Certain subgroups of patients are at greater risk for complications of hypertension and have lower blood pressure goals (i.e., patients with chronic kidney disease or diabetes mellitus should maintain blood pressures < 130/80 mm Hg).

B. Hypertension is an extremely **common disorder** in both outpatients and hospitalized patients. In general, hypertension in inpatients is a major concern primarily when patients present with hypertensive urgencies or emergencies.

II. CAUSES OF SECONDARY HYPERTENSION.

Although 95% of hypertensive patients have essential (primary) hypertension, causes of secondary hypertension must be considered in patients with characteristic signs or symptoms, onset of hypertension at a very young or old age, or when the blood pressure is refractory to medical therapy. The causes of secondary hypertension can be remembered using the following memory aid:

MNEMONIC **Causes of Secondary Hypertension**

One anatomic cause
Two renal causes
Three adrenal causes
Four CENTs
Calcium (hypercalcemia)
Ethanol abuse or **E**strogen use
Neurologic disease
Thyrotoxicosis

A. One anatomic cause. Aortic coarctation, a congenital disorder characterized by aortic constriction at the origin of the left subclavian artery, usually presents in children or young adults and can lead to hypertension.

B. Two renal causes

1. **Intrinsic renal disease.** Almost any parenchymal kidney disorder can lead to hypertension, usually as a result of increased intravascular volume, increased endothelial reactivity, and/or increased activity of the renin-angiotensin-aldosterone system.
2. **Renal artery stenosis,** a relatively common cause of secondary hypertension, is usually caused by atherosclerosis in older patients (most common) or fibromuscular dysplasia in young women (very infrequent). The stenosis leads to decreased renal blood flow, which leads to increased renin release and hypertension. Screening for renal artery stenosis is only indicated if an intervention would be performed as a result of diagnostic testing. Gold standard diagnosis is via renal angiography. An appropriate initial screen would use one of three methods: magnetic resonance angiography, computed tomography (CT) angiography, and Doppler ultrasonography. The choice of screening modality is usually based on patient- and hospital-specific factors.

Always consider renal artery stenosis as the cause of hypertension when a patient shows a dramatic increase in serum creatinine after starting angiotensin-converting enzyme (ACE) inhibitor therapy.

C. Three adrenal causes

1. **Primary hyperaldosteronism,** an uncommon cause of secondary hypertension, is caused by an aldosterone-secreting adenoma or bilateral adrenal hyperplasia.

Primary hyperaldosteronism should be suspected if a hypertensive patient is hypokalemic and not taking diuretics.

2. **Cushing's syndrome.** Excess glucocorticosteroids (as a result of any cause) will often cause the patient to be hypertensive. Usually, the other clinical manifestations of glucocorticoid excess will be present to aid in making the diagnosis.
3. **Pheochromocytoma** is a rare norepinephrine- and epinephrine-secreting tumor that may be malignant and can also lead to headaches and glucose intolerance. It is most commonly—but not always—located near the adrenals.

D. Four CENTs

1. **Calcium.** Hypercalcemia is an uncommon cause of hypertension but should be considered in those who have

underlying diseases apt to lead to hypercalcemia (see Chapter 77).

2. **Ethanol abuse, estrogen use,** or use of other drugs and toxins. The most common causes of secondary hypertension are the use of alcohol and oral contraceptives. Pregnancy can also lead to hypertension. Over-the-counter preparations, such as ephedrine-containing medications and other cold remedies, commonly raise blood pressure. Certain illicit drugs, such as cocaine and methamphetamines, are also common culprits.
3. **Neurologic disease.** Any process that leads to increased intracranial pressure can lead to the triad of hypertension, bradycardia, and irregular respiration (known as Cushing's triad).
4. **Thyrotoxicosis.** Patients with hyperthyroidism can also be hypertensive.

III. HYPERTENSIVE CRISES: URGENCIES AND EMERGENCIES

A. Hypertensive urgencies are situations in which the patient has systolic blood pressure greater than 220 mm Hg or diastolic blood pressure greater than 120 mm Hg and no evidence of end-organ damage. Urgencies are usually treated with **oral antihypertensive agents** (e.g., labetalol, clonidine, or captopril) in the emergency department. After blood pressure is lowered to an acceptable level, these patients can usually be discharged but warrant very close follow-up.

Sublingual or short-acting nifedipine should be avoided in almost all patients.

B. Hypertensive emergencies are those situations in which elevated blood pressure leads to end-organ damage.

1. **Examples.** The following situations qualify as hypertensive emergencies:
   a. **Hypertensive encephalopathy** (altered mental status)[1]
   b. **Intracranial hemorrhage**
   c. **Aortic dissection**
   d. **Myocardial infarction**
   e. **Unstable angina**
   f. **Hypertensive nephropathy** (progressive acute kidney injury with proteinuria and hematuria)

[1]Malignant hypertension is an outdated term that implies hypertension associated with encephalopathy (or neuropathy) and accompanied by papilledema. It is a form of hypertensive emergency.

2. **Treatment** for hypertensive emergencies usually requires admission to the intensive care unit (ICU) and the administration of **parenteral antihypertensives** (e.g., nitroglycerin, nitroprusside, labetalol). Typically, blood pressures should not be lowered by more than 25% over the first 1–2 days (i.e., not lower than 170/110 mm Hg) to minimize organ hypoperfusion.

REFERENCES

Chobanian AV, Bakris GL, Black HR, et al. Seventh Report of the Joint National Committee on Prevention, Detection, Evaluation, and Treatment of High Blood Pressure. Hypertension 2003; 42:1206. [Classic article].

Cutler J, Davis B. Thiazide-type diuretics and beta-blockers: as first line drug treatments for hypertension. Circulation 2008;117:2691–2705.

Approach to Fever

I. INTRODUCTION

A. Normal body temperature. Body temperature varies throughout the day. The nadir is usually in the early morning, and temperature peaks at 4–6 PM. This is the circadian temperature rhythm. The normal oral temperature is 36°C–37.4°C (average = 36.7°C).

1. In adults 18–40 years of age, the upper limit of normal temperature should be considered 37.2°C at 6 AM and 37.7°C overall.
2. The average rectal temperature is 0.5°C higher, and the average axillary temperature is 0.5°C lower than the oral temperature.

B. Fever reflects an upward shift in the body's temperature set point triggered by release of pyrogens. Hyperthermia reflects the body's inability to lower temperature by the usual mechanisms because of overheating or other causes.

C. Causes of fever. Fever may be a manifestation of infection, malignancy, connective tissue disorders, drug reactions, central nervous system (CNS) disorders, inflammatory diseases, or other diseases.

II. APPROACH TO THE PATIENT.

In many cases, the etiology of the fever is clinically obvious; other times, fever can be the initial manifestation of an elusive illness. This chapter provides a way to approach patients with recent onset of fever from an obscure source. If the fever persists for weeks without a diagnosis, a fever of unknown origin (FUO) may be present (see Chapter 51).

Remember:

- Patients who are elderly, immunocompromised, or, who are taking steroids or nonsteroidal anti-inflammatory drugs (NSAIDs) may not mount a fever, even in the presence of a severe infection.
- The degree of fever is of little predictive value in assessing the severity of an underlying illness in a given patient.
- Hypothermia may signal the presence of an overwhelming infection and should therefore be evaluated as thoroughly as hyperthermia.

A. Patient history

1. **Immune status.** Is the patient immunocompromised [e.g., as a result of leukemia, chemotherapy, steroid use, human immunodeficiency virus (HIV) infection, liver disease]?
2. **Medical history.** Patients with a known illness may have a fever caused by their underlying illness (e.g., tumor fever from lymphoma or a fever from a lupus flare); however, this is a diagnosis of exclusion, and infectious causes must be ruled out. Also, some illnesses predispose patients to certain infectious complications (e.g., abdominal abscess as a complication of Crohn's disease, endocarditis in a patient with an aortic valve replacement).
3. **Medication history.** What prescription or over-the-counter drugs is the patient taking? The medication history is aimed at discovering drugs that cause immunosuppression (e.g., steroids) and those that may result in drug fever (e.g., neuroleptics, anticholinergics, anesthetics, antibiotics).
4. **Social history.** What is the patient's travel history? Is there a history of injected drug use or other HIV risk factors? What is the patient's sexual history? Does the patient have pets or frequent animal contact? What are his or her occupation and hobbies? This information may lead to expanding the differential diagnosis to include diseases common in the developing world, HIV-related infections, sexually transmitted disease, tick-borne illnesses, endemic fungal disease, infectious complications such as endocarditis that are common in those using injected drugs, and so on.

Fever should be presumed to be secondary to an infection until proven otherwise because infections cause the majority of fevers and can be life-threatening.

B. Top-to-bottom approach. One way of determining the cause of a fever is to start at the patient's head and work your way down. Characteristic signs and symptoms (shown in parentheses) may increase your suspicion for the following disorders:

1. **Meningitis** (headaches, neck stiffness, photophobia)
2. **Sinusitis** (sinus tenderness)
3. **Otitis** (ear pain, diminished hearing)
4. **Pharyngitis** (sore throat, lymphadenopathy)
5. **Pneumonia** (cough, pleurisy, dyspnea)
6. **Endocarditis** (recent dental or other procedure, back pain, new skin lesions)
7. **Abdominal processes** (pain, change in bowel habits, nausea, vomiting)

8. **Urinary tract infection (UTI)** or **pyelonephritis** (dysuria, frequency, suprapubic or costovertebral angle tenderness)
9. **Pelvic infection** (discharge, dysuria)
10. **Prostatitis** (lower abdominal pain, tender prostate)
11. **Perirectal abscess** (pain, tenderness, swelling)
12. **Cellulitis** (erythema, pain, swelling)
13. **Joint infections** (pain, warmth, swelling)
14. **Local intravenous catheter site infection** (pain, pus)

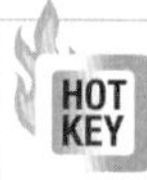

In patients exposed to antibiotics and presenting with diarrhea, always consider *Clostridium difficile* colitis.

C. Physical examination. A complete physical examination is critical and should cover all the areas mentioned in the review of systems.

Easily overlooked portions of the physical include a complete skin examination; a dental examination; careful evaluation of the joints, particularly the hips; a rectal and perirectal evaluation; and a pelvic examination. Each may provide critical clues that lead to the correct diagnosis.

D. Laboratory studies. The history and physical examination may provide enough information to make a diagnosis. Quite commonly, however, you may remain unsure about the etiology of the fever. The following laboratory tests will help you assess the likelihood of an infection and may also help to localize the source.

1. **Complete blood count (CBC) with platelets**
   a. **Neutropenia** with fever is a medical emergency and requires hospitalization and broad-spectrum antibiotics.
   b. A **leftward shifted white blood cell (WBC) count** often implies significant bacterial infection.
   c. A **low WBC count** may be just as worrisome as a high one; the WBC count may not be elevated in alcoholics, the elderly, HIV-infected patients, and other immunocompromised patients in the presence of a serious infection. Overwhelming infection can cause bone marrow suppression and a reduced WBC, which may be manifest before the presence of hemodynamic compromise. Many indolent infections may not be associated with elevations in the WBC. African-American patients normally have WBC counts slightly below the given "normal" range.

2. **Electrolytes with blood urea nitrogen (BUN)** and **creatinine.** The presence of an anion gap acidosis may indicate sepsis.
3. **Prothrombin time (PT)** and **partial thromboplastin time (PTT).** Abnormal coagulation studies may indicate disseminated intravascular coagulation (DIC), which may accompany serious infection.
4. **Liver tests** (e.g., bilirubin, alkaline phosphatase, and transaminase levels) help evaluate the possibility of hepatobiliary disease (e.g., cholecystitis, ascending cholangitis, liver abscess, hepatitis).
5. **Amylase levels** may be helpful if pancreatitis is suspected.
6. **Urinalysis** should always be done to evaluate the possibility of UTI.
7. **Urine pregnancy test.** A pregnancy test should be considered in all women of childbearing age.
8. **Cultures**
   a. **Blood cultures** provide the gold standard for diagnosing bacteremia. A minimum of two sets of blood cultures should be drawn. Depending on the organism, determining if a single positive blood culture represents true infection or skin contamination can be difficult. Patients at higher risk for endocarditis, such as those with prosthetic valves or a history of injected drug use, should always have blood cultures drawn.

Persistently positive blood cultures or multiple positive sets of cultures suggest an intravascular infection such as endocarditis, infectious aortitis, septic thrombophlebitis, or a vascular graft infection.

   b. **Urine culture with a urinalysis** should be obtained; however, bacteriuria in the absence of pyuria is unlikely to be the cause of fever.
   c. **Sputum evaluation** may be useful for patients with respiratory tract symptoms.
   d. **Throat culture** may be useful in patients with pharyngitis.
   e. **Cerebrospinal fluid (CSF) analysis** and **culture** is necessary in patients with meningeal symptoms or signs, altered mental status, or HIV infection and an unexplained fever.
   f. **Body fluid analysis** and **culture.** Patients with a fever accompanied by ascites, a pleural or joint effusion, or any other type of fluid collection need a diagnostic tap.

Patients who present with fever and rash should have a skin biopsy unless the diagnosis is straightforward.

E. **Radiographs**
   1. **Chest.** Posterior-anterior (PA) and lateral views should be taken on all patients with unexplained fever.
   2. **Abdomen.** Flat and upright views are useful when the patient has a fever and abdominal pain. Make sure to look for air–fluid levels, bowel distention, kidney stones, and free air.

F. **Ancillary studies.** At this point, you have systematically ruled out most of the possible infections from head to toe. If a diagnosis still has not been made, you need to consider the **easiest place for an infection to hide—the abdomen and pelvis.**
   1. **Computed tomography (CT).** A CT scan is the best radiographic test in this situation. It provides a thorough evaluation of the intra-abdominal organs and is more sensitive than ultrasound for detecting occult abscesses.
   2. **Ultrasound.** Abdominal ultrasound is often inadequate for ruling out intra-abdominal abscesses and other pathology, but may be better than a CT scan for evaluating the gallbladder and bile ducts (e.g., for cholecystitis or ascending cholangitis).
   3. **Other tests** [e.g., **bone marrow biopsy, liver biopsy, indium or positron emission tomography (PET) scans, bone scans]** may be obtained if the cause of the fever is still in question (see Chapter 51).

III. **TREATMENT.** If a potentially dangerous infection is suspected, or close follow-up is uncertain, admission to the hospital is warranted. Patients who are elderly, are immunocompromised, or have other organ system disease may also require admission.

A. **General measures**
   1. **Fluids** need to be administered to keep up with increased insensible losses.
   2. **Discontinuing medications** that may be responsible for a fever can be both diagnostic and therapeutic.

B. **Empiric antibiotic therapy**
   1. Nontoxic patients who are otherwise stable can be closely watched without antibiotics until a diagnosis is made.
   2. Patients hospitalized for fever and neutropenia, hospitalized for meningitis, or who are critically ill should be treated empirically pending culture results.
   3. A low threshold for giving empiric antibiotics should also be used for patients who are immunocompromised,

including those with HIV infection, diabetes, alcoholism, or liver or renal disease, and patients who are asplenic or taking steroids or immunosuppressants.

C. Antipyretic therapy

1. **Acetaminophen** (325–650 mg every 4 hours as needed) is given initially to provide symptomatic relief. It should preferentially be administered in response to fever rather than around the clock so the temperature curve can be monitored.
2. **Indomethacin** (25–50 mg every 8 hours) and cold sponge baths may be useful for persistent fevers.
3. **Evaporative cooling** is often used for patients with a temperature greater than 41°C. In this technique, the patient is sprayed with cool water while fans move ambient air across the body. Cooling blankets can be utilized as well.

REFERENCES

O'Grady NP, Barie PS, Bartlett JG, et al. Guidelines for evaluation of new fever in critically ill adult patients: 2008 update from the American College of Critical Care Medicine and the Infectious Diseases Society of America. Crit Care Med 2008;36(4):1330–1349.

Sipsas NV, Bodey GP, Kontoyiannis DP. Perspectives for the management of febrile neutropenic patients with cancer for the 21st century. Cancer 2005;103(6):1103–1113.

Speil C, Mushtag A, Adamski A, et al. Fever of unknown origin in the returning traveler. Infect Dis Clin North Am 2007;21(4):1091–1113.

49 Approach to Microbiology

I. OVERVIEW OF MICROBIOLOGY. The simplest way to approach microbiology is to divide the organisms into **six major categories** (based on Gram stain, morphology, and aerobic requirements) and consider the most important diseases each organism can cause.

A. Gram-positive cocci

1. ***Streptococcus***
   a. **Group A** streptococci cause "strep throat," scarlet fever, rheumatic fever, erysipelas, cellulitis, and pneumonia.
   b. **Group B** streptococci cause mainly perinatal infections and a variety of infections in adults [e.g., urinary tract infection (UTI), sepsis].
   c. ***S. pneumoniae*** causes pneumonia (usually lobar), bacteremia, meningitis, and endocarditis.
   d. **Viridans** streptococci are the most common cause of bacterial endocarditis.
   e. ***S. milleri*** originates from the gastrointestinal (GI) tract and causes abscesses, including pulmonary and central nervous system abscesses.
2. ***Enterococcus*** causes UTIs, intra-abdominal infections, endocarditis, and nosocomial infections. Infections caused by *Enterococcus* can be difficult to treat.
3. ***Staphylococcus***
   a. ***S. aureus*** (coagulase positive) causes skin infections, toxic shock syndrome, endocarditis, intravascular line infections, osteomyelitis, septic arthritis, pneumonia, and nosocomial infections. *S. aureus* is a virulent organism that has a propensity to cause "metastatic" infections.
   b. ***S. epidermidis*** (coagulase negative) causes intravascular line infections and prosthetic valve endocarditis.
   c. ***S. saprophyticus*** (coagulase negative) causes UTIs.

B. Gram-positive rods

1. ***Clostridium*** (anaerobic) can cause tetanus, botulism, food poisoning, antibiotic-associated colitis, cellulitis and skin infections, gas gangrene, abscesses, and septicemia.
2. ***Bacillus*** can cause cutaneous and pulmonary anthrax (woolsorter's disease, recently an agent of bioterrorism). Most cases in the United States are cutaneous; pulmonary

anthrax is usually fatal. *B. cereus* is a common cause of diarrhea.

3. ***Nocardia*** usually causes pulmonary disease that may disseminate (in immunocompromised hosts), leading to brain abscesses and subcutaneous nodules. *Nocardia* species are weakly acid-fast.
4. ***Actinomyces*** (anaerobic) causes cervicofacial infections (following dental infection or trauma), chronic pneumonia, abdominal infections (which may be confused with Crohn's disease), and pelvic inflammatory disease (PID) associated with the use of an intrauterine contraceptive device (IUD).
5. ***Listeria monocytogenes*** causes sporadic cases of meningitis and bacteremia as well as food-borne outbreaks in elderly or immunocompromised adults.
6. ***Erysipelothrix*** causes three types of human illness: erysipeloid (a localized skin lesion); a diffuse skin eruption accompanied by systemic illness; and bacteremia (usually associated with endocarditis). *Erysipelothrix* is acquired through skin abrasions following contact with infected swine, fish, turkeys, ducks, and sheep.
7. ***Corynebacterium***
   a. ***C. diphtheriae*** causes cutaneous, nasopharyngeal, and oropharyngeal infections. Infections of the respiratory tract are characterized by a thick, gray membrane over the pharynx and tonsils.
   b. ***C. jeikeium*** (group JK) causes sepsis, primarily in hospitalized, neutropenic cancer patients who are receiving multiple antibiotics and who have some type of skin disruption.
   c. **"Diphtheroids"** are common, nonpathogenic skin contaminants.

MNEMONIC **Gram-Positive Rods ("CLumsy BActeria NOrmally ACt LIke ERror-prone COrnballs")**

***Cl**ostridium*
***Ba**cillus*
***No**cardia*
***Ac**tinomyces*
***Li**steria monocytogenes*
***Er**ysipelothrix*
***Co**rynebacterium*

C. Gram-negative cocci

1. ***Neisseria***
   a. ***N. meningitidis*** causes meningitis (in children and young adults), meningococcemia (30%–50% of patients

have meningococcemia without meningitis), and sinusitis.

b. ***N. gonorrhoeae*** commonly causes urethritis (in both men and women) and endocervicitis, which may progress to PID or disseminated gonococcal infection (DGI). *N. gonorrhoeae* also causes pharyngitis and conjunctivitis.

2. ***Moraxella catarrhalis*** causes sinusitis, bronchitis, and pneumonia; however, it is often difficult to distinguish colonization from actual infection.

D. Gram-negative rods comprise the largest category of pathogenic organisms. Infections can involve many different systems, including the genitourinary, hepatobiliary, GI, and respiratory systems. Sepsis involving gram-negative rods is a major cause of mortality, especially for neutropenic or otherwise immunocompromised patients. A partial list of pathogens in this category follows.

1. ***Escherichia coli*** causes the majority of UTIs and can cause intra-abdominal and biliary infections—all of which may lead to sepsis.
2. ***Klebsiella*** causes the same diseases as *E. coli* as well as sinusitis and pneumonia (especially in alcoholics).
3. ***Pseudomonas*** is a destructive organism that can lead to sepsis following a variety of illnesses (e.g., skin, ear, sinus, eye, urinary tract, or lung infections). *Pseudomonas* infection is often nosocomial and usually occurs in the setting of local tissue damage or impaired host defenses.
4. ***Haemophilus influenzae*** causes pneumonia, bacteremia (especially in patients who have undergone splenectomy), cellulitis, otitis media, epiglottitis, sinusitis, chronic bronchitis, and meningitis (although less commonly now because of the availability of an effective vaccine).
5. ***Bordetella pertussis*** causes whooping cough (primarily in children) and prolonged bronchitis in adults.
6. ***Brucella*** causes an insidious febrile illness characterized by easy fatigability, headache, cervical and axillary lymphadenopathy, hepatosplenomegaly, and lymphocytosis. Acquisition of brucellosis is usually via animal contact or following ingestion of contaminated milk.
7. ***Francisella tularensis*** causes tularemia, a multisystem disorder (fever, headache, lymphadenopathy, prostration) usually acquired via rabbit or tick contact.
8. ***Yersinia pestis*** causes plague and is acquired via flea or rodent bites.
9. ***Salmonella, Shigella, Campylobacter, Yersinia enterocolitica,*** and ***Vibrio*** species can all cause infectious diarrhea.

E. Anaerobes. The anaerobes ***Actinomyces*** and ***Clostridium*** are discussed with the gram-positive rods. ***Bacteroides fragilis,***

B. (Prevotella) melaninogenicus, Peptostreptococcus, and ***Fusobacterium*** are also anaerobes.

1. In general, anaerobes are implicated (either alone or in combination) in gingivitis, sinusitis, otitis, abscesses (dental, brain, lung, intra-abdominal), aspiration pneumonia, empyema, skin and soft tissue infections, and pelvic infections.
2. As a rule of thumb, treatment of an abscess primarily depends on drainage and only secondarily depends on antibiotics.

F. Miscellaneous organisms

1. ***Rickettsia.*** Infections include Rocky Mountain spotted fever, murine (endemic) typhus fever, and louse-borne (epidemic) typhus fever.
2. ***Mycoplasma pneumoniae*** is the most common cause of pneumonia ("walking pneumonia") in young adults.
3. ***Chlamydiae.*** Infections include chlamydia (the most common sexually transmitted disease in the United States), lymphogranuloma venereum (LGV), trachoma, conjunctivitis, psittacosis, and pneumonia (in young adults).

II. ANTIMICROBIAL THERAPY. The best way to learn about antibiotics is to know the organisms that each antibiotic (or class of antibiotics) covers well and which organisms are missed. This information can be found in many antimicrobial guides.

III. APPROACH TO THE PATIENT

A. List approximately three of the most common or potentially lethal organisms that can cause the illness with which you are confronted.

B. Select an antibiotic that covers the organisms that are most likely responsible for the infection, making sure to consider cost, convenience, and coverage of potentially life-threatening pathogens.

If a patient is very ill, elegant antibiotic combinations are less important than broad coverage to protect against a potentially lethal organism.

REFERENCES

Catterall JR. Streptococcus pneumoniae. Thorax 1999;54(10):929–937 [Classic article].

Driscoll JA, Brody SL, Kollef MH. The epidemiology, pathogenesis, and treatment of Pseudomonas aeruginosa infections. Drugs 2007;67(3): 351–368.

Lowy FD. Staphylococcus aureus infections. N Engl J Med 1998;339(8):520–532 [Classic article].

Steer AC, Danchin MH, Carapetis JR. Group A streptococcal infections in children. J Pediatr Child Health 2007;43(4):203–213.

■ Fever and Rash

50

I. INTRODUCTION. Like chest pain, the symptom complex of fever and rash may represent an acute, life-threatening disease or a benign condition.

II. SEVEN KILLER CAUSES OF FEVER AND RASH. Although there are many causes of fever and rash, you must first consider the diseases that may kill the patient within hours. A SMARTTT physician can easily remember these seven killer causes:

MNEMONIC **Seven Killer Causes of Fever and Rash ("SMARTTT")**

Sepsis
Meningococcemia
Acute endocarditis
Rocky Mountain spotted fever
Toxic erythemas
Toxic epidermal necrolysis (TEN)
Travel-related infections

A. Sepsis. Fever accompanied by a generalized erythematous rash may signal impending sepsis (usually caused by gram-negative organisms).

B. Meningococcemia. Patients usually appear acutely ill. A petechial rash develops in most patients.

Disseminated gonococcal infection (DGI) is a less dangerous *Neisseria* infection that may also produce fever and rash. DGI often presents with palpable purpuric pustules and may be associated with fever, tenosynovitis, polyarthralgias, or septic arthritis.

C. Acute endocarditis should be considered in all patients with fever and a petechial rash. A careful cardiac examination is always necessary.

D. Rocky Mountain spotted fever. After 2–6 days of a flu-like febrile illness, a macular rash usually appears over the ankles or wrists. The rash spreads centrally and may evolve into a petechial rash.

E. **Toxic erythemas** include **toxic shock syndrome (TSS), staphylococcal scalded skin syndrome (SSSS), scarlet fever,** and **scarlatiniform eruptions.**

Common features of toxic erythemas include fever and an erythematous rash that is most significant in the flexural folds and later desquamates; mucocutaneous involvement occurs frequently.

1. **TSS** results in a diffuse erythematous rash that blanches easily; desquamation occurs after 1–2 weeks (see Chapter 90). Both *Staphylococcus aureus* and *Streptococcus pyogenes* can cause TSS.
2. **SSSS** results in generalized erythema and desquamation.
3. **Scarlet fever** follows *S. pyogenes* pharyngitis. Although it may not be immediately life-threatening, scarlet fever should always be considered when the patient presents with toxic erythema. Scarlatiniform eruptions resemble the rash of scarlet fever and are usually caused by *S. aureus.*

F. **Toxic epidermal necrolysis (TEN)** is caused by a reaction to **drugs.** It is a "SNAP" to remember the drugs that commonly cause TEN:

MNEMONIC **Drugs That Commonly Cause TEN ("SNAP")**

Sulfonamides
Nonsteroidal anti-inflammatory drugs (NSAIDs)
Allopurinol
Phenytoin

TEN results in large areas of erythema and desquamation and may be clinically indistinguishable from SSSS.

G. **Travel-related infections.** Fever and rash in a recent traveler should alert you to the possibility of a potentially life-threatening viral illness. Most of these dangerous viruses are acquired in Latin America, Africa, or Asia.
   1. **Hemorrhagic fevers** are the most worrisome and include Ebola, Lassa, and Hanta virus infection. These disorders are often characterized by petechiae or purpura as well as other types of bleeding, and are associated with a high mortality rate.

III. APPROACH TO THE PATIENT

A. **Rule out the seven killer causes of fever and rash.** In general, you will be able to rule out these life-threatening causes of fever and rash by paying attention to the patient history and the clinical manifestations of disease, including the rash.

1. **Patient history.** Always remember to obtain a **medication** and **travel history.** A negative drug and travel history usually rules out **TEN** and **hemorrhagic fever** as potential etiologies.
2. **Clinical manifestations**
   a. **Ill appearance.** Patients with **meningococcemia, Rocky Mountain spotted fever,** or **sepsis** usually appear systemically ill.
   b. **Cardiac murmur. Acute endocarditis** is usually accompanied by a cardiac murmur (see Chapter 54).
   c. **Rash**
      (1) **Desquamating rashes** often signal **toxic erythema** or **TEN.**
      (2) **Petechial rashes** should always alert you to the possibility of meningococcemia, Rocky Mountain spotted fever, or endocarditis.
3. **Helpful data**
   a. Laboratory evaluation to assess other organ systems may be necessary when toxic shock is still a consideration (e.g., in a patient who appears ill or has low blood pressure).
   b. Most of the toxic erythemas (with the exception of SSSS) can usually be ruled out on clinical grounds; however, a skin biopsy is always indicated to differentiate **SSSS** from **TEN.** A **s**plit epidermis (i.e., intraepidermal separation) is found in **S**SSS, whereas **t**otal epidermal separation (i.e., subepidermal separation) is seen in **T**EN.

B. Address other diagnostic possibilities.

1. **Types of lesions.** One way to establish a concise differential diagnosis of a fever and rash is to first determine the type of primary lesion (Table 50-1).
2. **Differential diagnoses.** Some common etiologies for each primary lesion associated with a fever are provided below.
   a. **Macules** and **papules** (or a **maculopapular rash**)
      (1) **Drug reactions** commonly present with a pruritic, confluent eruption over the trunk that usually occurs within 1 week of starting a new medication. Fever is usually absent.
      (2) **Viral infections** [e.g., measles and other childhood viral exanthems, infectious mononucleosis, primary human immunodeficiency virus (HIV)] usually result in rashes that are nonpruritic. Fever and other viral symptoms are often present.
      (3) **Toxic erythemas** are usually accentuated in the flexural folds, are not pruritic, and may have mucous membrane involvement.
      (4) **Connective tissue diseases** [e.g., systemic lupus erythematosus (SLE), Still's disease] often present

TABLE 50-1

TYPES OF CUTANEOUS LESIONS

Lesion	Description
Macules	Discolored, flat lesions
Papules	Raised lesions; <0.5 cm in diameter
Vesicles	Lesions filled with clear fluid; <0.5 cm in diameter
Bullae	Large vesicles (i.e., >0.5 cm in diameter)
Pustules	Pus-filled vesicles
Nodules	Raised lesions >0.5 cm in diameter and depth
Plaques	Raised lesions >0.5 cm in diameter, but without depth
Purpura	Purple, nonblanchable lesion
Petechiae	Purpuric lesions <3 mm in diameter
Ecchymoses	Purpuric lesions >3 mm in diameter

with rash in association with other characteristic symptoms (e.g., arthralgias).

(5) **Bacterial infections** are less likely causes.
   (a) **Lyme disease** may cause erythema chronicum migrans.
   (b) **Secondary syphilis** most often results in scaling papules that are present on the palms and soles.
   (c) **Typhoid fever** can cause "rose spots," which are usually seen as an individual papule on the trunk that fades with pressure.

b. **Vesicles** and **bullae** (see "VESICLES" mnemonic below).

MNEMONIC **Differential Diagnoses for Vesicles and Bullae Accompanied by Fever ("VESICLES")**

Viral infections (e.g., varicella-zoster, herpes simplex, Coxsackie)
Erythema multiforme
SSSS
Impetigo (bullous)
Contact dermatitis
LESs likely etiologies (e.g., porphyria cutanea tarda, bullous pemphigoid, pemphigus vulgaris, dermatitis herpetiformis)

c. **Pustules** (see "Very Full of PUS" mnemonic below).

MNEMONIC

Differential Diagnosis for Pustules Accompanied by Fever ("Very Full of PUS")

Viral infections (e.g., varicella-zoster, herpes simplex)
Fungal infections (e.g., candidiasis)
Pustular psoriasis
Urethritis related (i.e., DGI)
Syphilis

d. **Nodules** and **plaques**
   (1) **Nonpainful**
      (a) **Fungal infections**
      (b) **Lymphoma**
   (2) **Painful**
      (a) **Erythema nodosum** presents with tender nodules on the lower legs. It is often associated with another illness (e.g., tuberculosis, coccidioidomycosis, sarcoid, poststreptococcal infection) or pregnancy.
      (b) **Sweet's syndrome** should be suspected in patients with fever, neutrophilia, and red-brown lesions (usually on the head and upper extremities). The syndrome may be associated with leukemias (usually acute myelogenous leukemia), lymphomas, myelodysplasia, or other malignancies. Infiltration of neutrophils into the dermis is seen on biopsy.

e. **Purpura**
   (1) **Palpable purpura** is pathognomonic for **vasculitis** (see Chapter 76).
   (2) **Nonpalpable purpura.** Petechiae usually indicate a bleeding disorder (e.g., thrombocytopenia), and ecchymoses often result from vessel fragility (e.g., actinic purpura); however, overlap does exist [e.g., necrotic ecchymoses may occur with disseminated intravascular coagulation (DIC)].

Purpuric lesions in a patient with fever may be the harbinger of a life-threatening illness. Hemorrhagic fever, meningococcemia, Rocky Mountain spotted fever, endocarditis, sepsis, and vasculitis all need to be considered carefully and ruled out.

REFERENCES

Cunha BA. Rash and fever in the critical care unit. Crit Care Clin 1998;14:35–53 [Classic article].

Knowles SR, Shear NH. Recognition and management of severe cutaneous drug reactions. Clin Derm 2007;25(2):245–253.

Schlossberg D. Fever and rash. Infect Dis Clin North Am 1996;10:101–110 [Classic article].

51 Fever of Unknown Origin

I. INTRODUCTION. Fever of unknown origin (FUO) is defined as a temperature greater than 38.3°C for more than 3 weeks that eludes diagnosis even after 1 week of in-hospital evaluation. More recent authors have suggested that the duration of time in the hospital be modified to include patients whose illness remains undiagnosed after at least three outpatient visits or 3 days in the hospital. These definitions were designed to exclude common undiagnosed viral syndromes and to identify a homogenous population to describe in studies. This definition is arbitrary, and the following approach should be used in patients in whom the etiology of fever is obscure despite an initial work-up.

II. COMMON CAUSES OF FUO (Table 51-1)

A. Although the percentage of FUOs due to infectious etiologies is declining, infections still account for the majority of FUOs.

1. **Bacterial infections**
   a. **Intra-abdominal abscesses** (e.g., in the liver, spleen, or kidney) are especially common causes of FUO.
   b. **Osteomyelitis** and **sinusitis** are other localized infections that may elude initial diagnosis.
   c. **Bacteremias** from endocarditis, salmonellosis (typhoid fever), and brucellosis commonly cause FUO. Intravascular graft infections present with bacteremia and can be very difficult to diagnose.
   d. **Mycobacterial infections**
      (1) **Tuberculosis** is a common cause of FUO and is likely the most common cause worldwide. Human immunodeficiency virus (HIV)-infected patients have a higher rate of extrapulmonary tuberculosis.
      (2) ***Mycobacterium avium* complex infections** are the leading cause in the United States of FUO in patients with acquired immune deficiency syndrome (AIDS). CD4 counts are typically less than 50 in this setting.
   e. **Spirochetal infections. Secondary syphilis, leptospirosis,** and **Lyme disease** should be considered.
   f. **Rickettsial infections** include the typhus group (epidemic, endemic, and scrub typhus), the spotted fever group

TABLE 51-1

COMMON CAUSES OF FEVER OF UNKNOWN ORIGIN

Disease Category	Examples
Infectious	Bacterial, mycobacterial, viral, fungal, parasitic, spirochetal, rickettsial
Neoplastic	Lymphomas, leukemias, hepatic cancer, renal cancer, atrial myxoma
Connective tissue disorders	Systemic lupus erythematosus, rheumatoid arthritis, Still's disease, vasculitides
Miscellaneous	Inflammatory bowel disease, granulomatous hepatitis

(Rocky Mountain spotted fever, rickettsialpox, and tick fever), and other similar illnesses (trench fever and ehrlichiosis).

2. **Viral infections**
   a. **Cytomegalovirus (CMV) infection** is a common cause of FUO. Acute CMV infection in immunocompetent patients often presents without localizing signs.
   b. **Epstein-Barr virus infection** causes mononucleosis (especially in adolescents and young adults).
3. **Fungal infections**
   a. **Histoplasmosis** and **coccidioidomycosis** can cause FUO in immunocompetent or immunocompromised patients.
   b. **Candidiasis** and **aspergillosis** are opportunistic fungal infections that may cause FUO.
4. **Parasitic infections. Amebiasis, malaria,** and **toxoplasmosis** may cause FUO and are common causes of FUO in developing countries.

B. **Neoplasms.** Lymphomas, leukemias, hepatic and renal cancers, and atrial myxomas are often associated with febrile syndromes. Concurrent infection should always be ruled out.

C. **Connective tissue disorders.** Systemic lupus erythematosus (SLE), rheumatoid arthritis, Still's disease, giant cell arteritis, and the vasculitides (see Chapter 76) can all cause FUO.

D. **Other causes.** Inflammatory bowel disease, sarcoidosis, and granulomatous hepatitis may cause prolonged fever. Factitious fever and drug fever should also be considered.

III. **APPROACH TO THE PATIENT.** Because the cause of an FUO is elusive (by definition), there is a tendency to try to ''net the diagnosis'' by ordering every test under the sun. Proceeding in a logical, stepwise fashion will decrease the number of tests your patient must undergo, the cost of the total work-up, and the incidence of false-positive results. Before delving into an extensive evaluation, rule out factitious (patient-induced) fever by observing the elevated temperature reading yourself.

A. Go where the money is! The best bet for making a diagnosis is pursuing any symptoms, signs, or abnormal laboratory test results that present along with the fever. Make sure to always go down the list of possibilities from head to toe as outlined in Chapter 48. For example:

1. **Persistent headaches with a normal cerebrospinal fluid analysis.** A computed tomography (CT) scan or magnetic resonance imaging (MRI) may be indicated to rule out an intracranial abscess or sinusitis.
2. **Cardiac murmurs** associated **with negative blood cultures** may be evaluated with echocardiography (transthoracic or transesophageal).
3. **Hemoptysis** or **chronic cough** in the presence of an unremarkable chest radiograph may be further evaluated with a chest CT scan or bronchoscopy.
4. **Hematuria** may prompt an intravenous pyelogram or ultrasound to evaluate the possibility of renal carcinoma.
5. **Lymphadenopathy** may be evaluated by biopsy.
6. **Bone pain** can be pursued with radiographs and a bone scan.
7. **Cytopenias** can be evaluated by bone marrow biopsy.

In HIV-infected patients, you can use the **CD4 count** to help predict the disease processes a patient is likely to have (see Chapter 55). *Mycobacterium avium* complex infections and CMV infections are common causes of FUO in AIDS patients with low CD4 counts (<100 cells/μl).

B. Diagnostic studies

1. **Initial considerations**
   a. **Abdominal and pelvic CT scan.** There is no better place for an infection (e.g., an abscess) or malignancy (e.g., liver or renal carcinoma) to hide than in the abdomen or pelvis; therefore, performing this test early in the diagnostic work-up may be valuable.
   b. **Chest CT.** Although occult pulmonary infection is less common than occult abdominal abscess, unexpected findings (including infiltrates, cavitation, and lymphadenopathy) may lead to the diagnosis.
   c. **Screens for tuberculosis, Epstein-Barr virus,** and **syphilis** may be performed with a purified protein derivative (PPD) test, a heterophil antibody test, and a serum Venereal Disease Research Laboratory (VDRL) test, respectively.

d. **Rheumatologic work-up.** An antinuclear antibody (ANA) assay, a rheumatoid factor assay, and an erythrocyte sedimentation rate (ESR) are often requested early in the evaluation. Any rashes that are purpuric should be biopsied to rule out vasculitis (see Chapter 76).

e. **Other tests** may be ordered based on epidemiologic exposures. For example:

(1) **Thick and thin blood smears** examined every 8 hours for 2–3 days are appropriate if the patient has traveled to areas where malaria is endemic.

Fever in a traveler should be considered malaria until proven otherwise.

(2) **Stool for culture** or **ova and parasite (O&P) examination** is also useful in patients with an appropriate travel history.

(3) **Amebic titers** can help evaluate chronic intestinal amebiasis in patients with a remote travel history because O&P stool examination is usually negative in patients with chronic disease.

(4) **Toxoplasmosis titers** are approximately 85% sensitive for end-organ toxoplasmosis.

(5) **Specific serologies** or **cultures** for brucellosis, leptospirosis, Lyme disease, Rocky Mountain spotted fever, and other spirochetal and rickettsial diseases may be sent, depending on the geographic region, exposures to animals or the outdoors, and the clinical presentation.

(6) ***M. avium* complex** blood cultures may be performed in HIV-positive patients with low CD4 counts.

2. **Secondary considerations**

a. **Radionuclide studies**

(1) **Gallium scans, indium-labeled white blood cell (WBC) scans, and positron emission tomography (PET) scans** are often used when no etiology has been found. These tests are limited by low specificity.

(2) Bone scans may be performed to rule out osteomyelitis and primary or metastatic malignancies of bone.

b. **Invasive tests**

(1) **Bone marrow biopsies** are generally of low diagnostic yield, but are low risk and are often performed when the diagnosis is still in question.

(2) **Liver biopsies** have a higher yield in patients with abnormal liver tests.
(3) **Endoscopy** (upper and lower) should be performed earlier in the work-up if there are any gastrointestinal symptoms, signs, or suggestive laboratory abnormalities (e.g., a positive fecal occult blood test, iron deficiency anemia).
(4) **Temporal artery biopsy** may be revealing in elderly patients with FUO, even in the absence of localizing symptoms.
(5) **Bronchoscopy** should be performed in patients with suggestive abnormalities on chest radiograph or chest CT or by symptoms. In HIV-infected patients, bronchoscopy should be pursued as part of the standard work-up of FUO even in the asymptomatic patient.
(6) Exploratory laparotomy in the absence of abnormal findings on imaging studies no longer plays a significant role in the evaluation of FUO.

REFERENCES

Cunha BA. Fever of unknown origin: clinical overview of classic and current concepts. Infect Dis Clin North Am 2007;21(4):867–915.

Cunha BA. Fever of unknown origin: focused diagnostic approach based on clinical clues from the history, physical examination, and laboratory tests. Infect Dis Clin North Am 2007;21(4):1137–1187.

Hot A. Fever of unknown origin in HIV/AIDS patients. Infect Dis Clin North Am 2007;21(4):1013–1032.

Mourad O, Palda V, Detsky AS. A comprehensive evidence-based approach to fever of unknown origin. Arch Intern Med 2003;163(5):545–551 [Classic article].

Petersdorf RO, Beeson PB. Fever of unexplained origin: report on 100 cases. Medicine (Baltimore) 1961;40:1–30 [Classic article].

Safdar N, Abad CL, Kaul DR, et al. Clinical problem-solving: an unintended consequence. N Engl J Med 2008;358(14):1496–1501.

52

Skin and Soft Tissue Infections

I. INTRODUCTION

A. The **severity** of skin and soft tissue infections **can vary from insignificant to life-threatening** and is determined by both the causative organism and the depth of tissue involvement.

B. **Cellulitis** and **animal bites** are common reasons for emergency department visits and hospital stays.

C. **Pyomyositis** and **necrotizing fasciitis** are two clinical entities that may be difficult to distinguish from cellulitis but require different therapies. Necrotizing fasciitis is associated with a high mortality.

II. CELLULITIS

A. **Definition.** Cellulitis is an **infection of the dermal and subcutaneous tissues,** including the deep dermis and fat.

B. **Clinical manifestations.** Patients are often febrile and complain of pain at the affected site. On physical examination, erythema, warmth, tenderness, and edema are notable.

C. **Microbiology.** The most common etiologic agents are ***Staphylococcus aureus*** and **streptococcal species,** most commonly group A streptococcus. In specific settings, other organisms may cause cellulitis, including gram-negative bacilli and anaerobes.

D. **Approach to the patient.** Several historical features may provide important clues about the etiology of disease and may lead the physician to broaden empiric therapy or to watch for serious manifestations.

1. **Has any trauma occurred in the involved area?** Injections (e.g., diabetics requiring insulin, intravenous drug users) and skin tears can provide routes of entry for bacteria.
2. **Has the involved area been exposed to soil or fresh or salt water?** Soil exposure may increase the risk of anaerobes or gram-negative infections. Water exposure increases the risk of infection with organisms such as *Aeromonas hydrophila* or *Vibrio vulnificus.*
3. **Does the patient have any comorbid conditions?** Underlying diabetes or neoplasm may increase the risk of group B

streptococcal infection. Patients with cirrhosis are at increased risk of *V. vulnificus* infection after salt water exposure or eating raw shellfish.

4. **Is the cellulitis adjacent to a surgical wound or a diabetic foot ulcer?** Both these circumstances increase the risk of infection with gram-negative organisms or resistant gram-positive organisms [e.g., methicillin-resistant *S. aureus* (MRSA)].
5. **Did the cellulitis start in an area of an animal bite** (see III)?
6. **Does the patient's pain seem out of proportion to the examination? Is the area of cellulitis spreading over minutes to hours? Is there crepitus, or are there bullous lesions?** A positive answer to any of these questions should lead the physician to consider more serious diagnoses that require more aggressive intervention (see V).
7. **Is the border of the lesion raised and well demarcated? Is the involved area significantly edematous and indurated?** The presence of these findings likely indicates **erysipelas,** which is actually a more superficial infection than cellulitis. Erysipelas is almost always caused by group A streptococci.
8. **Is there an abscess?** The presence of an abscess suggests infection with **community-acquired MRSA** (CA-MRSA). The classic presentation of CA-MRSA is a cutaneous lesion that looks like a "spider bite" with development of surrounding cellulitis and abscess formation.

E. Treatment

1. **In the absence of several of the risk factors** discussed in II D (e.g., animal bite, surgical wound, presence of underlying diabetes mellitus or malignancy, contamination of the site with soil or environmental water), narrow coverage with an agent that covers streptococcal and staphylococcal species is preferred. Reasonable intravenous choices include nafcillin or cefazolin; good oral choices include cephalexin or dicloxacillin.
2. **If cellulitis is associated with a surgical wound,** vancomycin may be a more appropriate initial choice. Gram-negative coverage should be tailored to the appropriate organisms based on historical exposures.
3. **If CA-MRSA is suspected,** vancomycin is an appropriate intravenous choice. Good oral choices include linezolid, tetracycline, trimethoprim-sulfamethoxazole, or clindamycin. If an abscess is present, drainage is indicated.

III. ANIMAL BITES

A. Epidemiology. Animal bites are a common reason for emergency department visits. Patients often present acutely, within hours of the bite, or later after cellulitis or deeper infections have developed.

B. Microbiology. Infections due to bites from dogs and cats most often are caused by *S. aureus,* streptococcal species, gram-positive anaerobes, and *Pasteurella multocida.* Less common organisms include *Capnocytophaga canimorsus,* which causes fulminant disease in patients with liver disease or splenectomy; *Francisella tularensis* (tularemia); and rabies virus.

C. Approach to the patient

1. **Determine the history of the bite.**
   a. **What type of animal was it? Was the bite unprovoked?** The first responsibility of the treating physician is to determine whether the patient needs **rabies prophylaxis.** Rabies is uncommon in the United States, but it is fatal without appropriate prophylaxis. Bats and raccoons are known to harbor the rabies virus. Domesticated dogs are not a common source of the virus, but an unprovoked attack should lead to observation of the animal and consideration of prophylaxis.
   b. **How rapidly have symptoms developed after the bite?** Rapidly progressive cellulitis should lead to consideration of *P. multocida* infection.
   c. **Was the bite a cat bite and was it near a joint?** Cat bites can leave deep puncture wounds, which appear unimpressive but can inoculate organisms deep into a joint or tendon sheath, leading to septic arthritis, osteomyelitis, or tenosynovitis. Examination should be performed carefully to consider these complications, and patients with cat bites should be followed closely and treated aggressively.
2. **Culture the wound** if possible.

D. Treatment. In non–penicillin-allergic patients, the **treatment of choice is ampicillin/sulbactam** or **amoxicillin/clavulanate.** Ciprofloxacin plus clindamycin may be considered in the penicillin-allergic patient.

IV. PYOMYOSITIS

A. Definition. Pyomyositis is a bacterial infection of the muscle, which can mimic cellulitis.

B. Epidemiology. In the United States, pyomyositis occurs most often in immunocompromised patients (e.g., patients with diabetes or cirrhosis, individuals taking corticosteroids) and those with local trauma (e.g., intravenous drug users).

C. Microbiology. The most common etiology is *S. aureus.* Streptococci and gram-negative bacilli are much less common.

D. Approach to the patient. Typically, the onset is subacute. Pyomyositis progresses to a febrile illness with pain, erythema, and fluctuance at the involved site.

1. Pyomyositis should be considered in the differential diagnosis in patients with the following conditions:
   a. Risk factors (e.g., patients receiving systemic corticosteroids, presence of diabetes mellitus or cirrhosis, intravenous drug use, HIV infection)
   b. Slowly resolving cellulitis despite usual treatment
   c. "Cellulitis" in a less typical location (e.g., thigh) or with more induration or fluctuance than expected
2. Magnetic resonance imaging (MRI) or computed tomography (CT) of the affected area can aid in diagnosis.

E. Treatment. Adequate therapy requires both antistaphylococcal antimicrobial therapy (e.g., nafcillin) and adequate drainage (e.g., percutaneous aspiration or open surgical drainage).

V. NECROTIZING FASCIITIS

Necrotizing fasciitis is a **true clinical emergency** and has a mortality rate of 30%. Differentiation of necrotizing fasciitis from cellulitis in the early stages requires an astute clinician and close follow-up.

A. Definition. Necrotizing fasciitis is a necrotizing cellulitis that involves the superficial fascia and subcutaneous tissues.

B. Epidemiology. Patients at increased risk include those with diabetes or alcoholism, with immunosuppressed status, or with peripheral vascular disease.

C. Clinical manifestations

1. There is often a **preexisting history of trauma,** including recent surgery, but the insult may be minor (e.g., a small cut or site of injection).
2. The **most common involved areas** are the **extremities, perineum,** and **abdominal wall.**
3. **Spread of infection is rapid.** The initial stages are notable for **pain out of proportion to the examination,** with minimal or absent skin changes. Over hours to days, **loss of sensation can occur** due to tissue ischemia and nerve destruction. Erythema, edema, cyanosis, and bullous formation may develop. **Crepitus** (subcutaneous gas) is an ominous sign. Patients are ill-appearing, with high fevers, and become hemodynamically unstable.

D. Microbiology. Two primary types of necrotizing fasciitis have been described. The first is **polymicrobial** and may involve gram-positive and gram-negative organisms, including anaerobes. The second is caused by **group A streptococci.**

E. Approach to the patient

1. **Diagnosis of this condition in the early stages is difficult.** Serial clinical examinations are necessary in patients who appear to have cellulitis with atypical features **(too much pain, too high a fever, bullous lesions, hemodynamic instability)** and in those with **underlying immunosuppressive conditions** (diabetes, alcohol abuse, end-stage renal disease) or **recent trauma.** Marking the involved area with a pen is helpful to gauge progression over time.
2. **CT or MRI may be helpful** but should be reserved for stable patients. The diagnosis should be confirmed in the operating room in acutely ill patients.

If a diagnosis of necrotizing fasciitis is seriously being considered, it is never too early to ask for a surgical evaluation.

F. Treatment. Adequate therapy combines urgent **surgical debridement with antimicrobial therapy.** Blood cultures and surgical wound cultures can help guide therapy. Antimicrobial therapy should be broad and include anaerobic coverage until the etiologic organisms are identified. Many clinicians favor including clindamycin in the regimen because its mechanism (protein synthesis inhibition) leads to inhibition of bacterial toxin synthesis.

REFERENCES

Abrahamian FM, Talan DA, Moran GJ. Management of skin and soft tissue infections in the emergency department. Infect Dis Clin North Am 2008;22(1):89–116.

Anaya DA, Dellinger EP. Necrotizing soft tissue infection: diagnosis and management. Clin Infect Dis 2007;44(5):705–710.

Bisno AL, Stevens DL. Streptococcal infections of skin and soft tissues. N Engl J Med 1996;334:240–245. [Classic article].

Crum NF. Bacterial pyomyositis in the United States. Am J Med 2004;117(6):420–428.

Stryjewski ME, Chambers HF. Skin and soft-tissue infections caused by community-acquired methicillin-resistant *Staphylococcus aureus.* Clin Infect Dis 2008;46 Suppl. 5: S368–377.

53 Acute Rheumatic Fever

I. INTRODUCTION

A. Definition. Acute rheumatic fever is a systemic, immune-mediated disorder that occurs as a **sequela** to **group A streptococcal pharyngeal infection.** (Skin infections are not associated with rheumatic fever.)

B. Epidemiology. Acute rheumatic fever most commonly occurs in school-age children, 1–5 weeks (mean, 19 days) after an acute throat infection.

1. Acute rheumatic fever rarely occurs in patients younger than 5 years of age or older than 40 years of age.
2. It is uncommon in the United States but can be seen in recent immigrants.

C. Rheumatic fever **"bites the heart and licks the joints"** [i.e., chronic arthritis is not a sequela of rheumatic fever, but valve disease and congestive heart failure (CHF) can be]. The incidence of valve involvement varies depending on the valve.

1. The **mitral valve** is affected in the **majority** of cases.
2. The **aortic valve** is affected in **less than half** of cases (but almost never as the sole valve).
3. The **tricuspid** and **pulmonary valves** are affected in **less than 5%** of cases, usually in association with mitral valve involvement.

II. DIAGNOSIS

A. Jones criteria. Diagnosis of rheumatic fever is based on evidence of a preceding streptococcal pharyngitis [e.g., a positive antistreptolysin O (ASO) titer or culture], plus two major Jones criteria or one major and two minor Jones criteria.

1. **Major**
   a. **Arthritis.** The arthritis takes the form of a migratory polyarthritis that tends to involve the large joints sequentially; however, adults may have only single joint involvement. Arthritis resolves spontaneously within 1 month, and there are no residual joint deformities.
   b. **Heart involvement.** Evidence of carditis includes pericarditis, myocarditis, cardiomegaly, congestive heart failure, and mitral or aortic regurgitation.

c. **Nodules.** Small, firm, nontender subcutaneous nodules occur over areas of bony prominence and over tendons. Nodules are rarely seen in adults.

d. **Erythema marginatum** is the classic rash seen in less than 10% of cases. It is erythematous and nonpruritic. Individual lesions are evanescent with a serpiginous border.

e. **Sydenham's chorea (St. Vitus's dance)**—the most diagnostic of the major criteria—is characterized by involuntary choreoathetoid movements of the face, hands, and feet.

MNEMONIC **Major Jones Criteria ("J♡NES")**

Joints (arthritis)
♡ Involvement
Nodules
Erythema marginatum
Sydenham's chorea

2. **Minor**
   a. **Prolongation of the PR interval** on the electrocardiogram (ECG)
   b. **Increased erythrocyte sedimentation rate (ESR) and/or C-reactive protein (CRP)**
   c. **Fever**
   d. **Polyarthralgias**
   e. **Supporting evidence of antecedent group A streptococcal infection** including either a positive throat culture or rapid antigen test or an elevated or rising streptococcal antibody titer

B. Clinical presentation. Rheumatic fever usually presents in one of three ways:

1. **Insidious carditis**
2. **Acute-onset polyarthritis**
3. **Chorea** (least common)

III. TREATMENT

A. Bed rest. The patient should be confined to bed until the fever, tachycardia, and ECG changes resolve.

B. High-dose salicylates will rapidly decrease fever and joint swelling but do not affect the natural course of the illness. If salicylates do not provide symptomatic relief, steroids should be considered.

C. Antibiotics

1. **Prophylactic** antibiotics are recommended to prevent further streptococcal infections. The preferred regimen remains intramuscular penicillin every 4 weeks and should be

continued for a minimum of 5 years after the last episode *and* until the patient is in his or her mid-20s.

REFERENCES

Carapetis JR, McDonald M, Wilson NJ. Acute rheumatic fever. Lancet 2005;366(9480):155–168.

Cilliers AM. Rheumatic fever and its management. BMJ 2006;333(7579): 1153–1156.

Infective Endocarditis

54

I. INTRODUCTION

A. Once uniformly fatal, infective endocarditis (IE) continues to cause significant morbidity and mortality in the postantibiotic era. Early diagnosis by an astute clinician and proper therapy can improve outcomes substantially.

B. Before the availability of effective antibiotics, IE was classified as acute or subacute based on the organism and the clinical course. Today, these distinctions are less meaningful.

C. Certain subgroups of patients are at increased risk of IE development and should be evaluated carefully for evidence of disease. They include (1) persons with valvular abnormalities, including congenital bicuspid aortic valves and those with a history of rheumatic fever; (2) patients with prosthetic valves; and (3) intravenous drug users.

II. CAUSES OF INFECTIVE ENDOCARDITIS

A. Streptococci. Viridans streptococci (*Streptococcus salivarius, S. sanguis, S. mitis/mitior,* and *S. milleri*) remain the most common cause of IE. However, in recent years, staphylococcal species are increasing in importance. Other streptococcal species including **enterococci, *S. bovis*** (nonenterococcal group D streptococci), and occasionally ***S. pneumoniae*** are important causes of IE as well.

B. Staphylococci. IE caused by ***Staphylococcus aureus*** and ***S. epidermidis*** has increased in frequency and now is nearly as common as viridans streptococcal endocarditis. *S. aureus* is the most frequent cause of IE in those with a history of intravenous drug use and is an important cause of nosocomial endocarditis. *S. epidermidis* is the most common bacteria isolated in cases of prosthetic valve endocarditis.

C. Gram-negative bacteria can cause endocarditis, usually in association with genitourinary or gastrointestinal procedures, surgery, or intravascular catheters.

D. Fungi. Fungal endocarditis has a poorer prognosis than bacterial IE and is associated with injection drug use, long-term antimicrobial therapy, and chronic hyperalimentation therapy. *Candida* spp. account for the majority of cases of fungal IE.

E. Culture-negative endocarditis is most frequently encountered in patients who have received prior antibiotics leading to sterile blood cultures. Certain organisms may be difficult to detect in routine culture systems, however. These include:

1. **HACEK group organisms.** ***H****aemophilus,* ***A****ctinobacillus,* ***C****ardiobacterium,* ***E****ikenella,* and ***K****ingella* are gram-negative organisms that often grow slowly over weeks; therefore, ask the laboratory to save the blood cultures for a prolonged period if culture-negative endocarditis is suspected.
2. **Nutritionally variant streptococcal species (now known as *Abiotrophia* spp.)** require specific media supplementation for growth.
3. **Fungi.** Large vegetations are often found in patients with endocarditis associated with fungal infection. An intravascular source is frequently noted (e.g., an indwelling intravenous catheter). *Candida* species are easily isolated in routine cultures; however, *Aspergillus* is almost never recovered from cultures. Other rare fungal causes of IE, including *Histoplasma capsulatum,* may require special fungal cultures (lysis-centrifugation system).
4. ***Legionella*, *Brucella* spp., *Coxiella burnetii*** (Q fever), ***Bartonella henselae*** (cat scratch disease), and ***Chlamydia* spp.** (including *Chlamydia psittaci*) are rare causes of culture-negative endocarditis.

III. CLINICAL MANIFESTATIONS OF INFECTIVE ENDOCARDITIS.

The clinical manifestations of endocarditis are variable, but most closely depend on which organism is involved and whether the patient has left-sided (aortic or mitral) or right-sided (usually tricuspid) disease.

A. Fever occurs in almost all patients; however, elderly patients, patients with congestive heart failure or renal failure, and patients taking steroids or nonsteroidal anti-inflammatory drugs (NSAIDs) may be afebrile. Other systemic symptoms such as **anorexia** and **malaise** are common.

B. Murmurs. Although a cardiac murmur is a classic sign of endocarditis, a murmur may be absent in as many as 15% of patients, and a new or changing murmur is present in only 3%–5% and 5%–10% of patients, respectively.

C. Low back pain, arthralgias, and **myalgias** are very common and may be the patient's presenting symptoms.

D. Splenomegaly may be seen in one-quarter to one-half of patients.

E. Classic findings, including **Osler's nodes, Janeway lesions, Roth spots** (retinal hemorrhages), **petechiae of the palate or conjunctivae,** and **subungual splinter hemorrhages** are often not found, probably because of early treatment of disease in the antimicrobial era.

Although Osler's nodes are typically violaceous nodules located on the pads of the fingers or toes and Janeway lesions are typically erythematous and found on the palms or soles, the predominant distinction between the two is that **Osler's nodes** are **painful,** whereas **Janeway lesions** are **painless.**

IV. COMPLICATIONS OF INFECTIVE ENDOCARDITIS

A. Congestive heart failure (CHF). Pulmonary edema and hypotension may occur with significant left-sided (aortic and mitral) valve dysfunction, whereas peripheral edema may result from right-sided (tricuspid) disease.

B. Myocardial abscess formation can lead to bundle branch block (aortic valve abscesses) or heart block (mitral valve abscesses). Perivalvular abscesses are common in patients with prosthetic valve endocarditis.

C. Emboli. Left-sided endocarditis may result in visceral infarcts, including splenic, hepatic, renal, central nervous system, and mesenteric infarcts as well as cutaneous infarcts. Right-sided endocarditis may cause septic pulmonary emboli with pulmonary infarction, abscess formation, or both.

D. Hematogenous seeding of other sites may occur, including bone (vertebral osteomyelitis), joint (septic arthritis), and other vessels (mycotic aneurysms).

V. APPROACH TO THE PATIENT

A. Patient history

1. IE is a diagnosis that is often missed; therefore, always make sure to include endocarditis in the "head to toe" approach to fever (see Chapter 48).
2. Be sure to ask the patient about risk factors for endocarditis (i.e., intravenous drug use, known valvular disease, recent procedures or surgery).

B. Physical examination. In addition to performing a complete physical examination, pay special attention to the:

1. **Funduscopic examination** (to search for Roth spots)
2. **Cardiovascular examination** (to detect murmurs or evidence of CHF)
3. **Skin and mucous membrane examination** (to search for Osler's nodes, Janeway lesions, splinter hemorrhages, and conjunctival or palatal petechiae)
4. **Bone and joint examination** (to detect septic joints or osteomyelitis)

C. Laboratory studies. Patients who have an unexplained fever, have a low clinical probability of endocarditis, and are conscientious concerning follow-up can sometimes be evaluated as outpatients. Patients with fever and a prosthetic valve, history of intravenous drug use, or examination findings concerning for endocarditis and no obvious alternative source of infection are almost always admitted to rule out endocarditis.

1. **Blood cultures** are the **gold standard** for diagnosis. **A minimum of two sets** of aerobic and anaerobic cultures are usually obtained; however, three sets may increase the sensitivity to greater than 90%.
   a. Different venous sites are usually used to avoid confounding skin contamination.
   b. Cultures should always be taken before initiating empiric antibacterial therapy.
2. **Urinalysis.** Abnormal urinalysis findings are common in endocarditis. Hematuria or proteinuria is common; red blood cell casts suggestive of glomerulonephritis should be sought.
3. **Echocardiography.** Because the duration of therapy may differ depending on which side of the heart (left or right) is involved, echocardiography is often performed to define which valve is infected and to identify complications of disease such as myocardial abscesses. Transthoracic echocardiography is often performed first, followed by transesophageal echocardiography in cases in which the diagnosis is still in question; however, the cost-effectiveness of this approach is unclear.
   a. **Transthoracic echocardiography (TTE),** with a sensitivity of approximately 60%, is not sensitive enough to rule out endocarditis. In addition, TTE is notoriously poor for ruling out mitral valve disease and evaluating prosthetic valves.
   b. **Transesophageal echocardiography (TEE)** increases the sensitivity to approximately 95% and is significantly better for evaluating the mitral valve.

VI. TREATMENT

A. Empiric therapy. Empiric therapy should be initiated only when the patient appears unstable or acutely ill. Patients with stable symptoms for days to weeks should be watched carefully while not taking antibiotics until a causative agent is discovered. Ill patients should receive vancomycin and gentamicin pending cultures. Penicillin and gentamicin is an appropriate empiric regimen in patients suspected of having viridans streptococcal endocarditis, but often these patients are not acutely ill, and the diagnosis can be made with blood culture data before urgently starting therapy.

The benefits of added gentamicin include the following:

- Synergy against *S. aureus,* which decreases the duration of bacteremia
- Broader coverage against gram-negative and multiorganism infections, an important advantage in intravenous drug users

1. **Suspected prosthetic valve endocarditis** may be treated with vancomycin, rifampin, and an aminoglycoside. This regimen will cover methicillin-resistant *S. epidermidis* (a common offender) while treating possible enterococcal infection as well.

B. Organism-specific therapy. The duration of therapy may vary depending on the causative organism, the severity of the illness, and whether disease is right or left sided.

1. **Viridans streptococcal infections** are usually treated with penicillin or ceftriaxone with or without an aminoglycoside. Therapy most commonly lasts for 4 weeks.
2. **Enterococcal infections** usually require prolonged combination therapy and are often treated with ampicillin or vancomycin and an aminoglycoside for 4–6 weeks.
3. **Staphylococcal infections**
   a. **Methicillin-sensitive *S. aureus* (MSSA) infections** may be treated with nafcillin or oxacillin.
   b. **Methicillin-resistant *S. aureus* (MRSA) infections** may be treated with vancomycin.
   c. **Prosthetic valve staphylococcal infections** should be treated with combination therapy with rifampin and 2 weeks of an aminoglycoside in addition to the aforementioned agents when possible.

C. Surgery. Valve replacement is often indicated when:

1. Fungal infection is strongly suspected.
2. A prosthetic valve is infected.
3. Complications have developed (e.g., myocardial abscess, acute valvular dysfunction with refractory CHF).
4. There is uncontrolled infection (inability to clear blood cultures).
5. The patient has experienced more than one embolic event.

VII. FOLLOW-UP

A. Frequent examinations are essential. Listen carefully for a new or changing murmur, look closely for embolic phenomena, and watch for widening of the pulse pressure (which should alert you to possible aortic regurgitation).

1. **Bilateral disease.** Although intravenous drug users more commonly have right-sided disease, they may also have left-sided or bilateral endocarditis. You should therefore continue to assess possible left-sided involvement.
2. **Persistent fever.** Defervescence occurs within 1 week in 72% of patients. Prolonged fever is an important prognostic sign. Drug reactions are the most common cause of persistent or recurrent fever, but myocardial and metastatic abscess formation should always be considered.

B. Electrocardiogram (ECG). Lengthening of the PR interval or a new bundle branch block should prompt an echocardiogram to evaluate possible myocardial abscess formation. (TEE is more sensitive.) An ECG should be obtained on admission and often on a frequent basis thereafter.

REFERENCES

Baddour LM, Wilson WR, Bayer AS, et al. Infective endocarditis: diagnosis, antimicrobial therapy, and management of complications: a statement for healthcare professionals from the Committee on Rheumatic Fever, Endocarditis, and Kawasaki Disease, Council on Cardiovascular Disease in the Young, and the Councils of Clinical Cardiology, Stroke, and Cardiovascular Surgery and Anesthesia, American Heart Association: endorsed by the Infectious Diseases Society of America. Circulation 2005;111(23):e394–434.

Durack DT, Lukes AS, Bright DK. New criteria for diagnosis of infective endocarditis: utilization of specific echocardiographic findings. Duke Endocarditis Service. Am J Med 1994;96(3):200–209 [Classic article].

Hermans PE. The clinical manifestations of infective endocarditis. Mayo Clin Proc 1982;57(1):15–21 [Classic article].

Houpikian P, Raoult D. Blood culture-negative endocarditis in a reference center: etiologic diagnosis of 348 cases. Medicine (Baltimore) 2005; 84(3):162–173.

55

CD4 Counts and Complications of HIV Infection

I. INTRODUCTION. In human immunodeficiency virus (HIV)-positive patients, a physician must consider many different possible diagnoses when the patient presents with a new symptom. These diagnoses include causes of disease present in nonimmunocompromised patients as well as those opportunistic infections and malignancies that present more frequently in patients with HIV. Furthermore, HIV-infected patients may present with protean symptoms such as fever and weight loss instead of classic manifestations of disease that may be produced by a vigorous inflammatory response. The list of possible diagnoses can often be simplified because patients infected with HIV acquire opportunistic infections and malignancies at relatively predictable CD4 counts. Therefore, a recent CD4 count may help you exclude etiologies of disease more likely at greater degrees of immunosuppression. Remember, however, that patients with very low CD4 counts may get any of the conditions noted as occurring at any higher CD4 count.

Remember that a CD4 count obtained during an acute illness may be falsely low or falsely high. It is therefore best to use the most recent CD4 count before the development of acute illness if available.

II. DIFFERENTIAL DIAGNOSES ACCORDING TO CD4 COUNT. CD4 counts should only be used as a general guide because there is a great deal of variability among patients. Common diseases that occur as the CD4 count falls are discussed here.

A. CD4 count greater than 200 cells/μl

1. **Bacterial infection.** Pneumococcal pneumonias are common.
2. **Pulmonary tuberculosis.** Both primary tuberculosis and reactivation disease can be seen at relatively high CD4 counts. As CD4 counts drop below 200 cells/μl, less common manifestations such as extrapulmonary tuberculosis

and miliary tuberculosis are encountered more frequently. Extrapulmonary sites may include the central nervous system (CNS), peritoneum, lymph nodes, pleura, and bone and joints.

3. **Lymphoma.** B-cell lymphomas are more common in HIV-infected patients at any CD4 count, and diagnosis of B-cell lymphoma in any individual should prompt HIV testing even in the absence of known risk factors. In patients with CD4 counts in this range, lymphomas are systemic, not the primary CNS lymphomas that occur with lower counts.
4. **Kaposi's sarcoma.** Patients may have pulmonary and gastrointestinal involvement as well as the typical cutaneous lesions.
5. **Herpes zoster.** Herpes zoster may present with a multidermatomal or single dermatome distribution.
6. **Candidiasis**
   a. **Oral and vaginal candidiasis** are very common.
   b. **Disseminated disease** is more likely in patients with neutropenia or intravascular catheters, or in those taking broad-spectrum antibiotics.

B. CD4 count less than 200 cells/μl

1. ***Pneumocystis jirovecii* (formerly *carinii*) pneumonia** (see Chapter 56)
2. ***Cryptococcus* infection** is a common cause of meningitis.
3. **Coccidioidomycosis** may be manifested as pneumonia, meningitis, or skin and soft tissue infection.
4. **Histoplasmosis** can cause pulmonary disease or disseminate with pulmonary, hepatic, bone marrow, and CNS involvement as well as fungemia.
5. **Extrapulmonary or miliary tuberculosis.** See A 2.
6. **Progressive multifocal leukoencephalopathy (PML).** Caused by JC virus, PML can lead to focal neurologic deficits (see Chapter 58).

C. CD4 count less than 100 cells/μl

1. **Toxoplasmosis** often manifests with CNS disease (see Chapter 58).
2. **Cryptococcosis** most commonly causes meningitis, but patients may have pulmonary or cutaneous disease as well.
3. **Candida esophagitis.** Although other manifestations of candidiasis may present at higher CD4 counts, esophagitis tends to be seen in patients with more impaired immunity.

D. CD4 count less than 50 cells/μl

1. **Disseminated *Mycobacterium avium* complex (MAC) infection** usually causes fever, cytopenias, and cachexia.
2. **Cytomegalovirus (CMV) infection.** Retinitis, esophagitis, colitis, acquired immunodeficiency syndrome (AIDS) cholangiopathy, and polyradiculopathy may all be seen with CMV infection.
3. **Primary CNS lymphoma** (see Chapter 58)

REFERENCE

http://hopkins-hivguide.org. This website is maintained by Johns Hopkins University and contains an online HIV guide that can be downloaded to handheld, mobile devices. This and the book version (*Medical Management of HIV Infection*) are valuable and up-to-date resources about HIV infection.

Pulmonary Disease in HIV-Infected Patients

I. INTRODUCTION. At least two-thirds of patients with human immunodeficiency virus (HIV) have symptomatic pulmonary disease at some time during their lives. One way to approach respiratory complaints in HIV-infected patients is to:

A. Consider the organisms that can cause disease based on the patient's **CD4 count** (see Chapter 55).

B. Narrow the list of possible diagnoses by considering the appearance of the **chest radiograph** (Table 56-1). These patterns are not mutually exclusive, and each pattern can be caused by many disorders. When it comes to HIV disease, there are few absolute truths—use Table 56-1 as a starting point and modify it based on your clinical experience.

C. Further narrow the list based on the **clinical picture, laboratory data,** and results of **diagnostic testing.**

II. DIFFERENTIAL DIAGNOSIS OF PULMONARY INFILTRATES IN HIV

A. Bacterial. Bacterial pathogens remain the most likely cause of pneumonia in HIV-infected patients. Pneumonia due to *Streptococcus pneumoniae* is most common. Remember that *Haemophilus influenzae,* gram-negative bacilli (including *Pseudomonas*, particularly in late-stage HIV), *Legionella* species, and *Nocardia* can also be seen.

B. Mycobacterial. Tuberculosis and nontuberculous mycobacteria such as *Mycobacterium kansasii* are not uncommon. *M. avium* complex frequently colonizes sputum but is rarely viewed as a pathogen.

C. Fungal. Cryptococcosis, histoplasmosis, and aspergillosis all may present with pulmonary manifestations in HIV-infected patients.

D. Viral. The respiratory viruses including influenza, adenovirus, and respiratory syncytial virus must be remembered. A nasal swab for antigen testing can provide evidence of infection.

E. *Pneumocystis jirovecii.* See III.

F. Noninfectious. Both lymphoma and Kaposi's sarcoma may cause pulmonary disease.

TABLE 56-1

RADIOGRAPHIC PATTERNS IN HIV-ASSOCIATED PULMONARY DISEASE

Radiographic Pattern	Common Disease
Normal	*Pneumocystis jirovecii* pneumonia (PCP)
Diffuse interstitial infiltrates	PCP
	Disseminated fungal infection
	Tuberculosis
	Kaposi's sarcoma*
	Congestive heart failure (CHF)
	Viral and atypical pneumonia
Focal consolidation	Bacterial pneumonia
	Kaposi's sarcoma
	Tuberculosis
Pleural effusion	Tuberculosis
	Lymphoma
	Bacterial pneumonia
	Kaposi's sarcoma
	CHF
	Disseminated fungal infection

*Usually patchy infiltrates.

III. APPROACH TO THE HIV-INFECTED PATIENT WITH POSSIBLE *PNEUMOCYSTIS JIROVECII* PNEUMONIA. Whenever a patient with HIV disease presents with respiratory complaints, the diagnosis of *P. jirovecii* pneumonia (PCP) should always be considered because *P. jirovecii* is an extremely common pathogen.

A. The following questions are important to ask when considering PCP as a possible diagnosis:

1. What is the **CD4 count**? The CD4 count will indicate the patient's risk for PCP; those with CD4 counts greater than 200 cells/μl are at much less risk.
2. Is the patient receiving **PCP prophylaxis**? Patients taking trimethoprim-sulfamethoxazole or dapsone are less likely to have PCP.
3. What is the **clinical scenario?** Patients with PCP usually present with a subacute onset of shortness of breath (especially on exertion) that is associated with fever, fatigue, weight loss, and a dry cough. Community-acquired pneumonia, on the other hand, usually presents with the acute onset of a productive cough, fever, and evidence of consolidation on lung examination.

4. Does the physical examination reveal **evidence of a different disorder (e.g., tuberculosis, lymphoma,** or **Kaposi's sarcoma)?**
5. Does the chest radiograph reveal **diffuse interstitial infiltrates?** Diffuse interstitial infiltrates are the classic finding; patients may, however, present with minimal changes or atypical findings (e.g., pleural effusions, pneumothorax).

The radiographic appearance of the lung fields often looks much worse than predicted by auscultation in patients with PCP; however, a normal chest radiograph does not exclude PCP.

6. What is the patient's **alveolar-to-arterial (A-a) gradient**? The blood gas report allows definition of the degree of hypoxemia as well as evaluation for the necessity of steroid therapy in patients with PCP. (Patients with an A-a gradient >35 usually benefit when treated with corticosteroids.)

Oxygen saturation monitoring can be very useful. Patients who exhibit dramatic desaturation on ambulation may have PCP.

7. Is the **sputum purulent?** Finding *P. jirovecii* organisms is extremely difficult in purulent sputum. On the other hand, culturing sputum for routine pathogens and acid-fast bacilli (AFB) organisms may be diagnostic.

B. There are many ways to evaluate patients for the possibility of PCP. The algorithm in Figure 56-1 is one approach; it should be modified based on the sensitivity and specificity of the various tests available at your institution.

C. Treatment. First-line therapy for PCP in nonallergic patients is intravenous trimethoprim-sulfamethoxazole (TMP-SMX) 5 mg/kg intravenously (IV) every 8 hours. If the A-a gradient is greater than 35, corticosteroids (e.g., prednisone) should be added. The usual dose is 40 mg twice daily for 5 days followed by 40 mg once daily for 5 days, then a taper to zero over the ensuing 11 days. Treatment of PCP should be continued for 21 days. Patients may be switched to oral therapy once defervescence occurs and the patient is no longer hypoxic on ambulation at room air. Stable, reliable patients who are not initially hypoxic may receive their entire course of therapy orally. TMP-SMX two double-strength tablets orally three times per day is recommended. Options for TMP-SMX–intolerant patients include intravenous pentamidine, dapsone plus trimethoprim, or clindamycin plus primaquine.

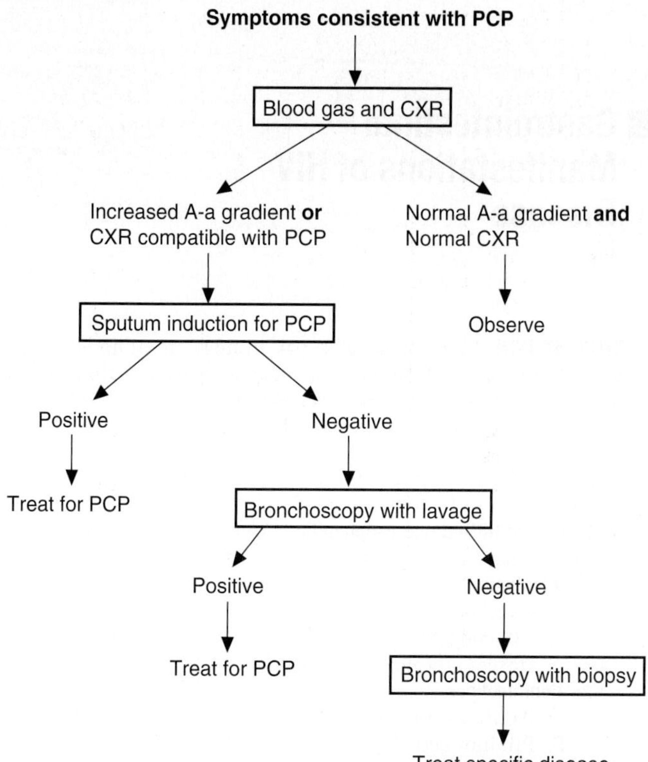

Figure 56-1 Algorithm for the assessment of patients with suspected *Pneumocystis jirovecii* pneumonia (*PCP*). *A-a gradient* = alveolar-to-arterial gradient; *CXR* = chest radiograph.

REFERENCES

Bartlett JG. Pneumonia in the patient with HIV infection. Infect Dis Clin North Am 1998;12:807–820 [Classic article].

D'Avignon LC, Schofield CM, Hospenthal DR. *Pneumocystis* pneumonia. Semin Respir Crit Care Med 2008;29(2):132–140.

Rosen MJ. Pulmonary complications of HIV infection. Respirology 2008; 13(2):181–190.

57

Gastrointestinal Manifestations of HIV Disease

I. INTRODUCTION. More than 50% of human immunodeficiency virus (HIV)-infected patients develop a gastrointestinal illness during the course of their disease. Esophagitis, enterocolitis, and hepatobiliary disease are commonly seen.

II. ESOPHAGITIS usually presents with dysphagia, odynophagia, or a substernal sensation of pain or burning.

A. Causes of HIV-related esophagitis. Common causes include the following:

1. **Infectious**
   a. *Candida*
   b. Cytomegalovirus (CMV)
   c. Herpes simplex virus (HSV)
2. **Noninfectious**
   a. Aphthous ulcers
   b. Pill induced

B. Approach to the patient

1. **Empiric antifungal therapy.** Patients with symptoms of esophagitis and oral thrush are usually treated empirically for candidal esophagitis. **Fluconazole** (often 200 mg orally once daily) may be administered for 2–3 weeks. A rapid improvement in symptoms is expected. Failure to improve should lead to further testing.
2. **Upper endoscopy** is usually indicated for patients without oral thrush and for those who are unresponsive to empiric antifungal therapy. Abnormal areas on endoscopy should be biopsied and sent for pathology as well as viral and fungal cultures. Viral and fungal esophagitis can coexist. Aphthous ulcers are an important consideration in those with negative cultures and pathology.

C. Treatment

1. **Fungal esophagitis**
   a. **Fluconazole** is usually the first-line treatment, unless fluconazole-resistant *Candida* is suspected. **Intravenous**

amphotericin (0.1–0.3 mg/kg/day) may be necessary in patients with resistant species. Itraconazole and amphotericin solution are also options, along with voriconazole.

b. **Maintenance therapy** may be given as one-half of the treatment dose (e.g., fluconazole 100 mg once daily).

2. **Viral esophagitis**

a. **CMV esophagitis** is usually treated with **ganciclovir** (often 5 mg/kg intravenously twice daily for 2–3 weeks). The maintenance dose is often 5 mg/kg intravenously daily. Oral agents (valganciclovir) also have a role in maintenance therapy.

b. **HSV esophagitis** is usually treated with **acyclovir.** Intravenous therapy may be necessary in patients who are unable to swallow and in those who are very ill (e.g., in patients with esophageal bleeding or fevers).

3. **Noninfectious esophagitis including aphthous ulcers** may be treated with **steroids** (often prednisone, 40 mg orally daily for 2 weeks followed by a taper) or **thalidomide.**

III. ENTEROCOLITIS. More than 50% of HIV-positive patients develop diarrhea at some time during their illness.

A. Causes of HIV-related enterocolitis

1. **Opportunistic infection**

a. **Bacteria.** ***Salmonella, Shigella, Yersinia, Escherichia coli,*** and ***Campylobacter*** are common causes of acute diarrhea in HIV-positive patients. ***Clostridium difficile*** is an important consideration even in patients without recent exposure to antibiotics.

b. **Protozoa.** Commonly implicated organisms include ***Entamoeba histolytica, Giardia lamblia, Cryptosporidium, Microsporidia,*** and ***Isospora belli.***

c. **Viruses. CMV** and **adenovirus** are common causes of enterocolitis in HIV-infected patients.

d. ***Mycobacterium avium* complex (MAC)** can cause diarrhea; however, stool is frequently colonized with this organism in the absence of disease.

2. **Acquired immunodeficiency syndrome (AIDS)-associated enteropathy** is a diagnosis of exclusion. It is not known whether this entity is directly caused by HIV itself.

B. Approach to the patient

1. **Laboratory studies**

a. **Fecal white blood cell (WBC) count.** A fecal WBC should be performed.

b. **Stool culture** should be performed to rule out bacterial infection.

c. **Stool ova and parasites (O&P).** Three samples are generally sent to increase the yield. The evaluation for *Cryptosporidium* and *Microsporidia* is enhanced by an **acid-fast stain** and a **modified trichrome stain,** respectively.

d. **Enzyme-linked immunosorbent assay (ELISA) for *C. difficile* toxin.** *C. difficile* may be a commonly missed diagnosis.

e. **Routine blood cultures** for *Salmonella* should be considered. In patients with CD4 counts less than 50 cells/μl, mycobacterial blood cultures for **MAC** should be obtained.

2. **Endoscopy** is often necessary when symptoms continue, and no etiology has been identified.
   a. CMV is a very common pathogen that is often missed by the initial screening studies.
   b. Colonoscopy with biopsy (followed by upper endoscopy with small bowel biopsy if colonoscopy findings are normal) should be performed.

C. Treatment

1. **Specific therapy** depends on the causative organism. Most bacterial causes of enterocolitis are fluoroquinolone susceptible, but increasing resistance is being reported, particularly with *Campylobacter.* Oral metronidazole is first line for *C. difficile.* Tinidazole or nitazoxanide is now considered first line for *Giardia. Isospora* responds to trimethoprim-sulfamethoxazole. Amebiasis can be treated with metronidazole plus paromomycin. Cryptosporidium can be treated with nitazoxanide and fumagillin and microsporidia with albendazole; but these infections tend to respond poorly.

IV. HEPATOBILIARY DISEASE. Abnormal transaminases, alkaline phosphatase, and bilirubin are common among HIV-infected patients. These abnormalities may be clinically insignificant and asymptomatic, but may be the initial indication of opportunistic infections and neoplastic disease or dangerous drug toxicity.

A. Causes of HIV-related hepatic parenchymal disease

1. **Viruses,** including **hepatitis B, hepatitis C,** and **CMV**
2. ***M. avium* complex** and less commonly, ***M. tuberculosis* infection**
3. **Fungal infections** including **histoplasmosis**
4. **Malignancy** including **lymphoma, Kaposi's sarcoma,** and **hepatocellular carcinoma**
5. **Medications**
   a. **Sulfa drugs, isoniazid, rifampin,** and **fluconazole** are well-known causes of hepatitis.
   b. All **antiretroviral medications** have been associated with transaminase elevations. Of these, the most serious is

hepatitis due to **nevirapine** (a nonnucleoside reverse transcriptase inhibitor), which can lead to fulminant hepatic failure.

c. **Nucleoside reverse transcriptase inhibitors** can cause hepatic steatosis in association with lactic acidosis leading to a transaminitis. If not recognized early, the lactic acidosis may be fatal.

6. Peliosis hepatis from ***Bartonella henselae*** or ***B. quintana***

B. Causes of HIV-associated obstructive biliary tract disease

1. **Sclerosing cholangitis** (i.e., **AIDS cholangiopathy**) often presents with right upper quadrant pain accompanied by significant elevation in alkaline phosphatase level that is out of proportion to transaminase elevations. Biliary involvement with CMV or *Cryptosporidium* is commonly associated with AIDS cholangiopathy, while *Microsporidia* and MAC are less common causes.
2. Remember that the protease inhibitors **indinavir** and **atazanavir** can cause an asymptomatic unconjugated hyperbilirubinemia.

C. Approach to the patient

1. **Patient history.** A medication history should be obtained to search for potentially hepatotoxic medications. Pain should be carefully characterized, including location and relationship to food.
2. **Physical examination.** As always, a careful physical examination should be performed, looking for cutaneous and other manifestations of disease such as drug rash, skin lesions suggestive of Kaposi's sarcoma or fungal infection, and lymphadenopathy.
3. **Laboratory studies**
   a. **Liver studies** [aspartate aminotransferase (AST), alanine aminotransferase (ALT), alkaline phosphatase, fractionated bilirubin]
   b. **Hepatitis A, B,** and **C serologies** should be obtained.
   c. **Blood cultures** for ***M. avium* complex, fungi, and *Bartonella* species** may be ordered.
   d. If hepatic steatosis with lactic acidosis is a consideration, obtain a **serum lactate** level.
   e. A **urine histoplasmosis antigen** may be diagnostic of disseminated histoplasmosis.
   f. **Serum quantitative CMV** studies should be obtained [CMV DNA by polymerase chain reaction (PCR)].
   g. **Stool studies** for *Cryptosporidium* and *Microsporidia*
4. **Imaging studies.** Although initial evaluation may uncover a potential etiology, it is often unclear whether that disease is an incidental finding or the cause of the hepatobiliary

process. Imaging studies are often performed to rule out other disorders (e.g., lymphoma).

a. **Ultrasound** may be especially useful for evaluating the bile ducts and is therefore often chosen for patients suspected of having biliary obstruction.
b. **Computed tomography (CT).** A CT scan provides better resolution of the liver parenchyma and is useful for patients suspected of having parenchymal disease.
c. **Endoscopic retrograde cholangiopancreatography (ERCP)** may be used for the diagnosis and treatment of sclerosing cholangitis. In this disease, intraluminal irregularities of the bile ducts are often accompanied by distal narrowing of the common bile duct (i.e., papillary stenosis). Biliary brushings for culture and cytology can be obtained during the procedure.

5. **Liver biopsy** may be considered for patients with a negative evaluation and persistent symptoms.

D. Treatment depends on the cause. In patients with sclerosing cholangitis, **papillary sphincterotomy** may provide symptomatic benefit.

After obtaining the history, performing the examination, and obtaining initial liver chemistries, think about whether the patient is presenting predominantly with obstructive or infiltrative disease (elevations of alkaline phosphatase out of proportion to transaminases) or hepatitis (transaminases elevated out of proportion to alkaline phosphatase) and whether the process is acute or chronic. This can help direct the remainder of your work-up. As a rough guideline, drugs and viral hepatitis tend to present with hepatitis, whereas many of the other listed etiologies are more likely to show an alkaline phosphatase–predominant pattern.

REFERENCES

Cohen J, West AB, Bini EJ. Infectious diarrhea in HIV. Gastronterol Clin North Am 2001;30(3):637–664 [Classic article].

Mahajani RV, Uzer MF. Cholangiopathy in HIV-infected patients. Clin Liver Dis 1999;3(3):669–684 [Classic article].

Sidiq H, Ankoma-Sey V. HIV-related liver disease: infection versus drugs. Gastroenterol Clin North Am 2006;35(2):487–505.

Zaidi SA, Cervia JS. Diagnosis and management of infectious esophagitis associated with HIV infection. J Int Assoc Physicians AIDS Care 2002;1(2):53–62.

58 Neurologic Manifestations of HIV Disease

I. INTRODUCTION. Human immunodeficiency virus (HIV)-infected patients frequently develop neurologic disorders, which can be divided into five clinical categories: meningitis, space-occupying lesions, encephalopathy, myelopathy, and peripheral neuropathy.

II. MENINGITIS

A. Causes of meningitis. The following are common causes of meningitis in HIV-positive patients.

1. **Bacteria** (see Chapter 88)
2. **Viruses. Herpes simplex virus (HSV) and cytomegalovirus (CMV)** may cause aseptic meningitis and encephalitis. **HIV** itself may cause a slight cerebrospinal fluid (CSF) pleocytosis and elevated CSF protein even without clinical meningitis.
3. **Fungi.** Cryptococcal meningitis is common, often presenting as fever and headache without neck stiffness or photophobia. A lumbar puncture with no pleocytosis does not rule out cryptococcal meningitis. When this infection is in the differential diagnosis, an opening pressure should always be obtained.
4. **Spirochetes.** The incidence of central nervous system (CNS) syphilis is increased in HIV-infected patients.
5. **Mycobacteria.** Tuberculosis is the most common mycobacterial cause of CNS disease in HIV-positive patients.
6. **Malignancy.** Lymphomatous meningitis is the most common malignant etiology.

B. Approach to the patient. In general, the approach to an HIV-positive patient with suspected meningitis is the same as that for other patients (see Chapter 88 V). However, the increased likelihood of certain etiologies leads to a few specific considerations for HIV-infected patients with possible meningitis.

1. Serum and CSF **cryptococcal antigen (CRAG) titers** should be obtained in HIV-infected patients who are being evaluated for possible meningitis. The sensitivity of these tests exceeds 95%.

2. Serum and CSF **Venereal Disease Research Laboratory (VDRL) tests** are often performed to evaluate the possibility of neurosyphilis.
3. The presence of an unexplained CSF lymphocytic pleocytosis or evidence of a basilar meningitis (e.g., meningitis with cranial nerve findings) usually raises suspicion of meningitis related to tuberculosis, endemic fungal infections, or lymphoma.
   a. **CSF analysis.** Multiple CSF samples should be sent for cytology, fungal, and acid-fast bacillus staining and culture.
   b. A **tuberculin purified protein derivative (PPD) skin test** may be performed to evaluate exposure to tuberculosis; however, a negative test does not exclude the diagnosis.
   c. **Magnetic resonance imaging (MRI)** is often useful to look for basilar meningitis; a biopsy of the brain or meninges is sometimes necessary for definitive diagnosis.

C. Treatment depends on the cause.

1. **Bacteria.** Treatment of routine bacterial meningitis is not different from that in an immunocompetent patient.
2. **Viruses.** HSV and CMV are treated with acyclovir and ganciclovir as first-line agents, respectively. See Section IV for details on therapy of disease caused by JC virus.
3. **Fungi.** Combination therapy with amphotericin B (0.7 mg/kg/day) and 5-flucytosine (25 mg/kg PO q6h) is recommended for initial treatment of cryptococcal meningitis. After 14 days, these drugs are discontinued and fluconazole (400 mg/day) is initiated orally. After 8 weeks, or when the CSF is sterile, the dose may be reduced for maintenance therapy to 200 mg/day. The duration of this therapy depends on the patient's CD4 count and HIV viral load over time but may be lifelong.
4. **Spirochetes.** Intravenous penicillin G for 14 days is recommended for patients with CNS syphilis.
5. **Mycobacteria.** Standard regimens for tuberculosis are used for CNS tuberculosis, but the duration of therapy is extended and corticosteroids may be beneficial.
6. **Malignancy.** HIV infection is not a contraindication to chemotherapy or radiation therapy, and the appropriate treatment of the underlying malignancy should be pursued.

III. SPACE-OCCUPYING LESIONS may present as headaches, seizures, focal sensory or motor deficits, visual field defects, or altered mental status.

A. Causes of space-occupying lesions. Although all the following causes should be considered in a patient who presents with signs and symptoms of a space-occupying lesion, the first two are the most common in HIV-positive patients.

1. **Toxoplasmosis**
2. **Primary CNS lymphoma**
3. **Bacterial abscess**
4. **Cryptococcoma**
5. **Histoplasmoma**
6. **Tuberculoma**
7. **Nocardiosis**

B. Approach to the patient

1. **Imaging studies. A computed tomography (CT)** or **MRI scan** is often useful for evaluating suspected CNS disease in HIV-infected patients.
   a. **CT scan.** Many space-occupying lesions are better seen with contrast enhancement, which should be used in the absence of contraindications.
   b. **MRI** is generally a more sensitive test and may reveal multiple lesions when only a single lesion is seen on CT scan.
2. **Laboratory studies**
   a. A **serum CRAG titer** is frequently ordered.
   b. **Blood cultures** and a **PPD test** may also be obtained, depending on the clinical situation.
   c. **Toxoplasmosis IgG titers.** A *Toxoplasma gondii* IgM titer has limited utility because nearly all cases of toxoplasmosis in HIV-infected patients are due to reactivated disease. Determining whether a patient has been exposed to *T. gondii* in the past (e.g., a positive toxoplasmosis IgG serology) can help determine if the patient is at risk of reactivation. Individuals receiving prophylaxis for toxoplasmosis are also at decreased risk of developing CNS disease. Daily trimethoprim-sulfamethoxazole is the first-line prophylaxis regimen for patients with CD4 counts less than 100 cells/μl.
   d. **CD4 counts.** The patient's risk of disease depends on the degree of immunosuppression. Bacterial abscess, tuberculoma, and lymphoma can be seen at relatively high CD4 counts, whereas cryptococcomas and toxoplasmosis more commonly occur in patients with CD4 counts less than 100 cells/μl.

Lumbar punctures are rarely useful for evaluating space-occupying lesions in HIV-infected patients and are contraindicated in patients with mass effect or posterior fossa lesions.

3. **Stereotactic brain biopsy.** This procedure should be performed early in the diagnostic work-up if the patient does not have a high likelihood of CNS toxoplasmosis, including:
   a. Those with negative toxoplasmosis IgG serologies
   b. Those with an increased risk for processes other than toxoplasmosis (e.g., intravenous drug users, who have an increased risk of brain abscess)
   c. Those with single lesions on MRI (because finding a single lesion makes toxoplasmosis less likely)
   d. Those with progressive neurologic deficits or mass effect on imaging (because appropriate treatment is needed immediately)
   e. Those who do not have regression of the space-occupying lesion or lesions after 2 weeks of empiric toxoplasmosis therapy

C. Treatment depends on the cause. In individuals believed to be at high risk for toxoplasmosis, empiric therapy is often given for 2 weeks, followed by repeat imaging to evaluate for response. Standard therapy is sulfadiazine (or high-dose clindamycin) combined with pyrimethamine.

IV. ENCEPHALOPATHY

A. Any alteration in mental status requires a thorough evaluation to rule out reversible causes (see Chapter 82). An **imaging study** (preferably an MRI) and **spinal fluid analysis** are necessary to rule out infectious or malignant processes. **Neuropsychiatric testing** is frequently performed to help rule out depression.

B. Progressive multifocal leukoencephalopathy (PML) due to JC virus is a common cause of cognitive impairment and focal neurologic deficits in patients with late-stage HIV infection. Imaging studies reveal patchy periventricular and/or subcortical white matter lesions best seen on MRI. A PCR for JC virus may be positive even in the absence of a CSF pleocytosis. No definitive therapy exists. Highly active antiretroviral therapy (HAART) may improve symptoms.

C. Some patients are ultimately diagnosed as having **HIV-associated dementia,** an illness that occurs late in the course of HIV infection and is often characterized by memory deficits, gait difficulty, behavioral changes including depression, and psychomotor slowing. CT scanning may reveal brain atrophy. MRI findings include symmetric subcortical white matter lesions with high intensity on T2-weighted images. HAART has reduced the incidence of HIV-associated dementia but has not has not been shown to reverse dementia.

V. MYELOPATHY usually presents with progressive lower extremity weakness that may be accompanied by bladder or bowel incontinence. Evidence of upper motor neuron disease with spastic paraparesis and hyperreflexia are usually noted unless peripheral neuropathy is also present.

A. Causes of myelopathy. Spinal cord disease often results from infection, external compression injury (i.e., cord compression), or miscellaneous insults.

1. **Infection.** Viruses [CMV, HSV, varicella-zoster virus (VZV), and HIV]; fungi (*Cryptococcus*), spirochetes (*Treponema pallidum*); and parasites (*Toxoplasma*) can infect the spinal cord, leading to myelopathy.
2. **Cord compression** may result from epidural abscesses (e.g., from bacterial infection or tuberculosis) or from malignancy (e.g., CNS lymphoma).
3. **Miscellaneous causes**
   a. **Vascular insults** (e.g., vasculitis)
   b. **Vitamin B_{12} deficiency**
   c. **HIV-related vacuolar myelopathy** is a diagnosis of exclusion and usually occurs late in the course of HIV infection. Motor weakness and decreased proprioception often reflect preferential loss of myelin from the lateral and dorsal columns, respectively. Examination reveals a spastic paraparesis with lower extremity hyperreflexia. There is no proven therapy.

B. Approach to the patient

1. **Imaging studies. MRI** of the involved area of spinal cord helps to rule out spinal cord compression.
2. **Laboratory studies**
   a. **Spinal fluid analysis** with PCR for CMV, HSV, and VZV; **CRAG titers** (serum and CSF); and **VDRL** titers (serum and CSF) should be obtained.
   b. **Serology for CMV** may be useful to evaluate the possibility of **CMV polyradiculopathy** (see VI A).
   c. A **vitamin B_{12}** level should be obtained.

VI. PERIPHERAL NEUROPATHY is common in patients with acquired immunodeficiency syndrome (AIDS).

A. Causes of peripheral neuropathy. All causes of peripheral neuropathy should be considered (see Chapter 83); however, common causes and patterns of peripheral neuropathy in patients with AIDS are given here.

1. **Polyneuropathy**
   a. **Distal symmetric peripheral neuropathies** are the most commonly seen peripheral neuropathies in HIV-infected patients. Typically, patients present with painful dysesthesias. The etiologies are many but common causes

include antiretroviral medications (most commonly didanosine and stavudine) or HIV itself. The latter is seen in late-stage disease. In cases in which medication is the suspected cause, therapy should be changed (when possible) to agents not associated with neuropathy. **Symptomatic therapy** with tricyclic antidepressants or gabapentin may be helpful.

b. **Predominantly motor neuropathies**

(1) **CMV polyradiculopathy** may cause progressive lower extremity weakness associated with a CSF neutrophilic pleocytosis (in the absence of bacterial infection). Therapy with **ganciclovir** may result in clinical improvement.

(2) An **inflammatory demyelinating polyneuropathy** may result in severe motor weakness and significantly depressed nerve conduction velocities. The clinical scenario resembles that of the more acute Guillain-Barré syndrome. **Plasmapheresis** is often used as treatment.

2. **Mononeuritis multiplex** is much less common than polyneuropathy. Although HIV itself is an etiology, other infections (e.g., CMV, VZV) and malignancies (e.g., lymphoma) should be ruled out.

B. Approach to the patient. Other potentially reversible causes of peripheral neuropathy should be considered (see Chapter 83).

REFERENCES

Ferrari S, Vento S, Monaco S, et al. HIV-associated peripheral neuropathies. Mayo Clin Proc 2006;81(2):213–219.

Mamidi A, DeSimone JA, Pomerantz RJ. Central nervous system infections in individuals with HIV-1 infection. J Neurovirol 2002;8(3):158–167.

McArthur JC, Brew BJ, Nath A. Neurological complications of HIV infection. Lancet Neurol 2005;4(9):543–555.

59 Pancytopenia

I. INTRODUCTION. Pancytopenia is defined as a decrease in all blood cell lines.

II. CLINICAL MANIFESTATIONS OF PANCYTOPENIA

A. Pancytopenia usually presents with signs and symptoms that are related to a decrease in the particular cell line.

1. **Anemia**
   a. Defined as a hemoglobin less than 13.5 g/dl or a hematocrit less than 41% in men and a hemoglobin less than 12.0 g/dl or a hematocrit <36% in women
   b. Can result in increased fatigue, shortness of breath, lightheadedness, and pallor
2. **Thrombocytopenia**
   a. Defined as a platelet count of less than 150,000 cells/μl
   b. Patients with platelet counts greater than 100,000 cells/μl often have normal bleeding times (unless platelet function is abnormal) and are usually asymptomatic.
   c. Easy bruisability may be noted as the platelet count approaches 50,000 cells/μl.
   d. Counts below 10,000–20,000 cells/μl can be associated with petechiae, mucosal bleeding, and spontaneous internal bleeds.
3. **Neutropenia**
   a. Defined as an absolute neutrophil count of less than 1500 cells/μl
   b. Predisposes patients to bacterial infections (however, patients usually present with symptoms related to anemia or thrombocytopenia first)
   c. The risk of infection increases substantially once the neutrophil count falls below 500 cells/μl

B. Disease-specific symptoms (e.g., neurologic symptoms in vitamin B_{12} deficiency, cachexia in malignancy) may also be present.

Pancytopenia is a great reminder that even mild, nonspecific symptoms can be the harbinger of a serious illness. You should therefore consider getting a complete blood count (CBC) with a differential on all patients with a prolonged or recurring illness.

III. CAUSES OF PANCYTOPENIA. Many textbooks attempt to differentiate causes of decreased production from those of increased destruction. For pancytopenia, this distinction is not very useful because both processes are often involved. The mnemonic "PANCYTO" can help you remember the most common causes of pancytopenia.

MNEMONIC **Common Causes of Pancytopenia ("PANCYTO")**

Paroxysmal nocturnal hemoglobinuria (PNH)
Aplastic anemia
Neoplasms and **N**ear neoplasms
Consumption
Vitamin deficiencies (the "V" looks like a "Y")
Toxins, drugs, and radiation therapy
Overwhelming infections

A. PNH is a disorder of stem cells that results in an increased sensitivity for complement-mediated cell lysis. PNH can clinically manifest as chronic intravascular hemolysis, a hypercoagulable state, and/or bone marrow aplasia.

B. Aplastic anemia is one of the misnomers in medicine because it involves a disorder of stem cells and therefore affects all cell lines. The etiology of aplastic anemia is unknown, but an immune-mediated reduction in hematopoietic progenitors is probable. Exposures and disorders associated with aplastic anemia are listed below; many cases of aplastic anemia have no identifiable cause.

1. **Fanconi's anemia** is an autosomal recessive or X-linked disease that usually appears in childhood and is often associated with other congenital abnormalities (e.g., cardiac and renal malformations, hypoplastic thumbs, hyperpigmented skin). Fanconi's anemia is associated with an increased risk of solid tumors and leukemias, as well as aplastic anemia.
2. **Drugs** and **toxins**. Chemotherapeutic agents, chloramphenicol, sulfa drugs, gold, nonsteroidal anti-inflammatory medications, certain antiepileptic drugs, ionizing radiation, benzene, and various other drugs have been associated with aplastic anemia.

3. **Infections.** Parvovirus B19 is the most frequently documented viral cause of aplastic anemia. Hepatitis, human immunodeficiency virus (HIV) and, Epstein-Barr virus infections have also been seen; however, the specific type of hepatitis virus associated with aplastic anemia has not been identified.
4. **Immune disorders** and dysregulation may also play a role in the development of aplastic anemia.
5. **Idiopathic.** The cause remains unclear in a large number of patients. In these cases, the leading hypothesis is that a host immune response against hematopoietic progenitor cells leads to the aplastic anemia.

C. Neoplasms (e.g., **leukemia, metastatic malignancies**) and **near neoplasms** (i.e., **myelodysplasia**) can cause pancytopenia.

D. Consumption

1. **Hypersplenism** (see Chapter 31), regardless of the cause, can result in pancytopenia. Hepatitis B and C leading to cirrhosis can induce hypersplenism and pancytopenia.
2. **Immune-mediated destruction** usually results in decreases of one or two cell lines but can also cause pancytopenia.

E. Vitamin deficiencies (e.g., vitamin B_{12} and folate deficiencies) should always be considered in patients with pancytopenia.

F. Toxins, drugs, and **radiation therapy.** For example, ethanol use may result in pancytopenia.

G. Overwhelming infections. Sepsis, tuberculosis, or fungal infection can cause pancytopenia. HIV infection can also result in pancytopenia, from the infection itself, superimposed infections, or medications used to treat the infection.

IV. APPROACH TO THE PATIENT

Pancytopenia should be considered a primary bone marrow failure until proven otherwise.

A. Patient history. Inquire about medications, exposures, and HIV risk factors. Perform a review of systems, asking the patient about cachexia and other symptoms of an occult malignancy. Inquire about recent bruising, bleeding, or recurrent infections.

B. Physical examination. Carefully examine the spleen and lymph nodes. The presence of splenomegaly increases the likelihood of malignancy and essentially rules out aplastic anemia.

C. Laboratory studies. Although a bone marrow biopsy is indicated to help establish the diagnosis, there are some potential clues to the diagnosis that can be obtained on a routine peripheral blood smear. Other tests may also be indicated in certain patients.

1. **Peripheral blood smear**
   a. **Megaloblastosis** increases the likelihood of vitamin B_{12} or folate deficiency.
   b. **Blasts** implicate a possible myelodysplastic syndrome or acute leukemia.
   c. **Leukoerythroblastic smear.** A leukoerythroblastic smear, which reveals **early (nucleated) red blood cells (RBCs)** and **early white blood cells (WBCs)** (i.e., bands, metamyelocytes, myelocytes), implies marrow invasion by malignancy, fibrosis, or infection. **Teardrop cells** (i.e., RBCs shaped like a teardrop from being "squeezed" out of the bone marrow) are frequently seen with leukoerythroblastosis.
   d. **Pseudo Pelger-Huet anomaly** (i.e., neutrophils with bilobed nuclei) is seen in patients with myelodysplasia (see Chapter 70).
2. **Vitamin B_{12}** and **folate** levels are often obtained.
3. **HIV test.** An HIV test should be performed in patients with risk factors.
4. **PNH work-up.** PNH results in intravascular hemolysis that can be precipitated by infections or acidosis (e.g., while sleeping at night) resulting in hemosiderinuria; therefore, PNH should be evaluated in all patients with pancytopenia and especially those describing episodes of dark urine. The diagnostic test involves the flow cytometric evaluation for glycosylphosphatidylinositol (GPI)-anchored proteins including CD14, CD55, or CD59.

D. Bone marrow biopsy. Because a "dry tap" may occur (i.e., one in which bone marrow aspirate is unobtainable as a result of aplasia, fibrosis, or malignancy), a core biopsy is also essential to determine the etiology of pancytopenia. Patients with HIV and pancytopenia often still undergo bone marrow biopsy to rule out a contributing infection or malignancy.

1. **Increased cellularity** suggests peripheral destruction (hypersplenism or an immune-mediated disorder). Some forms of myelodysplasia, acute leukemia, and PNH can have either a hypercellular or hypocellular marrow.
2. **Decreased cellularity** is the common finding in aplastic anemia, but can also be seen in PNH, myelodysplasia, or, occasionally, a hypoplastic acute leukemia.
3. **Cytogenetic analysis** may help establish the diagnosis of a myelodysplastic syndrome or acute leukemia by finding a clonal abnormality. However, hypoplastic myelodysplasia can have a normal karyotype.

4. **Other findings.** Evidence of an infiltrative malignancy or cultures and/or molecular analyses for an infection can also be useful in establishing the cause of the pancytopenia.

V. TREATMENT

A. General treatment is aimed at preventing the complications associated with a decrease in each cell line.

1. **Packed RBC transfusions** are usually given to maintain the hematocrit above 25% in most symptomatic patients and 30% in older patients or those with known or suspected coronary artery disease. Younger patients may tolerate a lower hematocrit. For each unit of packed RBCs transfused, the hemoglobin is expected to rise by 1 g/dl and the hematocrit by 3%.
2. **Platelet transfusions** may be necessary to control bleeding or when the platelet count falls below 10,000 cells/μl to reduce the risk of spontaneous bleeding (see Chapter 60).
3. **Infection prevention and treatment**
   a. **Granulocyte colony-stimulating factor (G-CSF)** is sometimes used to increase neutrophil counts.
   b. **Neutropenic precautions** (e.g., **handwashing, minimizing injections, avoiding unpeeled fruit and fresh flowers**). The risk from neutropenia is highest when the patient's absolute neutrophil count is less than 500 cells/μl. Neutropenic precautions should be used for these patients. Prophylactic antibiotics in the absence of signs or symptoms of infection are not recommended.
   c. **Broad-spectrum antibiotics** should be used for patients with fever and neutropenia, which is a medical emergency.

B. Specific treatment is aimed at the underlying illness. Specific treatments for most of the causes of pancytopenia are found in the relevant chapters. Therapies for PNH and aplastic anemia will be briefly discussed here.

1. **PNH** carries approximately a 40% lifetime risk of thrombosis and the median survival is 10–15 years. Approximately 50% of patients with PNH die of either a thrombotic event or due to complications from cytopenias. Spontaneous remission may occur in approximately 15% of patients.
   a. The constant hemolysis and hemosiderinuria/hematuria can actually result in iron deficiency that may require replacement. Likewise, folate replacement is recommended in all patients with a chronic hemolysis.
   b. **Chronic anticoagulation therapy** is indicated for all patients with a history of thrombosis; patients should be managed similarly to other patients with a hypercoagulable state. Although still unproven in a randomized trial,

some suggest prophylactic anticoagulation in those individuals with more than 50% of their granulocytes lacking the GPI-anchored proteins (since this confers a higher risk for a thrombotic event).

   c. **Eculizumab** is a recently Food and Drug Administration (FDA)-approved monoclonal antibody that binds to the C5 component of complement and inhibits further complement activation. It has been demonstrated to reduce the rate of hemolysis, transfusion requirements, and thrombotic complications in patients with PNH.
   d. **Bone marrow transplantation** may be curative but carries significant morbidity and mortality.

2. **Aplastic anemia**
   a. **Removal of potential etiologies** (e.g., medications) is always important.
   b. **Transfusion support** and appropriate **antibiotic therapy** for infectious complications
   c. **Pharmacologic therapy.** Decisions regarding therapy depend on the severity of the aplastic anemia as well as the age of the patient. Treatment options include:
      (1) **Steroids** are sometimes useful for patients with mild aplasia but are generally not effective in patients with more severe disease unless added to antithymocyte globulin and/or cyclosporine as combination therapy.
      (2) **Antithymocyte globulin** is usually the first-line pharmacologic treatment for patients with severe aplastic anemia.
      (3) **Immunosuppressive agents** (e.g., cyclosporine) are also used in conjunction with antithymocyte globulin and increase the likelihood of remissions.
   d. **Bone marrow transplantation** may cure 80% of patients, but the morbidity and mortality increases with the age of the patient as well as with the use of matched unrelated donors versus related allogeneic donors. Because transfusions may increase the risk of rejection, transplant candidates should only receive transfusions when it is absolutely necessary. They should be leuko-"poor" to decrease the risk of human leukocyte antigen immunization as well as to reduce the risk of viral infections. If the patient is neutropenic, irradiating the blood product may lessen the chance of graft versus host reaction. Transfusions from potential donors should never be given.
   e. **Spontaneous recovery** is uncommon and usually is seen only in mild or moderate cases.

REFERENCES

Brodsky RA. Advances in the diagnosis and therapy of paroxysmal nocturnal hemoglobinuria. Blood Rev 2008;22(2):65–74.

Brodsky RA, Jones RJ. Aplastic anaemia. Lancet 2005;365(9471):1647–1656.

Halfdanarson TR, Walker JA, Litzow MR, et al. Severe vitamin B12 deficiency resulting in pancytopenia, splenomegaly and leukoerythroblastosis. Eur J Haematol 2008;80(5):448–451.

Young NS, Calado RT, Scheinberg P. Current concepts in the pathophysiology and treatment of aplastic anemia. Blood 2006;108(8):2509–2519.

Thrombocytopenia

I. **INTRODUCTION.** Thrombocytopenia, a common disorder in hospitalized patients, is defined as a **platelet count less than 150,000 cells/μl.**

II. **CLINICAL MANIFESTATIONS OF THROMBOCYTOPENIA.** Signs and symptoms are related to the degree of thrombocytopenia (in the absence of concomitant disorders of coagulation or platelet dysfunction).

A. **Platelet count 50,000–100,000 cells/μl.** Clinical manifestations are usually absent, but bleeding times may be prolonged on specific laboratory testing.

B. **Platelet count 30,000–50,000 cells/μl.** Patients may report easy bruisability, but spontaneous bleeding is usually not seen.

C. **Platelet count 10,000–30,000 cells/μl.** Patients are at increased risk for bleeding with minimal trauma and are at a small but measurable risk for spontaneous bleeding (e.g., petechiae, gastrointestinal bleeding).

D. **Platelet count less than 10,000 cells/μl.** Patients are at an increased risk for spontaneous bleeding and likely benefit from prophylactic transfusion support.

III. **CAUSES OF THROMBOCYTOPENIA.** It is easiest to remember the causes of thrombocytopenia if you classify them according to the underlying mechanism: decreased production, splenic sequestration, or increased destruction (Figure 60-1).

A. **Decreased production.** Because diseases of the bone marrow are involved, there is often a decrease in other cell lines as well. The causes of decreased platelet production are almost identical to those of pancytopenia (see Chapter 59).

1. **Paroxysmal nocturnal thrombocytopenia (PNH)** is more commonly associated with increased destruction but may also be associated with a production defect.
2. **Aplasia. Aplastic anemia** causes pancytopenia.
3. **Neoplasms** and **near neoplasms** include **leukemia, metastatic malignancies,** and **myelodysplasia.**
4. **Vitamin deficiencies,** including **vitamin B_{12}** and **folate deficiency,** are rare causes of isolated thrombocytopenia.

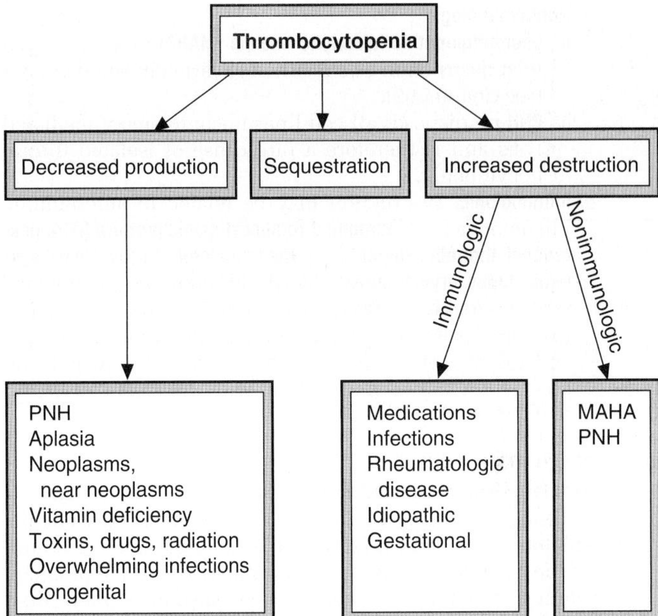

Figure 60-1 Causes of thrombocytopenia. *MAHA* = microangiopathic hemolytic anemia; *PNH* = paroxysmal nocturnal hemoglobinuria.

5. **Toxins, drugs,** and **radiation therapy. Ethanol, thiazide diuretics, interferon,** and **chemotherapeutic agents** can cause thrombocytopenia due to a decreased production.
6. **Overwhelming infections,** including sepsis, tuberculosis, fungal infection, and viral infections including the human immunodeficiency virus (HIV) disease, can cause thrombocytopenia.
7. **Congenital thrombocytopenia.** These include the May-Hegglin anomaly, Bernard-Soulier syndrome, Wiskott-Aldrich syndrome, congenital hypoplastic amegakaryocytic thrombocytopenia, and thrombocytopenia and absent radii (the TAR syndrome).

B. Increased splenic sequestration can result from **hypersplenism** of any cause, leading to thrombocytopenia (see Chapter 31).

C. Increased destruction is probably the most common cause of isolated thrombocytopenia. Disorders that cause increased destruction of platelets can be classified as nonimmunologic or immunologic.

1. **Nonimmunologic**
   a. **Microangiopathic hemolytic anemia (MAHA)** may cause platelet destruction as a result of shearing in small vessels (see Chapter 62).
   b. **PNH** predisposes all cell lines to complement-mediated lysis and is therefore a rare cause of isolated thrombocytopenia.
2. **Immunologic.** Destruction may be related to autoimmune phenomena [e.g., **immune thrombocytopenic purpura (ITP), gestational thrombocytopenia,** or **rheumatologic disease (e.g., systemic lupus erythematosus [SLE])**], alloimmune phenomena (e.g., **posttransfusion reaction**), or drug-dependent antibodies from **medications** (heparin, abciximab, quinine, gold salts, and valproic acid are commonly cited). There may be an association between infection with *Helicobacter pylori* and the development of ITP.

IV. APPROACH TO THE PATIENT

A. Exclude pseudothrombocytopenia. Pseudothrombocytopenia is an artifact of platelet clumping in the test tube in ethylenediaminetetraacetic acid (EDTA) anticoagulated blood. Examining the peripheral blood smear may alert you to the problem. Sending a citrate or heparinized specimen may limit the clumping in some cases or a manual count may be required.

B. Try to determine the cause of thrombocytopenia.

1. **Patient history.** Pay particular attention to the patient's medications. Risk factors for HIV or a history of substance abuse (e.g., alcohol) also deserve attention. A review of systems and asking about "B" symptoms (i.e., fevers, night sweats, and weight loss) may help reveal an occult malignancy. A bleeding history including questions about menstrual bleeding, surgical complications, and prior transfusions may help elucidate the chronicity of the problem. Family history may help establish a congenital pattern.
2. **Physical examination.** A complete physical examination is always necessary.
   a. Examination of the **spleen** is of particular importance (see Chapter 31 IV).
   b. A detailed skin examination for petechiae, purpura, and ecchymoses should be performed.
   c. In addition, a thorough examination for **lymphadenopathy** should be performed (see Chapter 68 II).
3. **Laboratory studies**
   a. **Peripheral blood smear.** A peripheral blood smear is absolutely essential.

(1) **Large platelets.** The finding of both normal-sized and large platelets implies increased destruction and early release from the bone marrow. ITP is classically associated with finding both normal and large platelets on the peripheral blood smear. The large platelets are young and hyperfunctional. As a result, patients with ITP may not have as high of an incidence of bleeding relative to their platelet count. Alternatively, a congenital thrombocytopenia typically has all large platelets.

(2) **Schistocytes.** The finding of fragmented red blood cells (RBCs) implies microangiopathic hemolytic anemia.

(3) **Other abnormalities** that may offer clues are discussed in Chapter 59 IV C 1.

b. Elevated **lactate dehydrogenase (LDH)** levels may be used to evaluate the possibility of a MAHA, although this finding is non-specific. **Prolonged prothrombin time (PT), partial thromboplastin time (PTT),** and fibrin degradation products (including D-dimer) are seen in **disseminated intravascular coagulopathy (DIC)**. **Blood urea nitrogen (BUN)** and **creatinine levels** should be obtained when hemolytic-uremic syndrome/thrombotic thrombocytopenic purpura (HUS/TTP) is a consideration.

c. **Serologic studies.** Serologic assays for HIV and other disease-specific serologies/molecular studies are useful for evaluating the possibility of immunologic destruction associated with SLE or infections with viruses.

(1) An HIV test is especially necessary in patients with HIV risk factors.

(2) Serologies and/or qualitative reverse transcriptase polymerase chain reaction (RT-PCR) assessments for Epstein-Barr virus (EBV), cytomegalovirus (CMV), hepatitis, and toxoplasmosis are most useful when the patient has systemic symptoms, lymphadenopathy, hepatomegaly, or splenomegaly on examination.

d. **Vitamin B_{12}** and **folate levels** and flow cytometry **tests for PNH** are sometimes performed, but these disorders are rarely associated with isolated thrombocytopenia.

e. **Antiplatelet antibody testing** is not sensitive or specific and should be avoided when considering the diagnosis of ITP.

4. **Bone marrow biopsy** is performed in many patients with thrombocytopenia. If the cause of thrombocytopenia is readily identifiable (e.g., thiazide diuretic therapy), a trial of removing the possible inciting agent may be both

diagnostic and therapeutic and may obviate the need for a bone marrow biopsy. Pertinent findings on bone marrow biopsy include the following:

a. **Decreased megakaryocytes** are diagnostic of one of the production problems. Evidence of the specific cause of the decreased production may also be found (e.g., malignancy, aplasia, infection).
b. **Increased megakaryocytes** are found when increased destruction or sequestration is the mechanism of thrombocytopenia. Increased megakaryocytes on bone marrow biopsy without other identifiable causes of increased destruction or sequestration is usually diagnostic for ITP.
c. **Evidence for myelodysplasia** can also be seen on bone marrow biopsy (see Chapter 70).

V. TREATMENT

A. General treatment

1. **Discontinue medications** that may cause thrombocytopenia.
   a. The platelet count will usually return to normal in 7–10 days.
   b. **Heparin-induced thrombocytopenia and thrombosis (HITT)** is a disorder in which immune-mediated thrombocytopenia and, paradoxically, systemic thrombosis coexist. Increasing the heparin dose in these patients is contraindicated; the therapy involves heparin withdrawal and systemic anticoagulation with a direct thrombin inhibitor to prevent further thrombotic complications.
      (1) Assessments for HITT should be made including a heparin-induced thrombocytopenia (HIT) enzyme-linked immunosorbent assay (ELISA) and/or a serotonin release assay.
      (2) A direct thrombin inhibitor such as lepirudin, bivalirudin, or argatroban may be used. Warfarin should not be reinstituted until the patient is stabilized on a direct thrombin inhibitor, and the platelet count is greater than or equal to 100,000 cells/μl.
2. **Platelet transfusions.** Unnecessary platelet transfusions should be avoided because they may induce immune resistance to future transfusions, especially in cases of TTP and ITP; if this complication occurs, single donor platelets or human leukocyte antigen (HLA)-matched platelets can be administered.
   a. Platelet transfusions are usually not indicated for patients with platelet counts greater than 20,000 cells/μl and no evidence of bleeding.

In general, platelet transfusions in asymptomatic patients with TTP should be avoided because transfusions may worsen the patient's condition.

b. **Indications.** Platelet transfusions are indicated in the following situations:
   (1) **Before surgery.** The platelet count is usually maintained above 50,000 cells/μl when minor surgery is to be performed. Although in patients with ITP, this may be both impossible and unnecessary. When neurosurgery or thoracic surgery is to be performed, the platelet count is usually maintained above 80,000 cells/μl in an attempt to minimize any bleeding risk.
   (2) **In a patient with active bleeding**
      (a) **Severe bleeding.** The platelet count is always maintained above 50,000 cells/μl and is sometimes increased to 80,000–100,000 cells/μl.
      (b) **Mild bleeding** or **petechiae.** The platelet count should be maintained above 20,000 cells/μl.
   (3) **To prevent spontaneous bleeding.** The platelet count is usually kept above 10,000–20,000 cells/μl, depending on physician preference.

B. Specific treatments for **ITP** (including HIV-associated ITP) are discussed here; specific treatments for other causes are discussed in relevant chapters.

1. **Observation** is often appropriate for patients with platelet counts greater than 20,000 cells/μl and no evidence of bleeding. Children frequently have an acute form of ITP that is usually related to a viral illness and resolves spontaneously over 3–6 months. In adults, ITP usually follows a chronic and recurrent course.
2. **Pharmacologic therapy**
   a. **Steroids** will benefit approximately 60%–80% of patients, leading to an increase in platelet count. Counts can increase as quickly as 3–7 days, but relapses occur in up to 50% of patients after the discontinuation of the therapy.
   b. **Intravenous gammaglobulin (IVIG)** or anti-Rh(D) (anti-D, WinRho) often increases the platelet counts in patients with steroid-refractory disease and can be combined with corticosteroids. Since the kinetics of the response can be quicker than with steroids, these therapies can be used to acutely raise platelet counts in medical

emergencies or prior to surgery. However, the relapse rate is significant. Anti-Rh(D) is used in patients that are Rh^+ with no preceding evidence of a Coombs-mediated hemolysis and no prior splenectomy. Response rates can be as high as 70%.

c. **Immunosuppressive agents** can be used for patients with ITP, including those associated with SLE or other connective tissue disorders, after the failure of steroids and/or IVIG. The most commonly used agents include cyclophosphamide, azathioprine, vincristine, or vinblastine.
d. **Danazol** is sometimes useful for male patients and nonpregnant female patients with ITP.
e. **Zidovudine** may be useful in patients with HIV-associated ITP. The key is to institute highly active antiretroviral therapy, and ITP typically improves as the viral load is reduced.
f. **Rituximab,** a monoclonal antibody directed against a B-cell antigen (CD20), has demonstrated responses in approximately 50% of patients with refractory ITP, with some responses lasting more than 5 years.
g. **Thrombopoietin receptor agonists** (including eltrombopag and romiplostim) have recently completed phase II/III clinical trials for patients with ITP as well as thrombocytopenia secondary to cirrhosis. Romiplostim recently received Food and Drug Administration (FDA) approval for the treatment of relapsed or refractory ITP.

3. **Splenectomy** is typically a second-line therapy for ITP, reserved for patients in whom steroid therapy fails or for those who experience relapse after a steroid taper. Although predicting which patients might benefit from splenectomy is not well established, it appears that the highest response rates are seen in younger patients or those responsive to IVIG. Immunization for *Streptococcus pneumoniae*, *Haemophilus influenzae* b, and *Neisseria meningitides* is required prior to splenectomy.

REFERENCES

Arnold DM, Kelton JG. Current options for the treatment of idiopathic thrombocytopenic purpura. Semin Hematol 2007;44(4 Suppl 5):S12–S23.

Stasi R, Sarpatwari A, Segal JB, et al. Effects of eradication of Helicobacter pylori infection in patients with immune thrombocytopenic purpura: a systematic review. Blood 2009; 113(6): 1231–40.

Warkentin TE, Greinacher A, Koster A, et al.; American College of Chest Physicians. Treatment and prevention of heparin-induced thrombocytopenia: American College of Chest Physicians evidence-based clinical practice guidelines (8th edition). Chest 2008;133(6 Suppl):340S–380S.

61 Thrombocytosis

I. INTRODUCTION. Thrombocytosis is defined as a **platelet count greater than 450,000 cells/μl.**

II. ETIOLOGY OF THROMBOCYTOSIS

A. Primary. If thrombocytosis is caused by a myeloproliferative neoplasm, the platelets are frequently abnormal and, the patient may be prone to both bleeding and clotting events.

B. Secondary. If thrombocytosis is secondary to another disorder (reactive), even patients with extremely high platelet counts (e.g., >1,000,000 cells/μl) are usually asymptomatic.

III. CAUSES OF THROMBOCYTOSIS

A. Primary causes. Any of the four **myeloproliferative neoplasms** can increase the platelet count through a clonal proliferation of a hematopoietic progenitor cell (see Chapter 70). A specific type of myelodysplastic syndrome, known as the $5q^-$ syndrome, can also be associated with a thrombocytosis.

B. Secondary causes. Reactive thrombocytosis is the most common cause of thrombocytosis.

1. **Malignancies**
2. **Infections** and **inflammatory disorders** (e.g., Crohn's disease)
3. **Postsurgical status**
4. **Connective tissue disorders**
5. **Iron deficiency anemia**
6. **Splenectomy**
7. **Recovery of the bone marrow from a stress** (e.g., chemotherapy or alcohol)

IV. APPROACH TO THE PATIENT

A. Patient history

1. A history of **gastrointestinal bleeding** may imply possible iron deficiency.
2. **Fevers, night sweats,** or **weight loss** may implicate malignancy or chronic infection (e.g., tuberculosis). A complete review of systems should be performed to help identify the presence of an occult malignancy or infection.
3. A history of recent **splenectomy** may provide a simple explanation for thrombocytosis.

4. Patients should be questioned regarding potential symptoms related to thrombocytosis including thrombosis, bleeding complications, and vasomotor symptoms of headache, visual symptoms, and **erythromelalgia** (burning pain of extremities associated with warmth and redness). Presence of these symptoms would point more toward a primary myeloproliferative neoplasm.

B. Physical examination. Perform a thorough physical examination, including pelvic and rectal examinations. Pay special attention to the spleen and lymph nodes because enlargement may signal malignancy or infection.

C. Laboratory studies can further narrow the differential diagnosis.

1. **Iron status** including the **transferrin saturation** and **serum ferritin** will help evaluate the possibility of iron deficiency anemia and is especially important in patients with a history of gastrointestinal bleeding, guaiac-positive stools, or a low mean corpuscular volume (MCV).
2. **Hematocrit** and **white blood cell (WBC) count.** The hematocrit and WBC count are often elevated in patients with myeloproliferative neoplasms, although essential thrombocytosis may result in an isolated elevation of the platelet count.
3. **Peripheral smear.** Rarely, automated hematology counters may count small fragmented red blood cells (RBCs) as platelets and report an elevated count. This spurious diagnosis of thrombocytosis can be confirmed by evaluating the peripheral smear. Howell-Jolly bodies, target cells, or abnormally shaped cells on the smear may suggest a postsplenectomy state as a cause of thrombocytosis.
4. **Molecular analysis for the *Janus Kinase-2* (*JAK-2*) mutation.** The *JAK-2* gene was independently identified to have a somatic activating mutation (V617F) in a significant proportion of patients with primary myeloproliferative disorders. However, its presence neither rules in nor rules out a myeloproliferative neoplasm.
5. **Bone marrow biopsy.** Primary myeloproliferative neoplasms often have characteristic morphologic changes seen on bone marrow aspirates and biopsies, including megakaryocytic hyperplasia, with clustering of megakaryocytes. This can also help exclude other secondary diagnoses.
6. **Other tests** may be performed if reactive thrombocytosis is suspected [e.g., a purified protein derivative (PPD) test for possible tuberculosis, a computed tomography (CT) scan for suspected intra-abdominal malignancy, or serologic testing for connective tissue diseases]. If a reactive cause is ruled out, a bone marrow biopsy may be necessary to look for a primary cause.

V. TREATMENT

A. Primary causes. Myeloproliferative neoplasms may predispose the patient to both bleeding and thrombosis as a result of abnormal platelet function. Risk stratification models for myeloproliferative neoplasms have been established and will assist in deciding appropriate therapeutic options. Immediate platelet apheresis should be considered in patients with acute thromboses or in patients experiencing symptoms due to the elevated platelet count. Low-dose aspirin is often indicated and can prevent thromboses as well as limit vasomotor symptoms. Hydroxyurea or anagrelide can be used for longer-term management of patients with significant thrombocytosis, with thromboses, or who are otherwise at high risk for complications due to the myeloproliferative neoplasm. However, anagrelide is associated with an elevated risk of arterial thrombosis, venous thrombosis, serious hemorrhage, or death from vascular causes compared with hydroxyurea.

B. Secondary causes. Most causes of reactive thrombocytosis do not require treatment to lower the platelet count. The platelet count usually returns to normal following treatment of the underlying disorder. Patients with reactive thrombocytosis rarely have associated thromboses, so anticoagulant therapy is usually not warranted.

REFERENCES

Harrison CN, Campbell PJ, Buck G. Hydroxyurea compared with anagrelide in high-risk essential thrombocythemia. N Engl J Med 2005;353(1): 33–45.

Levine RL, Gilliland DG. JAK-2 mutations and their relevance to myeloproliferative disease. Curr Opin Hematol 2007;14(1):43–47.

Tefferi A. Essential thrombocythemia, polycythemia vera, and myelofibrosis: current management and the prospect of targeted therapy. Am J Hematol 2008;83(6):491–497.

Levine RL, Gilliland DG. Myeloproliferative Disorders. Blood 2008; 112(6):2190–8.

Vannucchi AM, Barbui T. Thrombocytosis and Thrombosis. Hematology Am Soc Hematol Educ Program 2007; 2007:363–70.

Anemia

I. INTRODUCTION. Anemia is a common disorder among hospitalized patients.

A. Definition. Anemia is defined as a reduced absolute number of circulating red blood cells, yet this value is not practical to measure. Thus, anemia is often defined as a reduction in one or more of the major red blood cell (RBC) measurements: hemoglobin, hematocrit, or the RBC count. Anemia is often a manifestation of disease, rather than a disease in and of itself.

B. Normal values are both gender and age dependent.

1. In men, a hematocrit less than 41% is considered anemic.
2. In women, a hematocrit less than 36% is considered anemic.

C. Clinical manifestations of anemia. Patients with anemia may be asymptomatic or complain of **fatigue, dyspnea on exertion,** or **exertional angina.** Signs and symptoms of the underlying disorder may also be present.

D. Classification. Anemia may be classified as **microcytic, normocytic,** or **macrocytic** using the **mean corpuscular volume (MCV)** as a basis.

1. The **normal MCV** is **80–100 fL.**
2. If more than one disorder is present, the MCV may be an average of the different populations of RBCs, producing a normal MCV. In mixed disorders, the **red cell distribution width (RDW)** will be increased.
3. Other classification schemes stratify anemias according to the **Reticulocyte Index (RI)** (production of new red blood cells) and can be considered hypoproliferative (RI <2) or hyperproliferative (RI >2).
   a. The RI is a function of the reticulocyte percent, patient's hematocrit, normal hematocrit, and reticulocyte maturation time (RMT).
   b. The specific formula is:

$$\text{RI} = (\%\ \text{Reticulocytes} \times \text{Patient's hematocrit}) \div (\text{Normal hematocrit} \times \text{RMT})$$

where the normal hematocrit is 45 and the RMT depends on the patient's hematocrit per Table 62-1.

TABLE 62-1

CORRELATION BETWEEN HEMATOCRIT AND RETICULOCYTE MATURATION TIME (RMT)

Patient's Hematocrit	Reticulocyte Maturation Time
36–45	1.0
26–35	1.5
16–25	2.0
15 and below	2.5

c. Use of a medical calculator can be helpful (e.g., http://cpsc.acponline.org/enhancements/227rpiCalc.html)

II. MICROCYTIC ANEMIA (MCV <80 fL.)

A. Causes of microcytic anemia

1. **Iron deficiency** is a very common cause of microcytic anemia and is important to diagnose because it may be indicative of an underlying gastrointestinal malignancy.
2. **Thalassemia** ranges in severity. Patients with α- or β-thalassemia minor may even present with microcytosis without anemia.
3. **Anemia of chronic disease (ACD)** is associated with inflammatory diseases (e.g., rheumatoid arthritis, serious infection, carcinoma, chronic renal insufficiency).
4. **Sideroblastic anemias** are a heterogenous group of disorders that have in common various defects in the porphyrin pathway that lead to an increase in cellular iron uptake. Congenital sideroblastic anemia causes microcytosis, whereas other etiologies may lead to a variable MCV. Causes of sideroblastic anemia include:
   a. **Heredity** [e.g., X-linked, erythropoietic protoporphyria (EPP)]
   b. **Drugs** and **toxins** [e.g., **l**ead, **i**soniazid, **e**thanol (LIE)]. Heavy metal exposures should be evaluated.
   c. **Malignancy** [e.g., myelodysplasia (FAB subtype refractory anemia with ringed sideroblasts)]

B. Approach to the patient.

It is important to differentiate iron deficiency from the other causes of microcytic anemia.

1. **Iron deficiency versus thalassemia.** Iron studies are typically diagnostic for iron deficiency (decreased transferrin saturation and decreased ferritin), but iron deficiency can also be distinguished from thalassemia using the **thalassemia index** (Mentzer Index) [i.e., the **MCV (measured in fL) divided by the RBC count (measured in cells** $\times$ **10^6/mm^3)**]. A thalassemia index less than 13 suggests thalassemia; an index greater than 13 suggests iron deficiency.

2. **Iron deficiency versus other etiologies**
   a. **Determine the probability that a patient has iron deficiency.** The pretest probability is based on clinical factors. By estimating the pretest probability and using likelihood ratios for a given ferritin level (Table 62-2), you can estimate the posttest probability (see Chapter 2 III C 1).
   b. **Laboratory studies**
      (1) **Serum ferritin.** This test may be less helpful in patients with liver disease or other chronic inflammatory states because ferritin is an acute-phase reactant. Like most tests, ferritin is most useful when the pretest probability is approximately 50%.
         (a) If the serum ferritin is less than 15 ng/ml, it practically guarantees that the patient has iron deficiency.
         (b) Similarly, a value greater than 100 ng/m makes iron deficiency improbable.
      (2) **Serum transferrin** is occasionally helpful because it is usually elevated in iron deficiency and decreased in ACD. However, pregnancy and oral contraceptives can also elevate transferrin levels.
   c. **Bone marrow biopsy** remains the gold standard test to diagnose iron deficiency.

All forms of the microcytic anemias described above are hypoproliferative (i.e., RI < 2).

C. Treatment

1. **Iron deficiency anemia** therapy involves treating the underlying cause of blood loss and replacing lost iron. Oral iron is

TABLE 62-2

SERUM FERRITIN VALUES AND CORRESPONDING LIKELIHOOD RATIOS

Serum Ferritin (μ/L)	Likelihood Ratio
>100	0.1
25–100	Not helpful
15–24	10
<15	50

Based on data from Guyatt GH, Oxman AD, Ali M, et al. Laboratory diagnosis of iron-deficiency anemia: an overview. J Gen Intern Med 1992;7(2):145–153.

most commonly used; side effects include constipation, abdominal discomfort, and black discoloration of stools. Achlorhydria (i.e., patients on proton pump inhibitors or gastric bypass patients) or celiac disease may limit the ability to absorb iron; these patients can be given iron intravenously. With therapy, reticulocytosis should occur within a few days, and the hemoglobin should rise in 1–2 months.

2. **Thalassemia** treatment varies with disease severity. Patients may require no treatment, or may require frequent transfusions. Iron chelation therapy may be required for those patients receiving frequent blood transfusions. Severe disease can be treated successfully with bone marrow transplantation, but significant morbidity and mortality limits its widespread utilization.

III. MACROCYTIC ANEMIA (MCV >100 FL)

A. Megaloblastic anemias are caused by various defects in DNA synthesis that lead to hematologic abnormalities. Causes of megaloblastic anemia include:

1. **Vitamin B_{12} deficiency**
2. **Folate deficiency**
3. **Drugs** (e.g., hydroxyurea, methotrexate, azathioprine)
4. Miscellaneous (e.g., Lesch-Nyhan syndrome, thiamine-responsive or pyridoxine-responsive anemias)

B. Chronic liver disease causes a macrocytosis as a result of ineffective erythropoiesis.

The finding of hypersegmented polymorphonuclear neutrophils (PMNs) on the peripheral blood smear strongly suggests megaloblastic anemia.

C. Alcoholism produces erythrocyte membrane abnormalities, leading to macrocytic anemia.

D. Hypothyroidism causes macrocytic anemia via an unclear mechanism.

E. Reticulocytosis. An MCV greater than 110 fL is usually not due to reticulocytosis alone.

F. Myelodysplasia (see Chapter 70)

Practically all human immunodeficiency virus (HIV)-infected patients taking zidovudine and all patients receiving hydroxyurea will have an elevated MCV; therefore, this finding can aid in gauging compliance with medications.

IV. NORMOCYTIC ANEMIA. An **absolute reticulocyte count** is the initial test to order in a patient with normocytic anemia, because the RI allows the anemia to be classified as **hyperproliferative** or **hypoproliferative** (Figure 62-1).

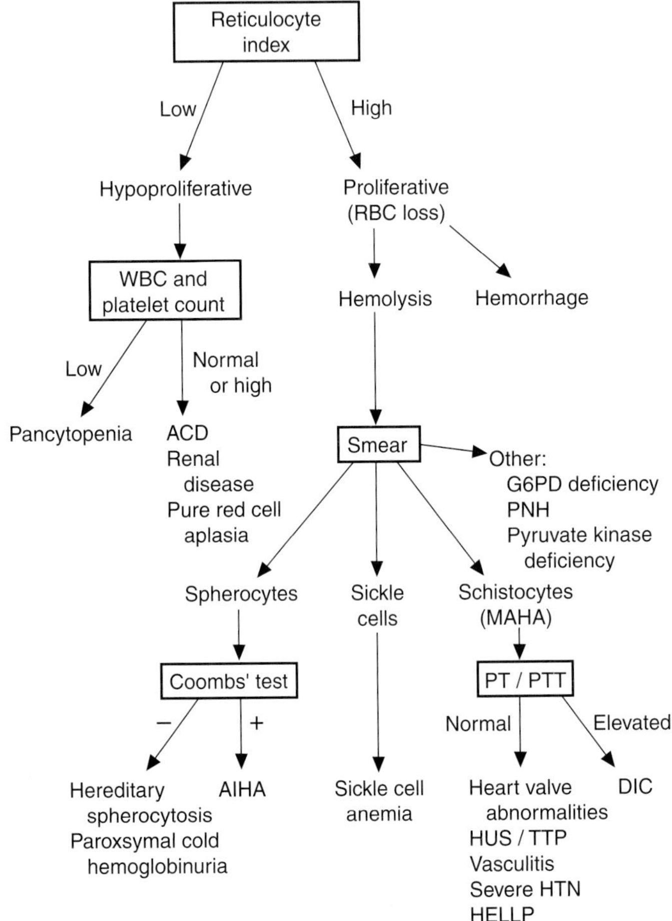

Figure 62–1 Determining the cause of normocytic anemia. *ACD* = anemia of chronic disease; *AIHA* = autoimmune hemolytic anemia; *DIC* = disseminated intravascular coagulation; *G6PD* = glucose-6-phosphate dehydrogenase; *HELLP* = hemolysis, elevated liver enzymes, and low platelet count syndrome; *HTN* = hypertension; *HUS/TTP* = hemolytic-uremic syndrome/thrombotic thrombocytopenic purpura; *MAHA* = microangiopathic hemolytic anemia; *PNH* = paroxysmal nocturnal hemoglobinuria; *PT* = prothrombin time; *PTT* = partial thromboplastin time; *RBC* = red blood cell; *WBC* = white blood cell.

A. **Hyperproliferative normocytic anemia** is characterized by erythrocyte loss.

1. **Hemolysis.** Clues that hemolysis may be present include elevated lactate dehydrogenase (LDH) and increased total bilirubin levels. If hemolysis is a concern, the **peripheral smear** must be examined. The cause of hemolytic anemia can be determined based on the morphology of the erythrocytes (e.g., schistocytes, spherocytes, or sickle cells). Two important causes of hemolysis include autoimmune hemolytic anemia (AIHA) and microangiopathic hemolytic anemia (MAHA).
   a. **AIHA** is caused by antibodies binding to RBCs. IgG autoantibodies are termed warm antibodies, and IgM autoantibodies are termed cold antibodies. Underlying etiologies include collagen vascular disorders, malignancy, infection (e.g., *Mycoplasma* and mononucleosis), drugs, prior allogeneic bone marrow transplant, or idiopathic causes.
   b. **MAHA** is characterized by intravascular shearing of RBCs, which leads to schistocyte formation. A few of the important causes of MAHA are listed here.
      (1) **Disseminated intravascular coagulation (DIC)**. In acute DIC, the major concern is bleeding, whereas in chronic DIC, thrombosis is more of a problem.

MNEMONIC **Causes of DIC ("MOIST")**

Malignancy
Obstetric complications
Infection
Shock
Trauma

(2) **Hemolytic-uremic syndrome (HUS)/thrombotic thrombocytopenic purpura (TTP).** The triad of HUS is hemolysis, uremia, and thrombocytopenia. TTP can contain the findings of the hemolytic-uremic syndrome plus fever and neurologic changes (although having all five findings is extremely rare). In certain patients, the neurologic abnormalities are the predominant feature and renal insufficiency is minimal. These patients are prototypical for TTP. Other patients will present with profound diarrhea and acute renal failure but with minimal neurologic changes. These patients likely represent HUS. However, there are many patients who overlap the spectrum of these two conditions.

(3) **Heart valve abnormalities**
(4) **Hemangiomas** (e.g., Kasabach Merritt syndrome)
(5) **Malignant hypertension**

2. **Hemorrhage.** If hemorrhage is suspected, the source of the blood loss (e.g., the gastrointestinal tract) must be determined.

B. Hypoproliferative normocytic anemia

1. **Pure red cell aplasia**
2. **Anemia of chronic disease**
3. **Renal failure**

C. Therapy

1. **AIHA.** Primary treatment includes steroids and/or splenectomy. Occasionally, immunosuppressive chemotherapy or immunotherapy (e.g., rituximab) may be required.
2. **MAHA** treatment should be aimed at correcting the underlying disorder if possible. Immediate therapy for TTP is critical and includes plasmapheresis. If unavailable, the patient can be temporized with fresh frozen plasma until transferred to a hospital with pheresis capability. Additional therapy with steroids, rituximab, or chemotherapy may also be required in refractory cases.
3. **Anemia of chronic disease or renal disease.** If anemia is profound enough to require intermittent transfusions, a trial of recombinant erythropoietin can be given. Erythropoietin should be titrated to raise the hemoglobin to a maximum of 12 g/dl and concurrent iron supplementation should be given if the ferritin is depressed.

REFERENCES

Franchini M, Zaffanello M, Veneri D. Advances in the pathogenesis, diagnosis and treatment of thrombotic thrombocytopenic purpura and hemolytic uremic syndrome. Thromb Res 2006;118(2):177–184.

Packman CH. Hemolytic anemia due to warm autoantibodies. Blood Rev 2008;22(1):17–31.

Petz LD. Cold antibody autoimmune hemolytic anemias. Blood Rev 2008;22(1):1–15.

Rund D, Rachmilewitz E. Beta-thalassemia. N Engl J Med 2005;353:1135.

Savona MR, Silver SM. Erythropoietin-stimulating agents in oncology. Cancer J 2008;14(2):75–84.

Polycythemia

I. INTRODUCTION. A hematocrit greater than 48% in women or 52% in men constitutes polycythemia. Likewise, a hemoglobin of greater than 16.5 g/dl in women or greater than 18.5 g/dl in men raises the suspicion for polycythemia.

A. Absolute polycythemia is characterized by an increase in red blood cell (RBC) mass.

B. Relative polycythemia is characterized by a decrease in plasma volume.

II. CLINICAL MANIFESTATIONS OF POLYCYTHEMIA

A. Patients are often asymptomatic if the hematocrit is lower than 60%. Higher hematocrits may cause:

1. Symptoms of **hyperviscosity** (e.g., headaches, dizziness, blurred vision)
2. Both **thrombosis** and **bleeding** may result from abnormalities in platelet function as the hematocrit rises.
3. Facial plethora (ruddy cyanosis) is a common finding.

B. Symptoms specific to polycythemia vera are described in Chapter 70.

III. CAUSES OF POLYCYTHEMIA. Polycythemia may be a secondary, physiologic response to another disorder (e.g., chronic hypoxia), or it may herald a primary myeloproliferative neoplasm like polycythemia vera.

A. Absolute polycythemia. There are six common causes of absolute polycythemia. Remember, "Hypoxia Can Cause Polycythemia Every Time."

MNEMONIC **Causes of Absolute Polycythemia ("Hypoxia Can Cause Polycythemia Every Time")**

Hypoxia (chronic)
Carboxyhemoglobinemia
Cushing's syndrome or **C**orticosteroids
Polycythemia vera
Erythropoietin-secreting **T**umors or post-renal **T**ransplant

1. **Hypoxia.** Chronic hypoxia, as a result of cardiopulmonary disease, sleep apnea, or high altitude, can lead to a secondary polycythemia.
2. **Carboxyhemoglobinemia** or **methemoglobinemia**. Carboxyhemoglobin and methemoglobin reduce the oxygen-carrying capacity of RBCs resulting in tissue hypoxia, which induces a secondary polycythemia. Smoking is a common cause of carboxyhemoglobinemia. Alternatively, high-affinity hemoglobin variants also cause a leftward shift of the hemoglobin–oxygen dissociation curve, cause decreased oxygen delivery to the tissues, and induce a compensatory polycythemia.
3. **Cushing's syndrome** or **corticosteroid therapy.** Corticosteroids have an erythropoietic effect, which can lead to polycythemia. Moreover, supplemental testosterone use can induce a secondary polycythemia by stimulating erythrocytosis through unclear mechanisms.
4. **Polycythemia vera** is a clonal myeloid neoplasm (myeloproliferative neoplasm) in which hematopoietic progenitor cells expand leading to elevated RBC indices (RBC count, hemoglobin, and hematocrit).
5. **Erythropoietin-secreting tumors** are primarily renal cell carcinomas, hemangioblastomas (of the cerebellum), uterine fibroids, or hepatocellular carcinomas.
6. **Post-renal transplant.** Due to unclear mechanisms, erythrocytosis can occur in up to 15% of patients after a renal transplant.

B. Relative polycythemia. There are two main causes of relative polycythemia.

1. **Dehydration** (e.g., from vomiting, diarrhea, excessive sweating, or diuretics) can deplete plasma volume, leading to a relative polycythemia.
2. **Stress erythrocytosis (Gaisböck's polycythemia)** actually results from contraction of the plasma volume and is therefore a misnomer. This benign disorder is seen most often in hypertensive, obese men.

IV. APPROACH TO THE PATIENT

A. Rule out hypoxemia, carboxyhemoglobinemia, and **methemoglobinemia.** These are relatively easy to evaluate. If abnormalities significant enough to result in polycythemia are found, the need for additional work-up may be eliminated. An arterial blood gas with oxygen saturation, carboxyhemoglobin, and methemoglobin levels is necessary for all patients and is more accurate than pulse oxygen saturation measurements (carbon monoxide values in excess of 5% are suggestive of this as the cause of the polycythemia). Moreover, while oxygen saturations may be adequate during the day, sleep apnea may be severe enough to lead to a secondary polycythemia, so consideration should be given to doing a sleep study if there is clinical suspicion.

B. Family history. If there is an associated family history of elevated blood counts, consider either polycythemia vera (see Chapter 70) or a high-affinity hemoglobin moiety, which may be evaluated by an oxygen dissociation curve.

C. Look at the patient's hematocrit.

1. **Greater than 60% in men or 55% in women**
   a. A hematocrit greater than 60% in men or 55% in women essentially rules out steroid excess, which usually causes a mild polycythemia. Furthermore, because an elevated RBC mass is found in 99% of these patients, decreased plasma volume is unlikely, and an RBC mass study is usually not necessary.
   b. A hematocrit greater than 60% in men or 55% in women usually reduces the list of possible diagnoses to either polycythemia vera (more common) or an erythropoietin-secreting tumor (less common). The following characteristics may provide clues to differentiating polycythemia vera from other secondary causes (see also Chapter 70 for the diagnostic criteria of polycythemia vera).
      (1) **Polycythemia vera**
         (a) Polycythemia can be associated with splenomegaly, leukocytosis, and thrombocytosis. These are factors used in the older Polycythemia Vera Study Group (PVSG) criteria for diagnosing polycythemia vera.
         (b) A history of bleeding or thrombotic complications points toward polycythemia vera.
         (c) Concomitant iron deficiency with elevated RBC indices, especially as determined by a bone marrow biopsy, is suggestive of polycythemia vera. Previously used tests—such as an increased leukocyte alkaline phosphatase score or an increased vitamin B_{12} level—are rarely employed today (see Chapter 70).
         (d) A decreased serum erythropoietin level is also useful (almost all patients with polycythemia vera have a level <20 mU/ml).
         (e) Molecular testing for the *Janus Kinase 2* (*JAK2*) gene mutation (V617F) has identified the change in approximately 95% of patients with polycythemia vera. However, it neither rules in nor rules out the diagnosis on its own.

(2) **Erythropoietin-secreting tumors**
   (a) An abdominal computed tomography (CT) scan may help rule out renal pathology (including cancer) and hepatic malignancies.
   (b) Brain imaging [preferably with magnetic resonance imaging (MRI)] may be performed if there is any clinical suspicion of a cerebellar lesion.

2. **Hematocrit less than 60% in men or 55% in women.** A **RBC mass study** should be performed to rule out a **decreased plasma volume,** which is responsible for polycythemia in approximately 50% of cases. In general, secondary causes will account for far more cases than polycythemia vera.

V. TREATMENT is aimed at the underlying disorder. Stress erythrocytosis requires no treatment other than encouraging weight loss and oral hydration. General therapeutic measures include the following:

A. Oxygen therapy is useful in patients with an arterial oxygen tension (PaO_2) lower than 60 mm Hg.

B. Smoking cessation is highly encouraged (especially in patients with carboxyhemoglobinemia).

C. Hydration is recommended for patients with evidence of dehydration.

D. An **ACE inhibitor** is used to treat post-renal transplant polycythemia.

E. Surgical consultation is recommended if an erythropoietin-secreting tumor is suspected.

F. Phlebotomy to lower the hematocrit is usually only indicated for patients with polycythemia vera (see Chapter 70 for management of polycythemia vera).

REFERENCES

Levine RL, Gilliland DG. Myeloproliferative disorders. Blood 2008;112(6): 2190–2198.

McMullin MF, Bareford D, Campbell P, et al. Guidelines for the diagnosis, investigation and management of polycythaemia/erythrocytosis. Br J Haematol 2005;130(2):174–195.

Tefferi A. Classification, diagnosis and management of myeloproliferative disorders in the JAK2V617F era. Hematology Am Soc Hematol Educ Program. 2006:240–245.

64

Leukocytosis

I. INTRODUCTION

A. The **circulating pool of white blood cells** (WBCs, leukocytes) consists of:

1. Neutrophils
2. Lymphocytes
3. Monocytes
4. Eosinophils
5. Basophils

B. Definitions

1. **Leukocytosis.** In leukocytosis, the total WBC count **exceeds 11,000 cells/μl.**
2. **Leukemoid reaction.** A leukemoid reaction occurs when the leukocyte count **exceeds 50,000 cells/μl.** There is often evidence of a "left shift"—early neutrophil precursors (myelocytes, metamyelocytes, and bands)—seen on the peripheral blood. This is not a formal diagnosis and etiologies such as primary bone marrow disorders must be evaluated. However, it may simply reflect a healthy bone marrow that is reacting to an external stimulus (e.g., trauma, inflammation, infection, malignancy).
3. **Leukoerythroblastosis.** This term is used when there is evidence of immature WBCs and nucleated RBCs on the peripheral smear, regardless of the total WBC count. Leukoerythroblastosis usually implies bone marrow infiltration either by a metastatic cancer, a hematopoietic malignancy, or an infection.

C. Because each cell type can be increased in response to various stimuli, determining the predominant cell type in patients with leukocytosis may offer some insight into the cause.

II. NEUTROPHILIA is defined as a neutrophil count that **exceeds 7700 cells/μl.**

A. Causes of neutrophilia. Neutrophilia can be caused by many of the major disease categories discussed in Chapter 1 (see Table 64-1).

B. Approach to the patient. When evaluating patients with neutrophilia, the most important initial consideration should be **infection.** If this and other benign disorders are excluded,

TABLE 64-1

COMMON CAUSES OF NEUTROPHILIA

Category of Disease	Specific Causes
Hematologic	Hemolytic anemia, splenectomy
Pregnancy related	Pregnancy-induced neutrophilia
Drugs/toxins	Corticosteroids, lithium, mercury, ethylene glycol
Metabolic/endocrine	Hyperthyroidism, ketoacidosis
Inflammatory	Rheumatoid arthritis, vasculitis, gout, acute myocardial infarcts, allergic reactions
Infectious	Bacteria, viruses, fungi, parasites
Neoplastic	Myeloproliferative neoplasms, myelodysplastic syndromes, acute myeloid leukemias, gastrointestinal or renal malignancy, melanoma, Hodgkin's disease
Trauma	Postsurgery, insect bites, jellyfish stings, crush injuries, electric shock

a search for malignancy (which may include a bone marrow biopsy) is usually warranted. Acutely infected or injured patients have elevated levels of endogenous glucocorticoids, which in turn will lead to low levels of eosinophils and basophils. The presence of eosinophils and basophils in acutely ill patients usually indicates one of the following:

1. **Concomitant adrenal insufficiency**
2. **Granulocyte-macrophage colony-stimulating factor (GM-CSF)-secreting tumor**
3. **Hematologic malignancy** [especially chronic myeloid leukemia (CML)]

III. LYMPHOCYTOSIS is defined as a lymphocyte count that **exceeds 4000 cells/μl.**

A. Causes of lymphocytosis (Table 64-2). The severity of lymphocytosis may indicate possible causes.

B. Approach to the patient

1. The first step in evaluating a patient with lymphocytosis is to look for **leukoerythroblastosis** on the peripheral smear. If leukoerythroblastosis is present, a bone marrow biopsy is necessary.
2. In patients without evidence of leukoerythroblastosis, a benign cause should be evaluated by history, examination, and laboratory testing.
3. **Flow cytometry.** Clonality of the lymphocytes should be evaluated by flow cytometry, and this may aid in assessing

TABLE 64-2

COMMON CAUSES OF LYMPHOCYTOSIS

Type of Lymphocytosis	Specific Causes
Mild to moderate (4000–15,000/μl)	Viral illness (mononucleosis, acute hepatitis A or B, HIV, varicella, influenza, or HTLV-1) Secondary to other infections (e.g., pertussis, tuberculosis, toxoplasmosis, syphilis) Postsplenectomy Malignancy (e.g., lymphoma, leukemia)
Severe (>15,000/μl)	Viral illness (mononucleosis, coxsackie and enteroviruses) Pertussis Malignancy (e.g., lymphoma, leukemia)

HIV = human immunodeficiency virus; *HTLV* = human T-lymphotropic virus.

for atypical expression of lymphoid or myeloid markers, which may facilitate a diagnosis of a malignancy.

4. Alternatively, a bone marrow biopsy and aspiration may be required to assess for an underlying hematopoietic process.

IV. MONOCYTOSIS is defined as a monocyte count that **exceeds 1000 cells/μl.**

A. Causes of monocytosis (Table 64-3). Monocytes are very important, not only in the killing of **obligate intracellular parasites** (e.g., fungi, parasites, yeast), but also in **granulomatous inflammation.**

B. Approach to the patient

1. A clinical history of infectious symptoms, sick contacts, or recent travel should be sought. Additionally, signs of inflammatory or connective tissue diseases should be reviewed.
2. A peripheral blood smear should be examined to look for signs of concurrent hematologic abnormalities. If the level of monocytosis is extremely high, a hematologic malignancy, including acute myelomonocytic (FAB-M4 AML) and acute monocytic leukemia (FAB-M5 AML), or chronic myelomonocytic leukemia (CMML) should be strongly suspected. Moreover, FAB-M4 and FAB-M5 AML have a predilection to infiltrate tissues, which may manifest as gingival hypertrophy, leukemia cutis, or leukostasis occurring with WBC counts as low as 50,000 cells/μl.

TABLE 64-3

COMMON CAUSES OF MONOCYTOSIS

Category of Disease	Specific Causes
Infectious	Tuberculosis, endocarditis, brucellosis, syphilis, fungal or protozoal infections, CMV, and varicella
Neoplastic	Hodgkin's disease, multiple myeloma, acute myeloid leukemia, myeloproliferative neoplasms, myelodysplastic syndromes including chronic myelomonocytic leukemia, carcinoma
Hematologic	Autoimmune hemolytic anemia, ITP, postsplenectomy, chronic neutropenia
Inflammatory	Inflammatory bowel disease, sarcoidosis, connective tissue diseases, myositis, celiac sprue

CMV = cytomegalovirus; *ITP* = idiopathic thrombocytopenic purpura.

V. BASOPHILIA is defined as a basophil count that **exceeds 200 cells/μl.**

A. Causes of basophilia (Table 64-4). Basophils have an important role in the control of parasitic infections, but also may have roles in mediating hypersensitivity reactions.

B. Approach to the patient

1. Evaluate the patient for new exposures to medications or new foods.
2. The patient should also be asked about infectious symptoms, sick contacts, or recent travel.
3. If no clear underlying etiology is found, consider a bone marrow biopsy and molecular testing for a myeloid leukemia or myeloproliferative neoplasm.

TABLE 64-4

COMMON CAUSES OF BASOPHILIA

Category of Disease	Specific Causes
Inflammatory	Food or drug allergy, inflammatory bowel disease, juvenile rheumatoid arthritis
Endocrinopathies	Diabetes mellitus, ectopic estrogen use, hypothyroidism
Infectious	Viral (varicella, influenza, or smallpox), tuberculosis, parasitic infections
Neoplastic	Myeloproliferative neoplasms, especially chronic myeloid leukemia, acute myeloid leukemia, carcinoma

REFERENCES

Abramson N, Melton B. Leukocytosis: basics of clinical assessment. Am Fam Phys 2000;62:2053–2060.

Landgren O, Kyle RA. Multiple myeloma, chronic lymphocytic leukaemia and associated precursor diseases. Br J Haematol 2007;139(5):717–723.

Macintyre EA, Linch DC. Lymphocytosis: is it leukaemia and when to treat. Postgrad Med J 1988;64(747):42–47 [Classic article].

Marti G, Abbasi F, Raveche E, et al. Overview of monoclonal B-cell lymphocytosis. Br J Haematol 2007;139(5):701–708.

Vignola AM, Gjomarkaj M, Arnoux B, et al. Monocytes. J Allergy Clin Immunol 1998;101:149–152 [Classic article].

65 Eosinophilia

I. INTRODUCTION

A. Eosinophils, a type of white blood cell (WBC), are a normal component of peripheral blood and certain tissues. However, their presence in other tissues is often a sign of a pathologic process. Eosinophils do the following:

1. Play a major role in defending the body against multicellular, helminthic parasites
2. Elaborate mediators that promote mucus secretion and alter vascular permeability in allergic diseases
3. Induce mast cells and basophils to release allergic mediators

B. Eosinophil count. The normal range of eosinophils in the blood is 0–400 cells/μl (0%–4%), and counts greater than 650 cells/μl are frequently abnormal. Counts can vary based on numerous factors including age, environmental factors, and the time of day (which may be due to the diurnal variation of cortisol production).

1. **Eosinopenia** is commonly seen in bacterial and viral infections and with exogenous corticosteroid use.
2. **Eosinophilia** is associated with many diseases (see II).

II. CAUSES OF EOSINOPHILIA

A. Pulmonary diseases. Many primary lung disorders can lead to eosinophilia, including Löffler's syndrome and eosinophilic pneumonia. Asthma can also be associated with eosinophilia.

B. Helminthic infections. The level of eosinophilia may reflect the burden of the helminthic infection, but the absence of eosinophilia does not rule out this type of infection

1. **Filariasis**
2. **Ascariasis**
3. **Schistosomiasis**
4. **Strongyloidiasis**
5. **Trichinosis**

Disseminated strongyloides sometimes does not cause eosinophilia because of the superimposed bacterial infection that may accompany parasitic dissemination.

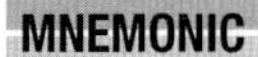

Causes of Eosinophilia

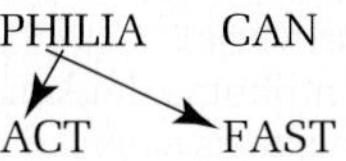

Pulmonary disease
Helminthic infections

Filariasis
Ascariasis
Schistosomiasis or **S**trongyloides infection
Trichinosis

Infections, other

Allergic bronchopulmonary aspergillosis
Coccidioidomycosis
Tuberculosis (especially chronic)

L-Tryptophan
Immunologic disorders
Addison's disease

Cutaneous disorder and **C**holesterol emboli
Allergic disorders
Neoplasms

C. Other infections

1. **Allergic bronchopulmonary aspergillosis (ABPA)**

Invasive aspergillosis does not cause eosinophilia.

2. **Coccidioidomycosis**
3. **Tuberculosis,** especially chronic tuberculosis
4. **Human immunodeficiency virus (HIV).** The eosinophilia may be associated with the viral infection itself or due to secondary infections seen in HIV or specific antiretroviral therapies.

D. Contaminated L-tryptophan can cause eosinophilia-myalgia syndrome.

E. Immunologic disorders [e.g., vasculitis (especially Churg-Strauss syndrome), severe rheumatoid arthritis, eosinophilic fasciitis]

F. Addison's disease

G. Cutaneous disorders (e.g., bullous pemphigoid, scabies, eosinophilic cellulitis)

H. **Cholesterol embolization**

I. **Allergic disorders** (e.g., asthma, allergic rhinitis, atopic dermatitis, drug reactions, acute urticaria)

J. **Neoplasms.** Solid tumors, lymphoma, leukemia, hypereosinophilic syndrome, and mastocytosis can lead to eosinophilia.

III. APPROACH TO THE PATIENT

A. History and physical examination

1. **New exposures** including dietary changes and new medications
2. **Travel,** including international travel, travel to the southwest United States, and exposure to unpurified water. Risks for specific infections may be tied to geographic boundaries and may direct the diagnostic testing. Asking about companions' symptoms may focus the evaluation of possible infectious causes.
3. **Focal symptoms** including rash, cough, shortness of breath, fever, connective tissue complaints, and gastrointestinal (GI) symptoms may focus the evaluation.

B. Laboratory exam

1. **Stool examination** including an examination for ova and parasites on several occasions may be required. Consideration for specific parasitic serologies (i.e., strongyloides IgG) or molecular testing may be helpful.
2. **Radiographic imaging** and **pulmonary testing** including bronchoscopy may be required to evaluate for pulmonary involvement of the eosinophilia as well as to establish the diagnosis of ABPA.
3. **Peripheral blood smear** may help identify specific pathogens (i.e., microfilariae) or may identify an acute leukemia associated with eosinophilia.
4. **Hypereosinophilic syndrome** is associated with a peripheral eosinophilia as well as tissue deposition of eosinophils into the lungs, heart, kidneys, and GI tract. Specific testing for tissue involvement may be required. Clonality can occasionally be proven in the eosinophilia, specifically by identifying a chromosomal abnormality. The most frequent abnormality involves an interstitial chromosomal deletion of chromosome 4q12 (called the CHIC2 deletion) resulting in the FIP1L1-PDGFR-alpha fusion. If clonal changes are found and the blast percentage is increased, consider the diagnosis of chronic eosinophilic leukemia.
5. **Mast cell disorders,** including cutaneous and systemic mastocytosis, can be associated with an eosinophilia and a diagnosis is based on either a tissue or bone marrow biopsy demonstrating an accumulation of an abnormal population of mast cells.

REFERENCES

Di Stefano F, Amoroso A. Clinical approach to the patient with blood eosinophilia. Eur Ann Allergy Clin Immunol 2005;37(10):380–386.

Rothenberg ME. Eosinophilia. N Engl J Med 1998;338:1592–1600 [Classic article].

Tefferi A. Blood eosinophilia: a new paradigm in disease classification, diagnosis, and treatment. Mayo Clin Proc 2005;80(1):75–83.

66 Bleeding Disorders

I. INTRODUCTION. A predisposition to bleeding can result from **problems with platelets** (either number or function) or **problems with coagulation** (factor deficiency or factor inhibitors).

II. CLINICAL MANIFESTATIONS OF BLEEDING DISORDERS

- **A. Recurrent bleeding** since childhood or a family history of bleeding suggests an **inherited problem.**
- **B. Mucocutaneous petechiae** or ecchymoses are usually indicative of **platelet problems.**
- **C. Spontaneous deep bleeding** into joints (hemarthroses) or **delayed bleeding** after surgery or trauma is suggestive of **coagulation problems.**

III. APPROACH TO THE PATIENT. Figure 66-1 summarizes the general approach to a patient with a bleeding disorder.

- **A. Platelet count.** Although affected by a number of variables, the platelet count is usually less than 100,000 cells/μl before the bleeding time becomes prolonged. Therefore, mildly decreased counts are not responsible for clinical bleeding, and a concurrent problem of platelet function or coagulation should be considered.
- **B. Prothrombin time (PT)/partial thromboplastin time (PTT).** There are three types of PT/PTT abnormalities: increased PT/normal PTT, increased PT/increased PTT, or normal PT/increased PTT.
  1. **Increased PT/normal PTT**
     - a. **Differential diagnosis**
       - (1) **Early disseminated intravascular coagulation (DIC)**
       - (2) **Liver disease**
       - (3) **Warfarin therapy**
       - (4) **Vitamin K deficiency**
       - (5) **Factor VII deficiency** (isolated factor VII deficiency is a rare cause of an elevated PT/normal PTT)
     - b. **Recommended work-up**
       - (1) **Patient history.** Ask about medications and note factors that may predispose a patient to vitamin K deficiency (e.g., malnutrition, pancreatic insufficiency, liver disease, recent antibiotic use).

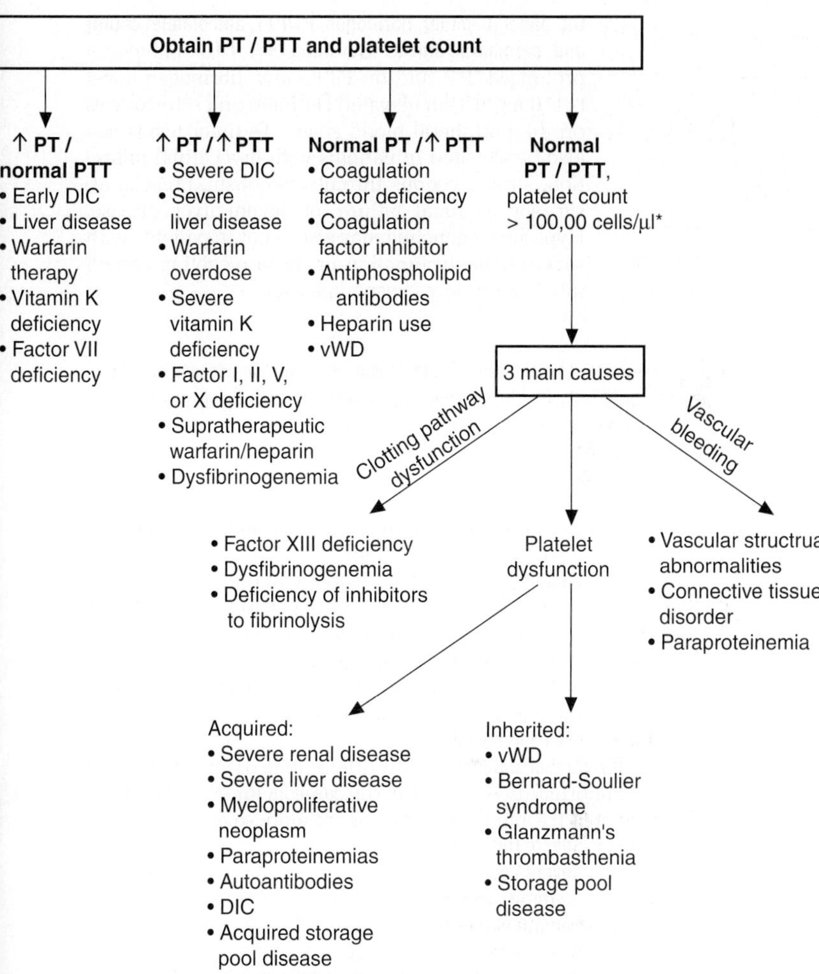

A platelet count less than 100,000 cells/μl may result in an increased bleeding time and a bleeding disorder. Patients with platelet counts greater than 100,000 cells/μl may still be thrombocytopenic (i.e., a platelet count less than 150,000 cells/μl), but this level of thrombocytopenia is usually not the cause of a bleeding disorder; therefore, other causes should be considered.

gure 66-1 Approach to the patient with a bleeding disorder. *DIC* = disseminated intra-scular coagulation; *PT* = prothrombin time; *PTT* = partial thromboplastin time; *vWD* = n Willebrand's disease.

(2) **DIC panel (D-dimer, fibrinogen, PT/PTT, and platelet count) and peripheral smear.** Evidence for DIC includes a prolonged PT and/or PTT, low fibrinogen level (<150 mg/dl), an elevated D-dimer, and schistocytes on the peripheral blood smear. D-dimer levels can also be elevated in patients with myocardial infarction, stroke, venous thromboembolism, preeclampsia, sepsis, renal failure, or severe liver disease. Hypofibrinogenemia may also occur in patients with severe liver dysfunction or those receiving certain medications (e.g., L-asparaginase).

Because of many overlapping findings between liver disease and DIC, the presence of schistocytes may be the only distinguishing feature for DIC in a patient with concomitant liver failure.

(3) **Liver tests.** Bilirubin, albumin, and transaminase levels are often obtained.

(4) **Vitamin K deficiency.** A decrease in the quantity of the vitamin K–dependant clotting factors II, VII, IX, and X can be used to assess for vitamin K deficiency.

(5) **Factor VII level.** An isolated factor VII level is rarely ordered but can be obtained if the cause of the increased PT is still unknown.

2. **Increased PT/increased PTT**

a. **Differential diagnosis.** The differential diagnosis for this abnormality is generally the same as for an isolated elevated PT, but the conditions are more severe.

(1) **Severe DIC**
(2) **Severe liver disease**
(3) **Warfarin overdose**
(4) **Heparin overdose**
(5) **Severe vitamin K deficiency**
(6) **Factor I, II, V,** or **X inhibitor or deficiency** (extremely rare causes of an elevated PT/PTT)
(7) **Dysfibrinogenemia**

b. **Recommended work-up.** The recommended initial evaluation is the same as that for increased PT/normal PTT. However, individual factor inhibitors or deficiencies can be identified with a mixing study and factor-specific quantitative analyses. Additionally, dysfibrinogenemia can be characterized through an assessment of both the fibrinogen antigen and activity levels as well as with the thrombin clotting time and reptilase time.

3. **Normal PT/increased PTT**
   a. **Differential diagnosis.** After excluding the obvious cause (i.e., heparin therapy), you need to consider four possibilities.
      (1) **Coagulation factor deficiency**
      (2) **Coagulation factor inhibitor**
      (3) **Antiphospholipid antibodies**
      (4) **von Willebrand's disease (especially type IIN and III)**
   b. **Recommended work-up**
      (1) **Patient history.** The patient history can provide valuable information. If the patient has a history of bleeding, a factor deficiency, a factor inhibitor, or von Willebrand's disease is most likely. If the patient has a history of clotting rather than bleeding, an antiphospholipid antibody may be present.
      (2) **Mixing study.** Only 50% factor activity is needed to have a normal PT or PTT. By mixing the patient's plasma with an equal amount of plasma with a normal PT and PTT, enough factor will be provided to correct for any factor deficiency, but often does not correct for an inhibitor of the specific clotting factor.
         (a) **If the PTT corrects,** a **factor deficiency** is diagnosed. The most common factor deficiencies are factor VIII **(hemophilia A),** factor IX **(hemophilia B),** and factor XI deficiencies; therefore, **factor VIII, IX,** and **XI levels** should be assessed after the mixing study corrects the PTT.
         (b) **If the PTT does not correct**, an **antiphospholipid antibody** may be present. Laboratory tests to identify an antiphospholipid antibody include analysis for a lupus anticoagulant, an anticardiolipin antibody, a β-2 glycoprotein 1 antibody, and assessment of the dilute Russell's viper venom time (see III D 1).
         (c) **A factor inhibitor** can also prolong the PTT and may be suspected with a prolonged PTT and a mixing study that does not correct. Some inhibitors function better at 37°C, and therefore, the mixing study always includes an immediate mixing value and one obtained after warming the sample to 37°C for 30 to 60 minutes. The results are reported as Bethesda units (BU), which indicates the number of titrations required to dilute out the inhibitor; a higher BU implies a higher amount of the inhibitor.
      (3) **von Willebrand's disease** (vWD) can result in a qualitative or quantitative decrease in proteins required to

form a functional clot. In **vWD type IIN**, there is a decreased ability of factor VIII to bind to the von Willebrand antigen resulting in a decreased level of factor VIII, which may prolong the PTT. Likewise, in **vWD type III,** there is a near absence of the von Willebrand antigen, resulting in a near absence of factor VIII.

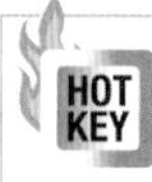

Because hemophilia A is an X-linked disorder, consider a type III vWD in females presenting with a near absence of factor VIII.

C. Patients with mucocutaneous bleeding and/or ecchymoses whose coagulation studies are normal may have a congenital or acquired platelet disorder or vWD. Historically, a **bleeding time** was used to assess for an underlying platelet disorder, but because this test is affected by a number of nonpathologic variables including skin temperature, age, sex, anxiety, cuff pressure, and depth of the incision, its use has diminished significantly. More recently, the **Platelet Function Analyzer (PFA-100)** has been used to screen for platelet disorders, mainly in the perioperative setting. However, the most accurate assessments include platelet aggregometry and agonist-induced platelet secretory testing, but this testing is limited to larger academic centers and cannot be sent to centralized centers.

1. If the coagulation tests are normal and the platelet count is greater than 100,000 cells/μl, platelet dysfunction, vWD, or vascular abnormality may be implicated.
   a. **Acquired platelet dysfunction**
      (1) **Differential diagnosis.** Acquired platelet disorders are usually systemic.
         (a) **Severe renal disease** (i.e., uremia)
         (b) **Severe liver disease**
         (c) **Malignancy.** Multiple myeloma and Waldenstrom's macroglobulinemia can both lead to platelet dysfunction due to the paraprotein interfering with platelet function but also due to hyperviscosity.
         (d) **Myeloproliferative neoplasms** can be associated with an increased risk of bleeding even when platelet levels are elevated.
         (e) **DIC.** The fibrin split products produced in DIC inhibit platelet function.
         (f) **Acquired storage pool disease.** Cardiopulmonary bypass surgery or vasculitis can cause platelets

to release all their granules, resulting in dysfunctional platelets.

(g) **Aspirin** irreversibly inhibits platelet function for the life of the platelet (7–10 days); other nonsteroidal anti-inflammatory drugs (NSAIDs) reversibly inhibit platelet function and the effect is more transient.

(h) **Additional medications. Clopidogrel, ticlopidine, abciximab,** and **eptifibatide** are increasingly being used in patients with cardiovascular disease and can be associated with an increased risk for bleeding.

(2) **Recommended work-up**

(a) **Patient history.** A history of renal, hepatic, or malignant disease should be sought. A medication history (including all over-the-counter drugs) should also always be elicited. Acquired storage pool disease is suspected if the clinical history and examination are appropriate.

(b) **Complete blood count (CBC) with platelets and differential.** A CBC will help evaluate the possibility of a myeloproliferative neoplasm (see Chapter 70) and may provide some evidence of a plasma cell dyscrasia (Chapter 72).

(c) **DIC panel.** A DIC panel can help evaluate the possibility of DIC.

(d) **Renal and liver tests [blood urea nitrogen (BUN), creatinine, aspartate aminotransferase (AST), alanine aminotransferase (ALT), protein, albumin, and alkaline phosphatase]** may help identify medical reasons for the bleeding disorder.

(e) **Serum protein electrophoresis with immunofixation, urine Bence Jones protein, or serum free light chain** analysis may be used to evaluate the presence of a paraproteinemia (see Chapter 72).

b. **Inherited platelet dysfunction.** Platelet activity in clotting is dependent upon their adherence, activation, aggregation, and release of granular products. Dysfunction in any of these steps may lead to clinical bleeding.

(1) **Differential diagnosis.** The first two disorders involve problems with platelet adherence, and the second two involve problems with platelet aggregation.

(a) **von Willebrand's disease.** von Willebrand's factor (vWF) is elaborated by megakaryocytes and endothelial cells but then undergoes extensive posttranslational modification. It then circulates in the plasma in multimers of varying size bound to factor VIII (which vWF stabilizes). vWF binds to the glycoprotein Ib receptor on platelets and helps platelets adhere to endothelium.

(i) In **type I vWD** (75% of vWD cases; autosomal dominant), there is a mild to moderate quantitative decrease in the amount of vWF.

(ii) In **type II vWD** (10%–15% of vWD cases; most are autosomal dominant), there is a qualitative decrease in vWF activity.

a. In **type IIA vWD** (autosomal dominant), there is an increased susceptibility to the cleavage of the vWF large multimers by the von Willebrand factor cleaving protease (ADAMTS 13), resulting in a relative decrease in the intermediate and large multimers of vWF, which are the more active forms in inducing platelet adhesion.

b. In **type IIB vWD** (autosomal dominant), there is an increased spontaneous binding of the high-molecular-weight multimers to platelets, resulting in a decrease in the free large multimers as well as a mild decrease in platelet numbers.

c. In **type IIM vWD** (autosomal dominant), there is a decreased binding of vWF to glycoprotein Ib with an apparently normal multimer analysis.

d. **Type IIN vWD** (autosomal recessive) results from an altered binding of factor VIII to the vWF, resulting in decreased factor VIII levels.

(iii) In **type III vWD** (autosomal recessive), vWF is almost completely lacking and results in a near complete absence of factor VIII. This is a very rare type.

(b) **Bernard-Soulier syndrome** results from a loss in the platelet receptor for vWF (glycoprotein Ib) and thus can be confused with type IIM vWD.

(c) **Glanzmann's thrombasthenia** results from the loss of the IIb–IIIa glycoprotein platelet receptor, which leads to decreased fibrinogen binding and, therefore, defective platelet aggregation.

(d) **Congenital storage pool diseases** are caused by defects in the formation of or the signaling mechanisms that induce the release of platelet granules. These include gray platelet syndrome (deficient α-granules), Wiskott-Aldrich syndrome (due to mutations in the X-linked WAS protein), Chediak-Higashi syndrome, and Hermansky-Pudlak syndrome.

(2) **Recommended work-up**

(a) **Patient history.** vWD is a largely autosomal dominant disorder, and Bernard-Soulier syndrome and Glanzmann's thrombasthenia are autosomal recessive disorders; therefore, obtaining the family history is important. Several of the storage pool diseases have coexisting physical findings including albinism (Chediak-Higashi and Hermansky-Pudlak) or coexisitng immune disorders (Wiskott-Aldrich).

(b) **vWD panel.** Screen for vWD first because vWD is the most common inherited disorder of platelet function. A vWD panel includes the following tests:

(i) **von Willebrand Factor antigen (vWF:Ag)** can be quantified utilizing a number of methods.

(ii) **von Willebrand antigen activity** is often assessed using the ristocetin cofactor activity (vWF:RCo). Ristocetin is an antibiotic that binds the platelet receptor glycoprotein Ib to vWF, especially the higher-molecular-weight multimers. The patient's plasma is mixed with normal platelets and ristocetin, which should cause the patient's vWF to bind to the platelet surface resulting in platelet aggregation. The absence of platelet aggregation implies a quantitative or qualitative decrease in vWF. Type II vWD with decreased large multimers (IIA and IIB) often have a depressed vWF:RCo compared to the vWF:Ag.

(iii) **Factor VIII antigen/factor VIII activity.** Since vWF binds factor VIII and stabilizes the protein, decreased vWF can lead to decreased factor VIII levels and thus decreased activity.

(iv) **Ristocetin-induced platelet aggregation (RIPA)** is an analysis of the affinity of binding of vWF to glycoprotein Ib. Interestingly, the vWF in type IIB binds to glycoprotein Ib with increased affinity, and it is the one vWD that has an elevated RIPA. Alternatively, Bernard-Soulier syndrome demonstrates a normal vWD panel but a decreased RIPA due to an absent glycoprotein 1b protein.

(v) **vWF multimer analysis** utilizes gel electrophoresis to visualize the size and quantity of the various vWF multimers.

Type I vWD often shows a **moderate parallel quantitative** decrease in all parts of the panel, whereas type III vWD demonstrates a **significant parallel quantitative** decrease in all parts of the panel. In type II vWD, there are **qualitative** changes in the von Willebrand pathways leading to changes in either the multimer analysis, vWF:RCo activity, or factor VIII levels.

(c) Platelet aggregometry, agonist-induced platelet secretory testing, and electron microscopy can be used to diagnose **Glanzmann's thrombasthenia** and many of the other congenital storage pool diseases.

(i) In many storage pool diseases, platelets will demonstrate an initial aggregation response to agonists, but then disassociate. Electron microscopy can help identify abnormal granule formation.

(ii) In Glanzmann's thrombasthenia, most platelet agonists other than ristocetin fail to induce any aggregation because the necessary IIb–IIIa receptor is missing.

2. **If there is a clinical history of bleeding** and the prior testing is normal, a few rare disorders still need to be considered. All these involve a defect in cross-linking of fibrin leading to a poor stability of the clot.
   a. **Differential diagnosis**
      (1) **Factor XIII ("fibrin-stabilizing factor") deficiency**
      (2) **Dysfibrinogenemia**
      (3) **Deficiency of inhibitors to fibrinolysis** (i.e., plasminogen activator inhibitor or α_2-plasmin inhibitor)
   b. **Recommended work-up**
      (1) **Increased clot solubility in urea, acetic acid, or monochloroacetic acid** is seen in factor XIII deficiency, but a quantitative analysis is required to finalize the diagnosis.

(2) **Increased thrombin time and reptilase time** is evidence of a possible dysfibrinogenemia.

(3) **Quantitative and functional assessments** of plasminogen activator inhibitor and α_2-plasmin inhibitor can be performed to diagnose deficiency of inhibitors to fibrinolysis.

D. Other tests

1. **Dilute Russell's viper venom time (dRVVT).** Russell's viper venom activates factor X, leading to activation of factor II (thrombinogen) and subsequently factor I (fibrinogen) but still requires phospholipid. The dRVVT may therefore be prolonged when **antiphospholipid antibodies** are present.
2. **Thrombin time** measures the time for the blood to clot after thrombin is directly added to plasma and therefore assesses thrombin's conversion of fibrinogen to fibrin. The thrombin time will be prolonged when thrombin is inhibited (as in **heparin therapy**), when there is low fibrinogen (as in **afibrinogenemia** or **DIC**), or when there is abnormal fibrinogen (as in **dysfibrinogenemia**).
3. **Reptilase time** is just like thrombin time, except it is not sensitive to the effect of heparin. If the thrombin time is prolonged but the reptilase time is normal, then a **heparin effect** is diagnosed. If the reptilase time is also prolonged, then afibrinogenemia, DIC, or dysfibrinogenemia should be considered.

E. Nonhematologic causes of bleeding. A number of vascular abnormalities noted in Figure 66-1 have been associated with clinically relevant bleeding. These include congenital or acquired structural and connective tissue disorders involving the vascular wall as well as vasculitides that result in increased blood vessel fragility or permeability. Diagnosis and treatment depend on the etiology identified, although some congenital disorders have no specific therapy available.

IV. TREATMENT

A. Platelet problems

1. **Quantitative problems.** The treatment of thrombocytopenia is discussed in Chapter 60.
2. **Qualitative problems** are usually only treated when the patient is acutely bleeding or surgery is planned. Specific therapies may include dialysis for uremia, myelosuppression for myeloproliferative neoplasms, or platelet transfusions for platelet storage pool diseases. Other commonly used treatments include:
   a. **Desmopressin (DDAVP)** (0.3 μg/kg/day) works presumably by increasing the release of stored vWF and factor VIII from endothelial cells and is useful as prophylaxis

before surgery in patients with type I vWD or hemophilia A. It may also be useful in other disorders of platelet dysfunction [e.g., uremia, drug-induced platelet dysfunction, and some storage pool diseases (Bernard-Soulier but not Glanzmann thrombasthenia)].

(1) A test dose of desmopressin given while the patient is not bleeding should always be administered to ensure adequate levels of vWF are induced 60 minutes and 3–4 hours after the infusion. Use in emergent situations without prior testing is not recommended as some patients will not respond.

(2) Stores of vWF are depleted in 2–3 days, so desmopressin is usually only effective as a short-term treatment. Moreover, desmopressin is an antidiuretic and prolonged use or use in children under the age of 2 can lead to hyponatremia and an increased risk of seizures.

(3) Desmopressin is ineffective in type III vWD. In type IIB vWD, abnormal large multimers of vWF have a high affinity to platelets, and treatment with desmopressin can trigger paradoxical thromboses and thrombocytopenia (from splenic removal). Therefore, the use of desmopressin should be avoided in patients with these subtypes.

b. **Intermediate purity factor VIII concentrates** also contain vWF and are coprecipitated with factor VIII and pasteurized to reduce the risk of viral transmission.

c. **Cryoprecipitate** (10–15 units every 12 hours) is effective in raising vWF levels 30%–50% (approximately 3% per unit), and therefore can be used in patients with vWD. However, cryoprecipitate carries an elevated risk of transmitting viral infections and has a higher risk of transfusion-associated allergic reactions, and therefore its use in hemophiliacs or in those with vWD has fallen out of favor.

d. **Platelet transfusions** can be used for refractory bleeding.

B. Coagulation problems

1. **Increased PT/normal PTT** and **increased PT/increased PTT**

a. **With significant acute bleeding**

(1) **Fresh frozen plasma** is given to correct the PT/PTT regardless of the underlying etiology.

(2) **Cryoprecipitate** can be used for patients with DIC to restore the fibrinogen level to greater than 150 mg/dl.

(3) **Vitamin K** (10 mg subcutaneously daily for 3 days) can be administered in cases where vitamin K deficiency plays a primary or contributing role in the patient's coagulopathy.

Fresh frozen plasma contains all factors but only small amounts of fibrinogen. Cryoprecipitate contains concentrated factor VIII, vWF, and fibrinogen.

b. **Without significant acute bleeding.** Treatment takes into account the underlying cause.
   (1) **DIC.** In patients with DIC but no acute bleeding, the elevated PT is not treated. Instead, treatment is aimed at correcting the cause of the DIC (e.g., antibiotics for sepsis).
   (2) **Warfarin therapy.** The mechanism used to correct the international normalized ratio (INR) is dependent upon both the degree of the elevation of the INR and the presence of bleeding.
      (a) If the INR is less than 5 and the patient is not bleeding, the warfarin dose is usually withheld temporarily, and the PT is rechecked daily.
      (b) If the INR is greater than 5 but less than 9 and the patient is not bleeding, the warfarin dose may be withheld temporarily and the PT is rechecked daily, or vitamin K (1–2.5 mg) may be given orally or subcutaneously until the INR is reduced.
      (c) If the INR is greater than 9 and the patient is not bleeding, the warfarin dose is withheld temporarily and vitamin K (2.5–5 mg) is given orally or subcutaneously until the INR is reduced.
      (d) If the patient is bleeding, fresh frozen plasma is given to correct the INR and vitamin K is also given (10 mg) orally, subcutaneously, or intravenously.

Remember, there is approximately a 2- to 3-day lag between the changes in warfarin dose and changes in the PT. If you have withheld the warfarin, do not wait until the PT is in the appropriate range to resume therapy because the PT will continue to drop. Therapy is best reinitiated when the PT is slightly higher than desired.

(3) **Vitamin K deficiency** or **liver failure.** Frequently, it is unclear whether the patient's elevated PT is from vitamin K deficiency, liver disease, or both (especially in alcoholics, who are prone to both disorders). Vitamin K therapy is often both diagnostic and therapeutic.

(4) **Factor deficiency** is not treated unless trauma has occurred, and there is a risk for bleeding, bleeding is occurring, or surgery is planned.

2. **Normal PT/increased PTT**
   a. **Factor deficiency** is only treated if trauma has occurred and there is a risk for bleeding, the patient is acutely bleeding, or the patient is about to undergo surgery. Hemophilia A and B are treated with **factor VIII** and **IX concentrates** (either plasma purified or recombinant), respectively; other factor deficiencies are typically replaced with **fresh frozen plasma** because many do not yet have a purified product available.
   b. **Factor inhibitors**
      (1) **Acute treatment.** Factor inhibitors associated with active bleeding can be extremely difficult to treat. Treatment algorithms have been created that take into account the concentration of the inhibitor (Bethesda units).
         (a) **Aggressive factor replacement** (to "overwhelm" a low-titer inhibitor) and/or **plasmapheresis** (to remove the low-titer inhibitor) can be used.
         (b) **Bypassing products** that circumvent the inhibitor can be used to stop bleeding but carry an increased risk for unwanted thromboses. Choices include prothrombin complex concentrates, activated prothrombin complex concentrates, or recombinant activated clotting factors.
      (2) **Chronic treatment.** Steroids, immunosuppressive chemotherapy (e.g., cyclophosphamide, rituximab), or immune tolerance induction may be used in an attempt to decrease the titer of the inhibitor.
   c. **Antiphospholipid antibodies** have a tendency to cause thromboses, not bleeding. Therefore, treatment is anticoagulation therapy if clotting occurs (see Chapter 67). Because the patient's PT or PTT may be abnormal at baseline, monitoring for therapeutic levels of anticoagulation may be difficult and typically require chromogenic factor assays.

REFERENCES

Bolton-Maggs PH, Pasi KJ. Haemophilias A and B. Lancet 2003;361(9371): 1801–1809.

Gomperts ED, Astermark J, Gringeri A, et al. From theory to practice: applying current clinical knowledge and treatment strategies to the care of hemophilia a patients with inhibitors. Blood Rev 2008;22(Suppl 1): S1–11.

Nichols WL, Hultin MB, James AH, et al. von Willebrand's disease (VWD): evidence-based diagnosis and management guidelines, the National Heart, Lung, and Blood Institute (NHLBI) expert panel report (USA). Haemophilia 2008;14(2):171–232.

Peyvandi F, Cattaneo M, Inbal A, et al. Rare bleeding disorders. Haemophilia 2008;14(Suppl 3):202–210.

Hypercoagulable States

67

I. INTRODUCTION

A. Definition. Hypercoagulable states are **clinical disorders of the blood that increase the patient's risk for developing thromboembolic disease.** A risk factor (inherited or acquired) for the development of a thrombus can be identified in more than 80% of patients with a clot, and there may be multiple factors present. An inheritable genetic abnormality may be found in approximately 30% of individuals presenting with a deep venous thrombosis (DVT).

B. Pathogenesis. Homeostasis in blood clotting is maintained by interrelationships between procoagulant and anticoagulant proteins and their interactions with the vascular endothelium. The pathogenesis of thrombus formation is summarized by **Virchow's triad:**

1. Defects in blood flow (stasis)
2. Defects in vascular endothelium
3. Defects in blood coagulation (leading to hypercoagulability)

II. CLINICAL MANIFESTATIONS OF HYPERCOAGULABLE STATES.

A hypercoagulable state should be suspected in a patient who develops:

A. Multiple or recurrent clots

B. Clots in unusual locations (e.g., the upper extremities, mesenteric vessels, arteries)

C. Thromboembolic disease at an early age

III. CAUSES OF HYPERCOAGULABLE STATES

CAUSES OF HYPERCOAGULABLE STATES are important to consider when a patient has a blood clot.

A. Inherited clotting disorders

1. **Factor V Leiden mutation** is the most common inherited factor associated with hypercoagulability. This mutation causes resistance of factor V to the cleaving action of activated protein C.
2. **Prothrombin G20210A mutation** is the second most common inheritable factor associated with hypercoagulability and results in an mRNA that has an increased half-life, leading to elevated levels of the prothrombin protein. When co-inherited with a factor V Leiden mutation, patients have

a substantially increased risk for the development of a clot as well as an increased risk for recurrent DVT.

3. **Protein C and/or S deficiencies** are uncommon but display a high penetrance for the occurrence of venous thromboembolism. These proteins normally function to reduce levels of factor Va and factor VIIIa leading to decreased thrombin generation. Patients with deficiencies fail to properly regulate the coagulation cascade.
4. **Antithrombin (or antithrombin III) deficiency** is a rare autosomal dominant disorder also with a relatively high level of penetrance for DVT. The normal protein functions as a protease inhibitor of factors IIa (thrombin) and factor Xa, and its activity is modulated by heparin, leading to the basis of its clinical use. Deficiencies in antithrombin lead to dysregulation of the clotting cascade.
5. **Rare disorders** include dysfibrinogenemia, plasminogen deficiency, heparin cofactor II deficiency, factor XII deficiency, and elevated clotting factor levels.

B. Acquired clotting disorders

1. **Malignancy,** known or occult, is a common cause of thrombosis. Common offenders include cancers of the lung, pancreas, colon, kidney, and prostate.
2. **Medications**
   a. **Heparin-induced thrombocytopenia and thrombosis (HITT),** an acquired disorder associated with the development of arterial or venous thrombi concurrent with the development of thrombocytopenia, occurs in 1%–5% of patients receiving intravenous or subcutaneous heparin therapy. If HITT is being considered, heparin should be stopped promptly, appropriate serologies sent for diagnosis, and anticoagulation with a direct thrombin inhibitor initiated until platelet levels improve.
   b. **Oral contraceptives** increase the risk of thrombosis independently and in conjunction with other risk factors. The amount of increased risk varies with the dose of estrogen, type of progesterone, and route of administration of the contraceptive.
   c. **Additional medications** (e.g., hormone replacement therapy, tamoxifen)
3. **Pregnancy** is associated with increased rates of thrombosis that may be secondary to vascular stasis due to the enlarged uterus compressing pelvic blood vessels, vascular injury at the time of delivery, and a progressive increase in a number of the clotting factors as pregnancy progresses.
4. **Chronic renal disease** including nephrotic syndrome as well as end-stage renal disease are associated with an increased incidence of thromboses through unclear mechanisms.

Alterations in levels of procoagulant proteins and anticoagulant factors as well as alterations in platelet activity may contribute to this risk.

5. **Trauma/surgery** causes increased risk of thrombosis for multiple reasons including decreased venous blood flow, increased levels of tissue factor, immobilization, and alterations in the balance of endogenous procoagulants and anticoagulants after the trauma. Orthopedic, vascular, and neurosurgical procedures are associated with a particularly elevated risk.
6. **Hyperhomocysteinemia** is both an inherited (due to polymorphisms in the *MTHFR* gene) and acquired (due to vitamin deficiencies) defect in which there are high serum levels of homocysteine. Although elevated homocysteine levels are associated with thromboembolic disease and atherosclerotic disease, modulating these levels with folate supplementation does not appear to reduce this risk.
7. **Myeloproliferative neoplasms** such as polycythemia vera, essential thrombocythemia, and primary myelofibrosis are associated with thrombophilia. Patients presenting with idiopathic hepatic or portal vein thromboses should be considered for screening for an underlying myeloproliferative neoplasm.
8. **Antiphospholipid antibody syndrome** is marked by the presence of antiphospholipid antibodies, hypercoagulability, recurrent spontaneous abortions, and thrombocytopenia.
9. **Immobilization**
10. **Other causes** such as rheumatologic disease, paroxysmal nocturnal hemoglobinuria, hyperviscosity, and heart failure are also associated with hypercoagulability.

C. The causes of the most important hypercoagulable states (both primary and secondary) can be recalled using the mnemonic "DAMN THROMBUS."

MNEMONIC **Causes of Hypercoagulable States ("DAMN THROMBUS")**

Deficiencies or alterations in coagulation factors (e.g., protein C, protein S, antithrombin III, factor V, prothrombin, fibrinogen, plasminogen, heparin cofactor, factor XIII)
Antiphospholipid antibody syndrome
Malignancy (e.g., Trousseau's syndrome)
Nephrotic syndrome
Trauma
Hyperhomocysteinemia or **H**eparin-induced thrombocytopenia and thrombosis or **H**emoglobinuria [i.e., paroxysmal nocturnal hemoglobinuria (PNH)]

Rheumatologic causes (i.e., vasculitis)
Oral contraceptives (and other medications)
Myeloproliferative disorders
Baby carriers (i.e., pregnancy)
Unknown
Surgery or postoperative states (particularly neurosurgical and orthopedic)

IV. APPROACH TO THE PATIENT

A. In a patient with a new DVT, the patient history (including prior venous thromboembolism), physical examination, location and extent of the thrombus, complete blood count (CBC), urinalysis, prothrombin time (PT), and partial thromboplastin time (PTT) are often used to initially evaluate for one of the more common acquired hypercoagulable states. Beyond the acute medical treatment of venous thromboembolism, the key in the management of patients with thromboses is deciding whether to screen the patient for a heritable or acquired hypercoagulable state. Because a heritable factor can only be found in about 30% of patients with a first DVT, there are a limited number of patients who would benefit from these expensive extensive tests.

1. Additional testing should be strongly considered in patients with the following characteristics:
   a. An unprovoked DVT or pulmonary embolism prior to the age of 50
   b. A patient with a first-degree family member with an unprovoked DVT or pulmonary embolism prior to the age of 50
   c. A recurrent DVT or pulmonary embolism
   d. A thrombus in an unusual location (hepatic or portal vein or upper extremity vein)
2. Additionally, the timing of the screening is important to consider because the presence of a thrombus as well as the utilization of anticoagulants can affect the levels or activity of a number of coagulation cascade proteins.
   a. Most hematologists recommend pursuing hypercoagulable evaluation—especially for antithrombin, protein C, and protein S—at least 2 weeks after the cessation of anticoagulation to limit false-positive results.
   b. When screening for thrombophilias in the setting of a pregnancy, a number of coagulation factors are altered including elevated factor VIII levels and decreased protein S levels. Therefore, the optimal time to assess for

thrombophilia is after the completion of the therapy for the thrombus as well as after delivery of the baby.

B. The following **laboratory studies** may help evaluate for specific factors associated with hypercoagulability:

1. Factor V Leiden mutation test
2. Prothrombin G20210A mutation test
3. Screening tests for the presence of antiphospholipid antibodies include the PTT, lupus anticoagulant assay, anticardiolipin antibodies, anti-β_2-glycoprotein-1 antibodies, and dilute Russell's viper venom test (dRVVT).
4. Homocysteine level (test after overnight fast)
5. Quantitative and functional assays for proteins C and S, antithrombin III, and fibrinogen
6. Rarer antigenic testing (plasminogen levels, heparin cofactor II levels, and factor XII levels) can be performed if the index of suspicion is high even though initial screening is negative.
7. Heparin-induced thrombocytopenia (HIT) enzyme-linked immunosorbent assay (ELISA) and confirmation with a serotonin release assay in patients with presumed HITT
8. Flow cytometry assessment (CD55 and CD59) for PNH in the proper clinical scenario

Acute thrombi can reduce levels of antithrombin and protein C and S. Heparin reduces antithrombin levels. Warfarin reduces protein C levels before those of all other vitamin K–dependent factors because protein C has the shortest half-life. Therefore, warfarin can lead to a falsely low result on a protein C assay, but can also affect protein S activity.

V. TREATMENT

A. Anticoagulation therapy

1. **Initial therapy** of a patient presenting with DVT or pulmonary embolism consists of **heparin or low-molecular-weight heparin** and consideration of **warfarin.** Because protein C has the shortest half-life of all the vitamin K–dependent factors, warfarin therapy alone can lead to a deficiency of protein C relative to the other procoagulant factors (i.e., factors II, VII, IX, and X). Patients with an underlying protein C deficiency who are given high-dose warfarin alone may be susceptible to a transient hypercoagulable state, leading to "Coumadin skin necrosis." Coumadin necrosis can be avoided by administering heparin or low-molecular-weight heparin as

a bridge to warfarin. In addition, because Coumadin will not be fully effective for 3–5 days, the concomitant use of a heparin-based product ensures that the patient's blood rapidly becomes anticoagulated, which may prevent further extension of the clot.

a. **Unfractionated heparin** is given by continuous intravenous infusion, and dosing is initiated and adjusted using a weight-based nomogram to a goal PTT that is 1.5–2.5 times the normal range.
b. **Low-molecular-weight heparin** is an alternative to unfractionated heparin. This subcutaneous depot form of heparin is dosed every 12–24 hours and can even be used in select patients for outpatient management of thromboembolic disease. Dosing is weight based but should be used with caution in patients with renal insufficiency. Blood testing is rarely needed but can be checked if desired by measuring antifactor Xa levels 4–6 hours after dosing.

2. **Long-term therapy.** Heparin or low-molecular-weight heparin may be continued along with warfarin until the PT reaches the therapeutic range [i.e., an international normalized ratio (INR) between 2 and 3], which usually takes about 5 days. Warfarin or low-molecular-weight heparin is usually continued for a minimum of 3–6 months, although the optimal total duration is not well established.
3. **Hypercoagulable states.** Patients identified as having a factor associated with a hypercoagulable state may benefit from prolonged or lifelong anticoagulation, although the degree of anticoagulation and the absolute length of therapy remains unknown.
4. **Recurrent DVT or pulmonary embolism.** Patients with recurrent thrombi are at an elevated risk for additional recurrences, and therefore, subsequent treatment is given for longer than 6–12 months. As with hypercoagulable states, the risk of recurrent thrombi must be balanced with the risk of bleeding complications from the anticoagulation.

B. **Inferior vena cava (IVC) filter.** An IVC filter may be placed in patients with active bleeding or at high risk for bleeding with anticoagulation therapy or in patients with recurrent pulmonary emboli despite therapy. However, the placement of IVC filters may lead to an increased risk of lower extremity DVT because of alterations in blood flow through the IVC.

C. **Thrombolytic therapy** can potentially normalize blood flow sooner compared with anticoagulation therapy alone but is typically considered only in patients with profound DVT or pulmonary embolism resulting in circulatory or hemodynamic compromise.

REFERENCES

Agnelli G, Becattini C. Treatment of DVT: how long is enough and how do you predict recurrence. J Thromb Thrombolysis 2008;25(1):37–44.

Cohn DM, Roshani S, Middeldorp S. Thrombophilia and venous thromboembolism: implications for testing. Semin Thromb Hemost 2007;33(6):573–581.

Dalen JE. Should patients with venous thromboembolism be screened for thrombophilia? Am J Med 2008;121(6):458–463.

Snow V, Qaseem A, Barry P, et al. Management of venous thromboembolism: a clinical practice guideline from the American College of Physicians and the American Academy of Family Physicians. Ann Intern Med 2007;146(3):204–210.

Lymphadenopathy

68

I. INTRODUCTION

A. Definition. Lymphadenopathy occurs when the **lymph nodes** are of an **abnormal consistency** or **increased size** (>1 cm in size). Lymphadenopathy can be **regional** (i.e., only one group or a few contiguous groups of nodes are involved) or **generalized** (i.e., involving more than two separate sites).

B. Lymphadenopathy **usually signals the presence of disease** and therefore warrants medical evaluation.

II. APPROACH TO THE PATIENT

A. First, **make sure the lymph nodes are truly abnormal.** Certain lymph nodes (e.g., the submandibular and inguinal nodes) are commonly palpable.

B. Once lymphadenopathy is deemed abnormal, **generate a differential diagnosis** based on the location of the lymphadenopathy, the human immunodeficiency virus (HIV) status of the patient, the clinical scenario, the duration of the adenopathy, and the physical attributes of the node. This information helps to guide the need for laboratory tests and other studies [e.g., complete blood count (CBC) and peripheral smear evaluation, Monospot test, hepatitis serologies, serum lactate dehydrogenase (LDH), erythrocyte sedimentation rate (ESR), Venereal Disease Research Laboratories (VDRL) test, and radiographic imaging].

1. **Location of the lymphadenopathy.** The location of the lymphadenopathy allows you to form an initial differential diagnosis.
   a. If the lymphadenopathy is **generalized,** the most likely etiologies can be remembered with the mnemonic "SHE HAS CUTE LAN."
   b. If the lymphadenopathy is **localized,** refer to Table 68-1.

MNEMONIC **Causes of Generalized Lymphadenopathy ("SHE HAS CUTE LAN")**

Syphilis
Hepatitis
Epstein-Barr virus infection

Histoplasmosis
AIDS/HIV infection
Serum sickness

Cytomegalovirus (CMV) infection/**C**astleman's disease
Unusual drugs (e.g., hydantoin derivatives, antithyroid medications, antileprosy medications, isoniazid)
Toxoplasmosis
Erythrophagocytic lymphohistiocytosis

Leishmaniasis
Arthritis (rheumatoid)
Neoplasm: lymphoma, leukemia, metastatic cancer

2. **HIV status** must always be considered whenever a patient has regional or generalized lymphadenopathy. In HIV-infected patients, generalized lymphadenopathy typically occurs early in the course of HIV disease. Lymphadenopathy can be caused either by the HIV itself or other systemic diseases that are common in HIV-infected patients.
3. **Clinical scenario.** Considering the patient's age and associated findings can help narrow the differential diagnosis.

TABLE 68-1

MAJOR CAUSES OF LOCALIZED LYMPHADENOPATHY

Affected Lymph Nodes	Causes of Lymphadenopathy
Cervical	Head and neck malignancy, bacterial infection, Epstein-Barr virus, cytomegalovirus, tuberculosis, lymphoma
Supraclavicular	Lung, breast, gastrointestinal, or genitourinary malignancy, lymphoma
Axillary	Hand or arm infections, trauma from bites, cat-scratch disease, lymphoma, brucellosis, breast cancer, reactive changes secondary to breast implants
Epitrochlear	Hand infections, lymphoma, tularemia, syphilis
Inguinal	Leg or foot infections, pelvic malignancy, lymphoma, sexually transmitted disease
Hilar/mediastinal	Sarcoidosis, tuberculosis, lymphoma, fungal infections, lung cancer
Abdominal	Lymphoma, tuberculosis, *Mycobacterium avium* complex infection, metastatic malignancy

a. **Patient age.** Lymphadenopathy in patients younger than 30 years of age is most often benign (and caused by an infection). In patients older than 30 years, the possibility of malignancy becomes much more worrisome.
b. **Signs and symptoms.** Symptoms of fever, chills, night sweats, and weight loss should always be sought and, if present, usually imply a serious systemic infection or malignancy. Symptoms or signs of a local infection (e.g., pharyngitis, conjunctivitis, otitis, skin infection, or trauma) usually imply an infectious etiology.
c. **Historical data.** Pertinent historical data should be ascertained including a history of smoking, tick bites, travel, high-risk behavior, tuberculosis exposure, and animal contact.

4. **Characteristics of lymphadenopathy on palpation.** The physical attributes of lymphadenopathy can help a little but may be misleading; therefore, these findings alone should not dissuade further evaluation. In general, abnormal nodes are greater than 1 cm in diameter, and the likelihood of a malignancy increases proportionally with the size of the node. The following tend to be true:
   a. **Infections** tend to cause **tender** lymphadenopathy because of rapid growth of the node and subsequent capsular stretching. The nodes tend to be **asymmetric** with erythematous skin overlying the node.
   b. **Lymphoma** classically leads to **large, firm, rubbery, nontender** lymphadenopathy.
   c. **Metastatic cancer** usually results in **very firm** (sometimes **"rock hard")**, **nontender** nodes that are **immobile** (i.e., fixed to the underlying tissue).

Infamous lymph nodes include **Virchow's node** (a left supraclavicular lymph node) and **Sister Mary Joseph's node** (a periumbilical lymph node), both of which can be seen with gastrointestinal malignancies.

C. Evaluation

1. **In cases of generalized lymphadenopathy,** an evaluation beginning with a CBC and differential, comprehensive metabolic panel, and an LDH are reasonable. Additional specific testing for HIV, tuberculosis, and syphilis may be considered in appropriate patients.
2. If **metastatic malignancy** is strongly considered, proceed to **fine-needle aspiration,** which is quite sensitive for metastatic malignancies (and infections) but not for lymphomas.

If **lymphoma** is a strong possibility, a **core biopsy or excisional biopsy** is required.

3. If **bacterial infection** is the most likely diagnosis, a **period of observation** (2–3 weeks, with or without antibiotics) is reasonable. If there is no evidence of resolution, fine-needle aspiration or core or excisional biopsy is usually required.
4. If the **etiology** of the lymphadenopathy is **unclear, close follow-up** is essential because a small but significant percentage of these patients develop lymphoma within 1 year.

III. TREATMENT varies considerably and depends on the underlying cause.

REFERENCES

Bazemore AW, Smucker DR. Lymphadenopathy and malignancy. Am Fam Physician 2002;66(11):2103–2110.

Brown JR, Skarin AT. Clinical mimics of lymphoma. Oncologist 2004;9(4):406–416.

Habermann TM, Steensma DP. Lymphadenopathy. Mayo Clin Proc 2000;75:723–732.

Lymphoma

I. INTRODUCTION

A. Definition. Lymphomas are a group of malignant neoplasms resulting from the transformation of normal lymphoid cells within preexisting lymphoid tissues.

B. Classification. While numerous classification schemes have been developed over the years, the two most frequently used today are the Revised European-American Classification of Lymphoid Neoplasms (REAL) and the World Health Organization (WHO) classifications. One can initially stratify lymphomas into two groups: Non-Hodgkin's lymphoma (NHL) and Hodgkin's lymphoma (HL) (Table 69-1).

1. **Hodgkin's Lymphoma.** Reed-Sternberg cells are usually present.
2. **Non-Hodgkin's lymphoma (NHL).** Reed-Sternberg cells are absent.

II. HODGKIN'S LYMPHOMA

A. Epidemiology

1. **Incidence.** Approximately **8000 cases** are reported per year in the United States.
2. **Patient profile**
    a. **Age.** Hodgkin's lymphoma has a **bimodal age distribution.** The incidence peaks in patients **aged 20–25 years** and again in patients **older than 55 years.**
    b. **Gender.** Except for the nodular sclerosis subtype, Hodgkin's lymphoma is more common in **men** than women.
    c. **Race.** Hodgkin's lymphoma is more common in Caucasians than African Americans.
    d. **Disease association.** As with many lymphomas, Hodgkin's lymphoma is increased in patients with human immunodeficiency virus (HIV) infection, but on average HIV patients with HL have higher CD4 counts than HIV patients with NHL.

B. Pathogenesis of Hodgkin's lymphoma. Based on available data, the cell of origin in most cases of Hodgkin's lymphoma is likely a germinal center or postgerminal center B cell. Disease progression is **orderly.** Initially, the malignancy spreads to anatomically adjacent lymph tissues. Hematogenous spread to the liver, bone marrow, and other viscera occurs only in advanced disease.

TABLE 69-1

COMPARISON OF HODGKIN'S LYMPHOMA (HL) AND NON-HODGKIN'S LYMPHOMA (NHL)

Disease	Etiology	Malignant Cell Line	Site of Origin	Spread	Mediastinal Involvement	Bone Marrow Involvement	Systemic ("B") Symptoms*	Best Prognostic Indicator(s)
HL	Unknown (viral etiology suspected)	Unclear Likely a B cell	Nodal	Contiguous	Common	Uncommon	Very common ESR[†] "B" symptoms	Stage
NHL	Unknown (Burkitt's lymphoma associated with Epstein-Barr virus)	90% B cell 10% T cell	Extranodal in up to 40% of patients	Noncontiguous	Rare	Low grade: very common High grade: more common in higher stage	Seen in <50% of patients	IPI[‡]

*"B" symptoms include weight loss of more than 10% of body weight during the 6 months prior to the diagnosis, recurrent temperatures above 38°C during the previous month, and recurrent drenching night sweats during the previous month.

[†]Erythrocyte sedimentation rate (ESR). An ESR greater than 50 mm/hr or an ESR greater than 30 mm/hr in the presence of B symptoms can be considered to carry a poorer prognosis stage for stage.

[‡]International Prognostic Index (IPI) including the traditional IPI, the age-adjusted IPI, or the Follicular Lymphoma International Prognostic Index (FLIPI)

C. Clinical manifestations of Hodgkin's lymphoma

1. **Painless, superficial adenopathy** (usually involving the neck or supraclavicular areas)
2. **Constitutional ("B") symptoms** (i.e., **fever, night sweats, weight loss**) are seen in one-third of patients.
3. **Severe pruritus** is often encountered at some point during the disease.
4. **Alcohol-induced pain** can occur at the site of enlarged lymph nodes within minutes of the ingestion of even small amounts of alcohol in approximately 10%–15% of patients.
5. **Characteristic laboratory findings** include:
   a. Anemia
   b. Leukocytosis (initially), thrombocytosis
   c. Eosinophilia
   d. Elevated erythrocyte sedimentation rate (ESR)
   e. Elevated alkaline phosphatase level

D. Approach to the patient

1. **Diagnosis.** Obtaining a core biopsy or excisional biopsy is essential because a fine-needle aspiration (FNA) will not allow for architectural findings and a proper diagnosis. The finding of Reed-Sternberg cells on lymph tissue biopsy is characteristic of Hodgkin's lymphoma.
   a. **Differential diagnosis.** Reed-Sternberg cells are also seen with phenytoin-induced lymphoid hyperplasia, some NHL or solid tumors, and mononucleosis.
   b. **Subtypes.** Initial stratification involves classifying the disease as either classical Hodgkin's lymphoma or nodular lymphocyte-predominant Hodgkin's lymphoma (NLPHL). Within the classical Hodgkin's lymphoma category, there are four main histologic subtypes, which are distinguished by the morphology of the Reed-Sternberg cells and the architecture of the surrounding cells (Table 69-2).
2. **Staging.** Survival is affected by multiple factors including the clinical stage, presence of "B" symptoms, elevated ESR, and bulk of disease.
   a. **Staging evaluation.** The vast majority of patients are staged clinically; rarely is pathologic staging (exploratory laparotomy including splenectomy, liver biopsy, and lymph node sampling) required.
      (1) **Radiographic imaging.** A chest radiograph can be the initial evaluation for mediastinal involvement, but almost all patients today receive computed tomographic (CT) scan of the chest, abdomen, and pelvis to document the size and location of all involved lymph nodes.
      (2) **Other studies.** Many patients will undergo positron emission tomography (PET) scanning prior to the

TABLE 69-2

HISTOPATHOLOGIC SUBTYPES OF HODGKIN'S LYMPHOMA

Histologic Subtype	Comments
Nodular lymphocyte predominant	5% of all cases; characterized by the presence of Reed-Sternberg cell variants (called popcorn cells); often treated similarly to non-Hodgkin's lymphoma; often responds to chemotherapy but high recurrence rate
Classical Hodgkin's lymphoma	
Mixed cellularity	15%–30% of all cases; intermediate prognosis; patients are older
Lymphocyte depleted	Less than 1% of cases; many Reed-Sternberg cells; worst prognosis; patients are older
Lymphocyte rich	Usually presents in an earlier stage; better prognosis; rare relapses after remission
Nodular sclerosis	65%–80% of all cases; female predominance; patients are younger; usually involves lower cervical, supraclavicular, and mediastinal nodes

initiation of therapy and at predetermined intervals during and after the completion of chemotherapy to assess "responsiveness." The clinical utility of assessing responses with CT versus PET scanning is currently being evaluated. Patients with higher-stage disease will often undergo **bilateral bone marrow biopsies** prior to therapy.

b. **Staging classification.** The staging system for Hodgkin's lymphoma is based on the **Ann Arbor classification system.** Like most oncologic staging systems, prognosis is best for stage I patients and worst for stage IV patients. Table 69-4 presents a simplified staging scheme based on the extent of lymph node and extranodal involvement. Within these stages are factors that may affect treatment and prognosis.
   (1) If patients have no "B" symptoms, the letter **"A"** is added to the stage.
   (2) If "B" symptoms **[weight loss (in excess of 10% of body weight), unexplained fevers >38°C,** or drenching **night sweats]** are present, the letter **"B"** is added. In general, those with symptoms have a poorer prognosis.

(3) Involvement of the spleen is designated by the letter "S."

(4) Contiguous lymph node masses greater than 10 cm in size may be designated by the letter "X" indicating bulky disease.

E. Treatment. In general, Hodgkin's lymphoma should be thought of as a curable cancer.

1. **Treatment depends on the stage.** General approaches follow; an oncology reference can provide detailed information regarding regimens.
   a. **Low-stage disease** (e.g., **stage I** and **IIa**) is divided into those with favorable versus unfavorable characteristics (bulky disease, "B" symptoms, patient's age, and elevated ESR). Those with favorable disease may be treated with an abbreviated course of chemotherapy followed by radiation versus chemotherapy alone. Those with unfavorable disease are typically treated with chemotherapy and occasionally receive consolidative radiation.
   b. **High-stage disease** (e.g., **stage IIIb** and **IV**) is usually treated with chemotherapy and may receive consolidative radiation if they presented with bulky disease or have residual disease after completion of their chemotherapy.
   c. Patients with aggressive disease that relapses after treatment may be candidates for high-dose therapy followed by **autologous bone marrow transplant.** Those with chemotherapy-refractory disease have only a small chance for long-term survival even with allogeneic bone marrow transplant.
2. **Long-term complications of treatment**
   a. **Chemotherapy** increases the risk for acute leukemia; this risk peaks 5 years after initiation of therapy and decreases after 10 years. The development of acute leukemia as a result of chemotherapy for Hodgkin's lymphoma is much more common in older patients.
   b. **Radiation therapy** leads to an increased incidence of solid tumors (e.g., breast, stomach, or thyroid tumors); this risk, unlike that of leukemia, continues to increase with time. Additionally, the risk of breast cancer in women is higher for those receiving radiation at a younger age.
   c. **Cardiovascular disease**. There appears to be an increased risk for heart failure as well as coronary artery disease in those receiving chemotherapy and radiation therapy.
   d. **Fertility.** Fertility can be affected by many anticancer therapies and the issue should be discussed prior to initiating chemotherapy to allow for possible gamete preservation.

III. NHL is the name given to a **heterogeneous group** of malignancies involving either B or T cells.

A. Epidemiology

1. **Incidence.** The incidence is much higher than for Hodgkin's lymphoma. There are approximately 60,000 new cases and almost 20,000 deaths from NHL annually in the United States. In addition, HIV infection has led to an increase in the incidence of NHL.
2. **Patient profile**
   a. **Age.** The median age at the time of diagnosis is **50 years.**
   b. **Gender.** NHL is 50% more common in **men** than women.
   c. **Race.** It is more common in Caucasians than African Americans or Asian Americans.
   d. **Other factors**
      (1) NHL is more common in patients with **altered immunity** (e.g., HIV-positive patients, those receiving immunosuppressive therapy, and those with congenital immunodeficiencies or autoimmune disease).
      (2) Some subtypes are associated with specific **chromosomal balanced translocations** (Table 69-3).

B. Pathogenesis of NHL. NHL involves the malignant transformation of either a B or T cell. The spread of the disease is often not contiguous, skipping over lymph node sites.

TABLE 69-3

COMMON CHROMOSOMAL TRANSLOCATIONS IN NON-HODGKIN'S LYMPHOMA

Translocation	Genes Involved
t(14;18)	The *bcl*-2 antiapoptotic gene on chromosome 18 is fused to the immunoglobulin heavy chain gene on chromosome 14. Found in 85% of follicular lymphomas
t(11;14)	The cell cycle regulatory protein bcl-1 (cyclin D1) on chromosome 11 is fused to the immunoglobulin heavy-chain gene on chromosome 14. This finding is nearly diagnostic for mantle cell lymphoma
Chromosome 8q24	*c-Myc* gene. Several translocations involving this locus are associated with highly aggressive B-cell lymphomas (Burkitt's lymphoma)
t(2;5)	The *nucleophosmin (*NPM*)* gene on chromosome 5 is fused to the *anaplastic lymphoma kinase (*ALK1) on chromosome 2. Seen frequently in anapestic large-cell lymphomas

C. Clinical manifestations of NHL. Presentations depend on the site and subtype of tumor.

1. **Common complaints** include:
   a. **Asymptomatic superficial lymphadenopathy**
   b. **"B" symptoms** (much less common in low-grade than in high-grade NHL)
   c. **Abdominal complaints** due to bulky lymph nodes pressing on vital structures
   d. **Bone pain** or **pathologic fracture**
   e. **Symptoms related to pancytopenia**
   f. **Skin changes** due to cutaneous involvement
   g. **Acute emergencies** (e.g., superior vena cava syndrome, spinal cord compression, airway compression)
2. **Characteristic laboratory findings** include:
   a. Complete blood count (CBC) ranging from normal to a decrease in all cell lines (i.e., pancytopenia) due to marrow involvement
   b. Elevated uric acid and lactate dehydrogenase (LDH) levels
   c. Elevated alkaline phosphatase levels

D. Approach to the patient

1. **Diagnosis.** Obtaining a core biopsy or excisional biopsy is essential because FNA will not allow for architectural findings and a proper diagnosis. The initial classification of the lymphoma will determine whether it is of a B-cell, T-cell, or NK-cell origin (WHO/REAL classification). Subtypes can then be grouped into **three categories** based on their typical clinical behavior: **indolent, aggressive,** or **highly aggressive.**
2. **Staging**
   a. **Staging evaluation.** Chest radiographs and abdominal and pelvic CT scans are often performed, and some

TABLE 69-4

STAGING SYSTEM FOR PATIENTS WITH LYMPHOMA

Stage	Definition
I	Limited to one lymph node region or one extranodal site (stage IE)
II	Two or more lymph node regions on one side of the diaphragm and involvement of a limited, contiguous extralymphatic site (IIE)
III	Lymph node involvement on both sides of the diaphragm, which may include the spleen (IIIS); a limited, contiguous extralymphatic site (IIIE); or both (IIIES)
IV	Disseminated involvement of more than one extranodal site with or without lymph node involvement

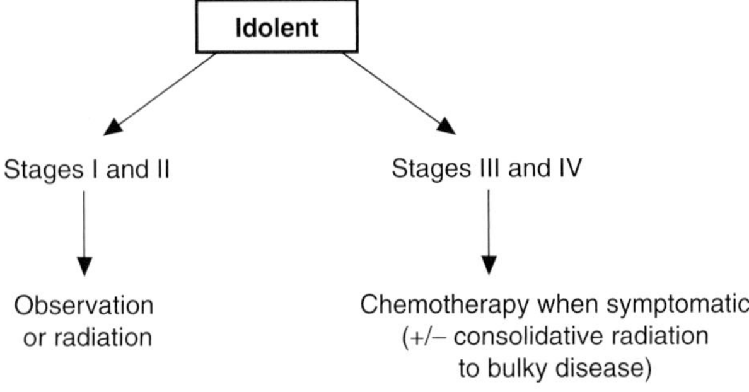

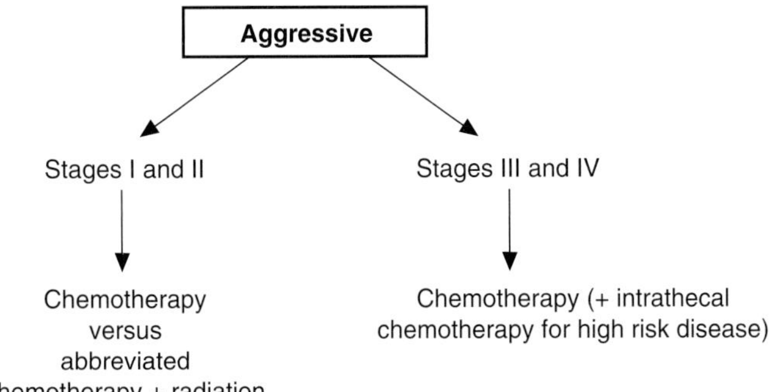

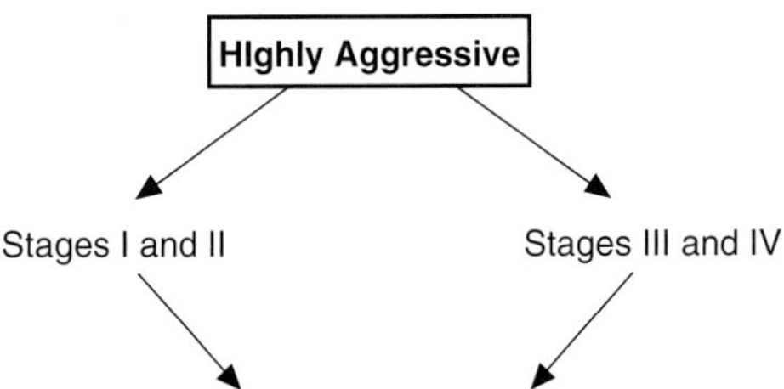

Figure 69-1 General therapeutic measures for patients with non-Hodgkin's lymphoma (NHL).

patients require lumbar puncture or a bone scan. Bilateral bone marrow biopsies are routinely performed. PET scanning is becoming increasingly employed in the staging and management of NHL. Staging laparotomy and lymphangiography are not usually indicated.

b. **Staging classification.** The Ann Arbor staging system is used for both Hodgkin's lymphoma and NHL (Table 69-4).

E. Treatment depends primarily on histology, the extent of disease, and patient characteristics. Treatment options are diagrammed in Figure 69-1. Most patients with B-cell NHL receive chemoimmunotherapy involving rituximab (a monoclonal antibody against the protein CD20) together with cytotoxic chemotherapy.

There exists a curious irony to NHL: Tumors that confer a favorable prognosis are the least likely to be cured because low-grade tumors are less responsive to chemotherapy. Patients with high-grade lymphomas generally have a poorer overall prognosis, but the chance of cure is increased.

REFERENCES

Armitage JO. How I treat patients with diffuse large B-cell lymphoma. Blood 2007;110:29–36.

Kwee TC, Kwee RM, Nievelstein RAJ. Imaging in staging of malignant lymphoma: a systematic review. Blood 2008;111:504–516.

Tsang RW, Hodgson DC, Crump M. Hodgkin's lymphoma. Curr Probl Cancer 2006;30(3):107–158.

Vitolo U, Ferreri AJ, Montoto S. Follicular lymphomas. Crit Rev Oncol Hematol 2008;66(3):248–261.

70

Myeloproliferative Neoplasms and Myelodysplastic Syndromes

I. **INTRODUCTION.** Myeloproliferative and myelodysplastic disorders are often confused. However, paying attention to the names will remind you that these are very different diseases.

A. **Myeloproliferative neoplasms** are a group of clonal myeloid neoplasms in which a hematopoietic progenitor proliferates leading to an increase in peripheral blood white blood cells (WBCs), red blood cells (RBCs), platelets, or a combination of these.

B. **Myelodysplastic syndrome (MDS)** are also a group of clonal myeloid neoplasms that result in ineffective hematopoiesis. This may lead to a hypercellular or hypocellular bone marrow with a concomitant **decrease** in WBCs, RBCs, platelets, or a combination of these. The hallmark of MDS is **dysplasia:** the unusual appearance of myeloid precursors in the bone marrow.

II. MYELOPROLIFERATIVE NEOPLASMS

A. Introduction

1. **Types of disorders.** There are four primary myeloproliferative neoplasms. They all involve clonal proliferation of a hematopoietic progenitor cell, leading to both qualitative and quantitative changes in all cell lines. While the type of disorder is characterized by the predominant cell line that is affected, more than one cell line is affected in most of these disorders.

   a. **Chronic myelogenous leukemia (CML)** is characterized by a prominent proliferation of myeloid progenitor cells leading to an expansion of the granulocytic series of cells resulting in a "left shift"—an increase in immature granulocytes of all stages of maturation in the peripheral blood and/or bone marrow.

   b. **Polycythemia vera (PV)** is characterized by prominent proliferation of erythroid progenitor cells leading to elevated red blood cell indices (RBC count, hemoglobin, and hematocrit).

c. **Essential thrombocytosis (ET)** is characterized by prominent proliferation of megakaryocytes leading to an elevated platelet count.

d. **Primary myelofibrosis (PMF)** is characterized by a proliferation of myeloid progenitor cells that leads to a prominent nonclonal proliferation of fibroblasts, resulting in the deposition of reticulin and collagen leading to fibrosis (scarring) of the bone marrow.

2. **General approach to the patient.** A myeloproliferative neoplasm is usually considered when elevated blood counts are found on the complete blood count (CBC).

   a. **Primary abnormality** (Table 70-1)

      (1) **In CML,** the predominant feature is usually a leukocytosis with a left shift. A mild anemia, normal to elevated platelet count, and peripheral blood basophilia are often seen.

      (2) **In PV,** the predominant features are elevated red blood cell indices (RBC count, hemoglobin, and hematocrit). Patients often also have a mild leukocytosis and thrombocytosis.

      (3) **In ET,** the predominant feature is an elevated platelet count. Patients often also have a mild leukocytosis and polycythemia.

      (4) **In PMF,** the predominant feature is evidence of extramedullary hematopoiesis in the form of hepatomegaly, splenomegaly, and lymphadenopathy. Patients often have a mild anemia, but their WBC and platelet counts can be quite variable. Myelophthisic changes [teardrops, nucleated RBCs, and early myeloid progenitors (blasts)] are often seen in the peripheral blood.

   b. **Multiple abnormalities.** More than one abnormality (e.g., an increased hematocrit and platelet count) can suggest a myeloproliferative neoplasm; however, most myeloproliferative neoplasms can present with multiple abnormalities. The following features can help suggest a specific myeloproliferative neoplasm:

      (1) **Massive splenomegaly** (see Chapter 31) implies either CML, PMF, or late-stage PV/ET.

      (2) A **decreased leukocyte alkaline phosphatase (LAP) score** is noted in CML, although this test is rarely used today.

      (3) **Nucleated RBCs, early WBCs,** and **abnormal RBC** morphology (i.e., **teardrop cells**) are characteristic of a **leukoerythroblastic smear** and are seen in PMF or in the fibrotic stages of ET or PV.

TABLE 70-1

2008 WORLD HEALTH ORGANIZATION (WHO) DIAGNOSTIC CRITERIA FOR MYELOPROLIFERATIVE NEOPLASMS*

	Polycythemia Vera (PV)†	Essential Thrombocytosis (ET)‡	Primary Myelofibrosis§
Major Criteria	1. Elevated red blood cell indices‖ or elevated red cell mass	1. Platelets $\geq$450 $\times$ 10^9 cells/L	1. Megakaryocytic proliferation with signs of atypia along with fibrosis or signs of trilineage expansion in the bone marrow
	2. *JAK-2* V617F+¶	2. Megakaryocytic expansion but normal granulocytic and erythroid numbers in the bone marrow	2. Not meeting criteria for PV, ET, chronic myelogenous leukemia (CML), or myelodysplastic syndrome (MDS)
		3. Not meeting criteria for PV, primary myelofibrosis (PMF), CML, or MDS	3. *JAK-2* V617F+¶ or no evidence of a reactive fibrosis
		4. *JAK-2* V617F+¶ or no other signs of a reactive thrombocytosis	
Minor Criteria	1. Bone marrow trilineage expansion		1. Leukoerythroblastosis
	2. Low serum erythropoietin level		2. Elevated lactate dehydrogenase
	3. EEC growth**		3. Anemia
			4. Splenomegaly

*Adapted from Tefferi A and Vardiman JW. Classification and diagnosis of myeloproliferative neoplasms: the 2008 World Health Organization criteria and point-of-care diagnostic algorithms. Leukemia 2008; 22(1); 14–22.

†Diagnosis of PV requires two major and one minor or the first major and two minor criteria.

‡Diagnosis of ET requires all four major criteria

§Diagnosis of Primary myelofibrosis requires all three major and two minor criteria.

‖The following constitute elevated red blood cell (RBC) indices: (a) a hemoglobin of >18.5 g/dl in men and 16.5 g/dl in women; (b) an elevated hemoglobin or hematocrit >99th percentile for age, sex, and altitude of residence; (c) hemoglobin >17 g/dl in men and 15 g/dl in women and an increase of $\geq$2 g/dl that was not associated with a correction of a vitamin/mineral deficiency; or (d) an RBC mass >25% of the upper limit of normal.

¶The *JAK-2* tyrosine kinase sequence is evaluated for the presence of the V→F mutation at codon 617. Additionally, mutations in exon 12 of JAK-2, c-Mpl mutations, or other signs of clonality may fulfill this criterion.

**EEC = endogenous erythroid colony formation.

B. CML

1. **Approach to the patient**
   a. **Patient history**
      (1) Common complaints include **fevers, sweats, fatigue,** and **abdominal fullness** (from splenomegaly).
      (2) Significant leukocytosis (e.g., a WBC count >300,000 cells/μl) may cause **leukostasis** in approximately 1% of patients with CML. Symptoms of leukostasis include **headaches, blurred vision, chest pain, respiratory distress,** and **priapism.**
   b. **Physical examination.** Significant splenomegaly is a common finding.
   c. **Laboratory studies**
      (1) **WBC count.** The WBC count can be significantly elevated. The WBC differential demonstrates a left shift with nearly all granulocytic precursors represented. **Basophilia** is often present.
      (2) **Peripheral blood smear.** Typically, myeloid forms in varying degrees of maturation are seen.
      (3) **Vitamin B_{12}** and **uric acid** levels may be increased as a result of increased transcobalamin secretion and high cell turnover, respectively.
   d. **Bone marrow biopsy.** A hypercellular marrow with left-shifted WBCs is usually seen. Basophilia can also be noted. When the disease progresses to the accelerated phase or blast phase, the peripheral blood or bone marrow has an elevated blast percentage (10%–19% for accelerated phase and ≥20% for blast phase). Profound fibrosis is also suggestive of progressive CML.
   e. **Cytogenetic studies.** The sine qua non of CML is the identification of the translocation of the *Abl* tyrosine kinase on chromosome 9 to a region within the Breakpoint cluster region (*Bcr*) of chromosome 22 resulting in the Philadelphia chromosome [t(9;22)] and the aberrant expression of the Bcr-Abl tyrosine kinase. The fusion can be identified by classical cytogenetics, fluorescence in situ hybridization (FISH) testing, or reverse transcriptase polymerase chain reaction (RT-PCR) analysis. It is essential to enumerate the karyotype as well as quantify the Bcr-Abl RT-PCR product at the time of diagnosis.
2. **Treatment**
   a. **Leukapheresis** is used if the patient has symptoms of leukostasis, which is a medical emergency.
   b. **Pharmacologic therapy**
      (1) **Hydroxyurea** is usually used to acutely lower the WBC count.

(2) **Interferon-α (IFN-α)** is a historic therapy that had a complete cytogenetic remission rate of approximately 7%–10%. It is rarely used today.
(3) **Selective tyrosine kinase inhibitors (TKIs)** including **imatinib (Gleevec), dasatinib (Sprycel),** and **nilotinib (Tasigna)** have become the mainstays in the treatment of CML. They work by selectively binding and inhibiting the Bcr-Abl tyrosine kinase. They have been shown to induce complete hematologic and cytogenetic remissions in most CML patients. Survival has dramatically improved; current 5-year survival is about 95%.

c. **Allogeneic bone marrow transplantation** offers the only possibility for cure. However, given the effectiveness of oral TKIs and the morbidity and mortality of transplant, this has generally been reserved for patients with relapsed or refractory disease.

3. **Prognosis.** With the introduction of the TKIs, 5-year survival is excellent. However, approximately 15%–20% of patients will be resistant or intolerant to the first TKI that they use. Second-generation TKIs (dasatinib or nilotinib) provide excellent treatment alternatives. Allogeneic transplantation also remains an option.

C. Polycythemia vera (PV)

1. **Approach to the patient**

a. **Patient history**

(1) Symptoms of **hyperviscosity** are common (e.g., **headaches, dizziness, blurred vision**).
(2) Both **thrombosis** and **bleeding** may result from abnormalities in platelet function.
(3) **Basophil/mast cell** release of histamine or alterations in prostaglandin production may account for the high incidence of both **pruritus** and **peptic ulcers.**
(4) **Facial plethora** (ruddy cyanosis) is a common finding.

Think of polycythemia vera when a patient is admitted with a bleeding peptic ulcer but continues to have a normal or elevated hematocrit.

b. **Physical examination.** Splenomegaly can be found on examination but is not as marked as in CML and PMF. Facial plethora, gouty arthritis and tophi, and skin excoriations can be indications of the hyperproliferative marrow.

c. **Laboratory studies** (see Table 70-1). The original diagnostic criteria for PV were established in the late 1960s by the Polycythemia Vera Study Group (PVSG). Newer molecular tests for the *Janus Kinase 2* (*JAK-2*) gene mutation (V617F) have been included in the 2008 WHO diagnostic criteria.

(1) **Hematocrit.** Elevated RBC indices are nearly universally found in polycythemia vera, but secondary causes of polycythemia must be ruled out first.

(2) **Mean corpuscular volume (MCV).** In approximately 25% of patients, there is an associated iron deficiency that causes a low MCV. Gastrointestinal bleeding from engorged vessels or peptic ulcer disease and increased demand from the elevated RBC mass are potential etiologies of the iron deficiency.

(3) **Erythropoietin level.** The erythropoietin level is usually low (<20 mU/ml).

(4) **Red blood cell mass assay** may help establish true PV versus a depressed plasma volume leading to an elevated hematocrit in secondary polycythemia.

(5) Although an elevated leukocyte alkaline phosphatase (LAP) score or an elevated serum B_{12} level can be seen in PV, neither are sensitive nor specific and are not often utilized in newer diagnostic guidelines (see Table 70-1).

d. **Bone marrow biopsy.** Although not essential for diagnosis, a bone marrow biopsy will reveal increased erythroid progenitors and megakaryocytes. Iron stores are decreased in 95% of patients. The procedure may help evaluate for other causes of abnormal blood counts as well as for progression of polycythemia (spent or fibrotic phases or even leukemic transformation).

e. ***JAK-2* mutational assessment.** A mutation in the *JAK-2* gene (V617F) has been identified in approximately 95% of patients with PV and may play a role in either the initiation or propagation of the disease. However, the presence or absence of the mutation does not rule in or rule out the diagnosis.

2. **Treatment.** The major goal of the treatment of PV is to reduce the thrombotic risk by lowering the hematocrit.

a. **Phlebotomy** may be performed weekly until the hematocrit has been lowered to approximately 45%; thereafter, maintenance phlebotomy may be performed as needed.

b. **Pharmacologic therapy**

(1) **Hydroxyurea** is sometimes added to phlebotomy in patients with elevated risk factors for thrombotic

complications from their PV, including age older than 70 years, prior thrombosis, platelet count greater than 1,500,000 cells/μl, or the presence of other cardiovascular risk factors.

(2) **Aspirin** in low doses (e.g., 81 mg/day) should be given to patients with PV assuming there is no medical contraindication.

(3) **Alkylating agents** and **radiophosphorus** can be leukemogenic and are increasingly avoided.

3. **Prognosis.** The average survival with treatment is 10–15 years. Polycythemia vera can progress to the spent phase with "normalization" of blood counts, followed by a fibrotic phase (i.e., post-PV myelofibrosis) and rarely acute myelogenous leukemia (AML).

D. Essential thrombocytosis

1. **Approach to the patient**

a. **Patient history**

(1) Abnormalities in platelet function can lead to both thromboses and bleeding. **Erythromelalgia** (i.e., intense, burning pain in dependent extremities often accompanied by skin warmth and mottling) results from microvascular occlusion. Although it can occur in all myeloproliferative disorders, erythromelalgia is especially common in patients with essential thrombocytosis. Other possible symptoms include headache, atypical chest pain, and livedo reticularis. It is important to document previous thrombotic events as well as symptoms related to a stroke or transient ischemic attack.

(2) Many patients (particularly young women) are **asymptomatic.**

b. **Physical examination.** Approximately one-fourth to one-half of patients will have splenomegaly, but it is not as common as in CML or PMF. Lymphadenopathy is rare.

c. **Laboratory studies**

(1) **Platelet count.** The platelet count is invariably greater than 400,000 cells/μl and often exceeds 1,000,000 cells/μl.

(2) **Peripheral blood smear.** The platelet morphology is frequently abnormal, with many small and many large platelets resulting in a high platelet distribution width (PDW).

(3) **Bleeding times** and **aggregation** studies may show abnormalities in platelet function. As platelet levels rise, the risk of an acquired type I von Willebrand's disease increases, potentially resulting in an increased risk of bleeding.

d. **Bone marrow biopsy.** This often reveals an increased number of large, hyperlobated megakaryocytes that tend to form clusters. This finding contrasts that of reactive thrombocytosis, in which the megakaryocytes have a normal morphology and random distribution.

e. ***JAK-2* mutational assessment.** A mutation in the *JAK-2* gene (V617F) has been identified in approximately 50% of patients with ET and may play a role in either the initiation or propagation of the disease. However, presence or absence of the mutation does not rule in or rule out the diagnosis. Other mutations in the *Mpl* gene (the receptor for thrombopoietin) have also been identified.

2. **Treatment.** The goal of therapy is to minimize thrombotic complications from the condition. Therefore, several strategies have been suggested to stratify an individual's risk factors for thrombosis and when to initiate treatment.

   a. **Low-risk patients** (age <60, no history of thrombotic events, no cardiovascular risk factors, and platelet counts $\leq$1,500,000 cells/μl) often require no therapy other than a low dose of aspirin.

   b. **High-risk patients** (age $\geq$60 years, previous history of thrombosis, or platelet counts $\geq$1,500,000 cells/μl) often require therapy. Treatment options include:

      (1) **Aspirin.** Small daily doses (e.g., 81 mg/day) may be indicated for both low- and high-risk patients and may help control vasomotor symptoms.

      (2) **Hydroxyurea** is often used as a first-line therapy for high-risk patients and can effectively reduce the risk of thrombosis.

      (3) **Anagrelide** is an effective oral agent to lower the platelet count. However, in a study comparing hydroxyurea with anagrelide, the composite endpoint of arterial or venous thrombosis, bleeding, or death from any causes was higher in patients treated with anagrelide. Therefore, it is usually a second-line therapy.

   c. **IFN-α** has been used to control thrombocytosis, but given numerous side effects, it is rarely used.

   d. **Alkylating agents** and **radiophosphorus** are increasingly avoided.

3. **Prognosis.** Essential thrombocytosis is an indolent disease. The average survival is usually at least 10–15 years.

Primary myelofibrosis is also called chronic idiopathic myelofibrosis or agnogenic myeloid metaplasia.

E. Primary myelofibrosis

1. **Approach to the patient**
   a. **Patient history.** Symptoms reflect anemia **(fatigue, dyspnea); night sweats**; thrombocytopenia **(easy bruisability); bone pain;** and marked splenomegaly **(abdominal distension and early satiety).**
   b. **Physical examination.** Splenomegaly is usually marked and hepatomegaly may also be present.
   c. **Laboratory studies**
      (1) **Hematocrit.** Anemia is seen in 50% of patients. There is more variability in the platelet and WBC counts with elevated or depressed values seen in equal numbers of patients.
      (2) **Peripheral blood smear.** The combination of **teardrop** cells, a **leukoerythroblastic smear** (nucleated RBCs and left-shifted WBCs), and **large, abnormal platelets** is often seen in PMF.
   d. **Bone marrow biopsy** is required to make the diagnosis and reveals an increase in the deposition of reticulin fibers in the early stages of disease and more severe fibrosis later in the course of the disease.
   e. ***JAK-2* mutational assessment.** A mutation in the *JAK-2* gene (V617F) has been identified in approximately 50% of patients with PMF and may play a role in either the initiation or propagation of the disease. However, presence or absence of the mutation does not rule in or rule out the diagnosis.
2. **Treatment.** The goal of therapy is to minimize symptoms related to the PMF. Prognostic scoring systems are often used to determine the appropriate treatment pathway.
   a. **Supportive measures** include blood and platelet transfusions as needed. Erythropoietin, androgens, and novel therapy such as thalidomide, lenalidomide, or etanercept may be given in an attempt to decrease transfusion requirements or control constitutional symptoms.
   b. **Hydroxyurea** can be useful in reducing spleen size or controlling thrombocytosis or leukocytosis.
   c. **Splenectomy** or **splenic irradiation** may be indicated for patients with refractory anemia or thrombocytopenia or in patients with recurrent pain from splenic enlargement.
   d. **IFN-α** may help control leukocytosis and thrombocytosis when other medications fail.
   e. **Allogeneic bone marrow transplant** currently offers the only chance for cure but has significant morbidity and mortality.
   f. Small molecule inhibitors of the *JAK-2* tyrosine kinase may show promise in the targeted therapy of this disease.

3. **Prognosis.** Average survival is quite variable, ranging from 13 months to 100 months. Predictive models based on hemoglobin, WBC count, absolute monocyte count, and platelet count have been used to counsel patients.

III. MYELODYSPLASTIC SYNDROME is a clonal myeloid neoplasm characterized by ineffective hematopoiesis. The bone marrow is variably cellular, and cytopenias are often noted on the peripheral smear. MDS is most often idiopathic but can be secondary to chemotherapy, chemical exposures, or radiation.

A. Classification. There are currently two frequently used classification schemes: the French-American-British (FAB) classification and the WHO classification (Table 70-2).

B. Approach to the patient

1. **Patient history.** Patients are **frequently asymptomatic** at diagnosis. If symptoms and signs are present, they result from one of the cytopenias and therefore include **fatigue, infection,** and **bleeding.**
2. **Physical examination.** Splenomegaly is rare except in chronic myelomonocytic leukemia (CMML).
3. **Laboratory studies.** Anemia can often be seen with occasional deficits in WBC or platelet counts.
   a. **RBC line.** Anemia is nearly universal, most with an increased MCV, macro-ovalocytes, and a decreased reticulocyte count.
   b. **WBC line.** Leukopenia is seen in 50% of patients with hypogranular neutrophils and the **pseudo-Pelger-Huet anomaly** (bilobed neutrophil nuclei).
   c. **Platelets.** Thrombocytopenia is seen in approximately 25% of patients and there may be hypogranular platelets.
4. **Bone marrow aspiration and biopsy** is necessary to diagnose and classify the myelodysplastic syndromes. According to the WHO classification, when more than 20% blasts are identified, **acute leukemia** is diagnosed. Cytogenetic findings from the aspirate are critical in the determination of the prognosis of MDS and likelihood of a response to certain therapies.

C. Treatment. The goal of therapy is to reduce symptoms related to the cytopenias and prolong life. Mortality is often related to infections as well as the transformation into acute myeloid leukemia. Treatment decisions are often based on the patient's prognosis, most commonly calculated by the International Prognostic Scoring System (IPSS), which includes number of cytopenias, percentage of blasts, and specific cytogenetic changes.

1. **Supportive therapy.** Blood and platelet transfusions are given as needed, but may eventually be complicated by

TABLE 70-2

FRENCH-AMERICAN-BRITISH (FAB) AND WORLD HEALTH ORGANIZATION (WHO) CLASSIFICATIONS OF MYELODYSPLASTIC SYNDROME (MDS)

FAB Classification of MDS*		WHO Classification of MDS[†]	
Category	**Diagnostic Findings**	**Category**	**Diagnostic Findings**
Refractory anemia (RA)	Anemia, <5% blasts, <15% ringed sideroblasts	Refractory anemia (RA)	Anemia, <5% blasts, <15% ringed sideroblasts
Refractory anemia with ringed sideroblasts (RARS)	Anemia, <5% blasts, ≥15% ringed sideroblasts	Refractory anemia with ringed sideroblasts (RARS)	Anemia, <5% blasts, ≥15% ringed sideroblasts
Refractory anemia with excess blasts	Multiple cytopenias, 5%–20% blasts	Refractory cytopenia with multilineage dysplasia (RCMD)	Multiple cytopenias and dysplasia, <5% blasts, <15% ringed sideroblasts
Refractory anemia with excess blasts in transformation[‡]	Multiple cytopenias, 21%–30% blasts	Refractory cytopenia with multilineage dysplasia and ringed sideroblasts (RCMD-RS)	Multiple cytopenias and dysplasia, <5% blasts, ≥15% ringed sideroblasts
Chronic myelomonocytic leukemia (CMML)[§]	Variable white blood cell (WBC) count, <20% blasts, monocyte count >1000 cells/μl	Refractory anemia with excess blasts-1 (RAEB-1)	Multiple cytopenias, 5%–9% blasts in the bone marrow
		Refractory anemia with excess blasts-2 (RAEB-2)	Multiple cytopenias, 10%–19% blasts in the bone marrow
		MDS-unclassified (MDS-U)	Multiple cytopenias with findings not classifiable in other categories
		MDS with del(5q)-[5q$^-$ syndrome]	Anemia, normal to elevated platelets, more common in females, isolated deletion of the long arm of chromosome 5 (5q)

(continued)

*Derived from Bennett JM, Catovsky D, Daniel MT, et al. Proposals for the classification of the myelodysplastic syndromes. Br J Haematol 1982;51(2):189–199.
†Derived from Bennett JM. A comparative review of classification systems in myelodysplastic syndromes (MDS). Semin Oncol 2005;32:S3–10; as well as Brunning RD, Bennett JM, Flandrin G, et al.: Myelodysplastic syndromes. In: Jaffe ES, Harris NL, Stein H, et al., eds.: Pathology and Genetics of Tumours of Haematopoietic and Lymphoid Tissues. Lyon, France: IARC Press, 2001. World Health Organization Classification of Tumours, 3, pp 61–73.
‡The WHO classification characterizes RAEB-T as acute myeloid leukemia (AML).
§The WHO classification characterizes CMML as an overlap MDS/myeloproliferative neoplasm (MPN) syndrome.

alloantibody formation, which increases the risk for a transfusion reaction and decreased platelet survival.

2. **Pharmacologic therapy**
   a. **Growth factors**
      (1) **Erythropoietin** may decrease the transfusion requirement in some patients. Serum erythropoietin levels and previous transfusion requirements can predict the likelihood of a response.
      (2) **Granulocyte colony-stimulating factor (G-CSF)** or **granulocyte-macrophage colony-stimulating factor (GM-CSF)** can increase neutrophil counts and decrease the incidence of associated minor infections, but no significant survival benefit has been demonstrated. G-CSF added to erythropoietin may also increase the RBC response compared to erythropoietin alone.
   b. **Pyridoxine** is nontoxic and improves anemia in a small number of patients with MDS with ringed sideroblasts.
   c. **Intensive chemotherapy** (with regimens similar to those for acute leukemia) have proven disappointing with significant morbidity and few long-term survivors.
   d. **New low-intensity chemotherapy regimens** including the methyltransferase inhibitors **azacytidine (Vidaza)** and **decitabine (Dacogen)** as well as the immunomodulatory drug lenalidomide (Revlimid) have demonstrated activity with significantly less morbidity than intensive chemotherapy. Recent studies have demonstrated improved overall survival in those receiving azacytidine.
3. **Allogeneic bone marrow transplantation** offers the only possibility of cure for the small group of eligible patients. Decisions regarding the timing of the transplant are often made based on the IPSS score.

D. Prognosis is based on a variety of features included in the IPSS score (which attempts to predict an overall tendency to evolve into AML). Patients with mild cytopenias and favorable cytogenetics can survive for many years. Patients with higher blast percentages and a poor-risk karyotype have an increased risk of transforming to AML and a significantly shorter median survival.

REFERENCES

Goldman JM. How I treat chronic myeloid leukemia in the imatinib era. Blood 2007;110(8):2828–2837.

Goldman JM, Melo JV. Chronic myeloid leukemia–advances in biology and new approaches to treatment. N Engl J Med 2003;349(15):1451–1464.

Levine RL, Gilliland DG. Myeloproliferative disorders. Blood 2008;112(6): 2190–2198.

Nimer SD. Myelodysplastic syndromes. Blood 2008;111(10):4841–4851.

Acute Leukemia

71

I. INTRODUCTION

A. Leukemia results from the clonal proliferation of white blood cells (WBCs). Leukemias can be classified according to the **cell line** involved (**lymphoid** or **myeloid**) as well as the **maturity of the malignant cell** [acute (immature blasts) or chronic (mature cells)].

B. Acute leukemia is often considered a hematologic emergency and patients are commonly hospitalized for chemotherapy and for complications associated with the leukemia itself (or the chemotherapy treatment).

II. ACUTE LEUKEMIA

ACUTE LEUKEMIA results from a clonal hematopoietic progenitor cell losing its ability to differentiate while replicating uncontrollably. It is typically diagnosed when greater than 20% blasts (immature hematopoietic cells) are seen in either the peripheral blood or bone marrow.

A. Classification

1. **Acute lymphoblastic leukemia (ALL).** The progenitor cell is a **lymphocyte precursor.** ALL can be classified according to:
   a. **Morphology**
      (1) L1 = small lymphoblastic
      (2) L2 = large lymphoblastic
      (3) L3 = undifferentiated
   b. **Immune subtype**
      Many immunophenotypic markers (cytoplasmic or surface expression) are used to differentiate lymphoid leukemias based upon their degree of differentiation:
      (1) pro-B ALL: CD22, CD79a, TdT
      (2) early pre-B ALL (formally common ALL): CD19, CD10, TdT
      (3) pre-B ALL: CD10, CD19, TdT, cytoplasmic mu heavy chain
      (4) mature B cell ALL: CD10, CD19, surface immunoglobulin
      (5) T cell: TdT, acid phosphatase, CD2, CD3, CD7
2. **Acute myelogenous leukemia (AML),** also known as **acute nonlymphocytic leukemia,** is diagnosed when the progenitor cell is a **myeloid precursor.** AML can be classified according

TABLE 71-1

CLASSIFICATION OF ACUTE MYELOGENOUS LEUKEMIA (AML)

FAB Classification*		WHO Classification†
Subtype	Common Name	1. AML with recurrent cytogenetic abnormalities including t(8;21), t(15;17), inv (16), t(16;16), or 11q23
M0	Minimally differentiated	2. AML with multilineage dysplasia
M1	Myeloblastic without maturation	3. Therapy-related AML
M2	Myeloblastic with maturation	4. AML not otherwise catergorized‡
M3	Promyelocytic	
M4	Myelomonocytic	
M5	Monocytic	
M6	Erythroleukemia	
M7	Megakaryoblastic	

*Derived from Bennett JM, Catovsky D, Daniel M-T, et al. Proposed revised criteria for the classification of acute myeloid leukemia: a report of the French-American-British Cooperative Group. Ann Intern Med 1985;103:626–629.

†Derived from Vardiman JW, Harris NL, Brunning RD. The World Health Organization (WHO) classification of the myeloid neoplasms. Blood 2002;100(7):2292–2302.

‡The subtypes included in this group are identical to the corresponding subtypes in the French-American-British (FAB) classifications (M0–M7).

to the microscopic/cytochemical reactivity of the cells [French-American-British (FAB) classification], or based on morphologic/cytogenetic information [World Health Organization (WHO) classification] (Table 71-1).

B. Epidemiology

1. **ALL** represents 80% of childhood cases of acute leukemia (peak age: 2–5 years) and approximately 10%–20% of adult cases; 85%–90% of childhood ALL cases have an FAB L1 classification.
2. **AML** represents approximately 80% of adult leukemias; the average age at onset is 67 years.
3. **Biphenotypic leukemia.** In another 2%–20% of adult cases, the immunophenotype of the leukemia has features of both ALL and AML.

C. Risk factors for acute leukemia include prior radiation or chemotherapy; chemical exposures (e.g., benzene); myelodysplasia; myeloproliferative neoplasms; aplastic anemia; and congenital chromosomal disorders (e.g., Down's syndrome, Turner's syndrome, Klinefelter's syndrome, Fanconi's anemia). In most cases, no obvious predisposing condition is found.

D. Clinical manifestations of acute leukemia. Patients usually seek medical attention within days or weeks of the start of their illness. The pathologic processes outlined as follows (particularly pancytopenia) give rise to the most common findings on presentation.

1. **Pancytopenia** may result in **petechiae, fatigue** and **pallor,** or **clinically apparent infections** (e.g., cellulitis, pneumonia).
2. **Blast cell proliferation and invasion**
   a. **ALL. Bone pain, arthralgias, lymphadenopathy,** and **hepatosplenomegaly**, are common with ALL. **Central nervous system** (CNS) involvement is more frequent in ALL than in AML, and patients can present with cranial nerve palsies.
   b. **AML.** Bone pain is common; adenopathy is rare. AML **type M5** is associated with **gingival, skin,** and less frequently **CNS** involvement.
3. **Leukostasis** [i.e., vaso-occlusion by white blood cells (WBCs)] may occur with a leukocyte count as low as 50,000–75,000 cells/μl but is more frequently seen with WBC counts greater than 100,000 cells/μl. CNS disorders **(headaches, strokes)** and pulmonary findings **(dyspnea, hypoxia)** are common manifestations of leukostasis.
4. **Disseminated intravascular coagulation (DIC)** may occur in all acute leukemias, but especially with AML FAB-M3. It usually results in **excessive bleeding** rather than clotting.

M3 causes DIC.

E. Approach to the patient

1. **Laboratory studies**
   a. **Complete blood count (CBC). Pancytopenia** is usually present but may also be found in a variety of other disorders (see Chapter 59). Alternatively, the patient may present with leukocytosis, anemia, and thrombocytopenia.
   b. **Peripheral blood smear**
      (1) **Blasts** are usually, but not universally, found on the peripheral blood smear.
      (2) **Auer rods,** eosinophilic rods that may be seen in the cytoplasm of blasts, are **pathognomonic for a myeloid neoplasm.** FAB-M3 AML often contains multiple Auer rods (Faggot cell).
   c. **Coagulation tests.** If DIC is present, a prolonged prothrombin time (PT) and partial thromboplastin time (PTT), decreased fibrinogen level, and elevated levels of fibrin degradation products (D-dimer) may be seen.

d. **Electrolyte panel.** Metabolic abnormalities may result from spontaneous **tumor lysis syndrome** or, more commonly, with therapy-induced tumor lysis. High cell turnover and lysis can result in hyperuricemia, hyperkalemia, hyperphosphatemia, hypocalcemia, and/or acidosis.
e. **Cerebrospinal fluid (CSF)** analysis may show abnormalities in patients with carcinomatous meningitis, which is most often associated with ALL and AML type M5.

2. **Radiography.** A **chest radiograph** may show an anterior mediastinal mass in patients with ALL (especially the T-cell variety).
3. **Bone marrow biopsy.** The diagnosis of acute leukemia relies on the presence of **more than 20% blasts** in the peripheral blood or bone marrow. Morphology; histochemical stains [i.e., peroxidase, periodic acid-Schiff (PAS)]; surface markers [i.e., terminal deoxynucleotidyl transferase (TdT) and CD markers]; and cytogenetics can all help determine whether the leukemia is ALL or AML as well as aid in the choice of treatments and counseling the patient on his or her prognosis.
   a. **ALL.** Remember that you "ALL PAST ('passed')" the test by using this mnemonic:

MNEMONIC **Differentiating ALL from AML ("ALL PAST")**

ALL is associated with a positive **PAS** stain and a positive **T**dT enzymology. (TdT is positive in 95% of ALL cases.)

   b. **AML** can be associated with a positive myeloperoxidase (MPO) (myeloperoxidase stains the myeloid granules) or nonspecific esterase (NSE) stain.
   c. Cytogenetics are critical in the prognosis of both AML and ALL. Specific translocations can also be identified by fluorescence in situ hybridization (FISH) or by polymerase chain reaction (PCR) testing.
      (1) Specific chromosomal changes are associated with individual diagnoses. (FAB-M3 AML is associated with the PML-RARα translocation involving chromosomes 15 and 17 [t(15;17)].)
      (2) Poorer responses to therapy and higher risks of relapse are seen with specific chromosomal alterations.
      (3) Additionally, specific changes alter treatment decisions.

(a) t(15;17) in AML: includes the addition of all-trans retinoic acid (ATRA) to chemotherapy

(b) t(9;22) in ALL or AML: addition of an oral tyrosine kinase inhibitor like imatinib (Gleevec)

F. Treatment

1. **Types of therapy**

   a. **Induction chemotherapy** is high dose, usually kills more than 99.9% of leukemic cells and is meant to induce a **complete remission (CR).** A patient is in CR if there are fewer than 5% blasts in the bone marrow, no blasts in the peripheral blood, no evidence of extramedullary disease, normal cytogenetics, and normalization of the blood counts.

   b. **Consolidation (early intensification) therapy** is usually needed to prevent relapse.

   c. **Maintenance therapy,** which entails lower doses, may be indicated and is often continued for several years (only in ALL).

2. **General approaches to therapy**

   a. **ALL**

   (1) **Chemotherapy**

   (a) **Induction chemotherapy** (often with a backbone of daunorubicin, vincristine, and prednisone) can induce a CR in most patients with ALL.

   (b) **CNS prophylaxis** with cranial irradiation and intrathecal methotrexate is usually administered after remission because leukemic meningitis is a common site of relapse in up to 30%–50% of patients who do not receive prophylactic therapy. This rate is reduced to less than 5% for those receiving prophylactic therapy.

   (c) **Late intensification/maintenance therapy** is often given for 2–3 years.

   (2) **Bone marrow transplantation.** With standard therapy, approximately 70%–95% of children and 50% of adults will be cured. Because these rates are comparable to those observed with allogenic transplantation during the first remission, bone marrow transplantation is usually reserved for patients with poor prognostic features or for **relapsed patients who achieve a second remission.**

   b. **AML**

   (1) **Chemotherapy**

   (a) **Induction chemotherapy** [usually with an anthracycline (Daunorubicin) and cytarabine] given over 3 days and 7 days respectively (the "3 + 7" regimen) produces a CR in approximately two-thirds of patients, but less than one-half are cured.

(b) **CNS prophylaxis.** Patients with symptoms suggestive of leukemic meningitis undergo a CSF evaluation to rule out leukemic meningitis. The use of prophylactic CNS therapy varies but is rarely utilized.

(c) **Consolidation therapy** is required to prevent systemic relapse. This typically involves abbreviated cycles with the same agents used in induction or high-dose cytarabine alone. Individuals above the age of 60 do not appear to benefit from consolidative therapy because of higher risks for complications from the therapy. In contrast to the management of ALL, **maintenance therapy is not indicated.**

(d) **ATRA** is used in addition to standard chemotherapy for M3 AML. These leukemic cells bear a characteristic translocation [t(15:17)] involving the retinoic acid receptor α gene. ATRA induces differentiation in M3 AML and improves both initial remission rates as well as overall survival.

(2) **Allogeneic bone marrow transplantation** may be preferable **following the first remission** in patients with poor-risk AML because cure rates may be increased.

III. COMPLICATIONS ASSOCIATED WITH ACUTE LEUKEMIA

A. Leukostasis with symptoms is more common in patients with AML than those with ALL and may necessitate emergent leukapheresis.

B. Tumor lysis syndrome may occur de novo (most commonly with M3 or M5 AML) or with the initiation of therapy. Preventive and therapeutic measures usually include **vigorous hydration, allopurinol therapy, calcium replacement,** and **sodium bicarbonate administration** (to treat acidosis and hyperkalemia and facilitate the excretion of uric acid). Rasburicase can be given to acutely lower uric acid levels.

C. Anemia and **thrombocytopenia** should be managed as described in Chapter 59 (V) and Chapter 60, respectively. Menstruation can be suppressed to prevent excessive bleeding.

D. DIC is frequently seen in FAB-M3 AML. Close monitoring of fibrinogen levels, coagulation parameters (PT and PTT), and platelet levels with strict blood product replacement is required.

E. Fever and **neutropenia.** The risks associated with neutropenia are highest when the absolute neutrophil count is less than

500 cells/μl. Neutropenic precautions should be taken (see Chapter 59 V A 3). Patients should be thoroughly evaluated for the source of their fever (see Chapter 48), and **broad-spectrum intravenous antibiotics** should be instituted as soon as blood cultures are drawn.

F. Complications associated with bone marrow transplant

1. **Graft versus host disease (GVHD)** may accompany allogenic bone marrow transplant. The perceived benefit of an allogeneic transplant is likely due to a graft versus leukemia effect, but this has not been successfully differentiated from the graft versus host effect.
   a. **Acute GVHD** is typically seen within the first 100 days following transplant and may be manifested by a rash, diarrhea, shortness of breath, or liver enzyme abnormalities. Immunosuppression with various combinations of medications including **prednisone, methotrexate, cyclosporine, tacrolimus,** and/or **mycophenolate** is used to suppress acute GVHD.
   b. **Chronic GVHD** can be manifested by skin changes, joint changes, dry eyes and mouth, and chronic shortness of breath. This is often treated with **prolonged immunosuppression.**
2. ***Pneumocystis jiroveci* pneumonia (PCP)** is usually treated with **trimethoprim-sulfamethoxazole (TMP/SMX).**
3. **Cytomegalovirus (CMV)** infections are increasingly recognized as complications of chemotherapy-induced immunosuppression and are actively screened for by reverse transcriptase PCR in previously exposed patients. Treatment is commonly with **valganciclovir.**
4. **Herpes virus infections,** including herpes simplex virus and varicella-zoster virus reactivations, may be prevented and/or treated with either oral or intravenous **acyclovir** or oral **valacyclovir.**
5. **Fungal infections,** including aspergillosis and candidiasis, confer an especially poor prognosis. Infections may be prevented or treated with fluconazole, itraconazole, voriconazole, or posaconazole.

REFERENCES

Estey E, Döhner H. Acute myeloid leukaemia. Lancet 2006;368(9550): 1894–1907.

Jordan CT, Guzman ML, Noble M. Cancer stem cells. N Engl J Med 2006;355:1253–1261.

Pui CH, Evans WE. Drug therapy: treatment of acute lymphoblastic leukemia. N Engl J Med 2006;354:166–178.

Pui CH, Relling MV, Downing JR. Mechanisms of disease: acute lymphoblastic leukemia. N Engl J Med 2004;350:1535–1548.

72 Plasma Cell Dyscrasias

I. INTRODUCTION

A. Definition. Plasma cell dyscrasias (a monoclonal proliferation of plasma cells producing a clonal immunoglobulin protein = monoclonal gammopathies = paraproteinemias) are derived from malignant B lymphocytes. Common plasma cell dyscrasias include **multiple myeloma** and **Waldenström's macroglobulinemia.**

B. Clinical manifestations of plasma cell dyscrasias

1. The clinical manifestations of all plasma cell dyscrasias result from:
   a. Proliferation of the neoplastic cells and invasion of various organs
   b. Secretion of cell products (either immunoglobulins or their subunits)
   c. The host's response to the tumor
2. Patients with plasma cell dyscrasias often have an **M (monoclonal) protein** (clonal immunoglobulin) in their serum.
   a. The M component represents the immunoglobulin (or solitary light or heavy chain) that is being secreted and can be quantitated by performing an immunofixation on a **serum protein electrophoresis.** Qualitative assessment can also be made with this assay (classification of the type of heavy and light chains). Quantification of the light chain can also be performed using a serum free light-chain assay.
   b. M components are **not specific to plasma cell dyscrasias.** They are also seen in leukemia, lymphoma, sarcoidosis, cryoglobulinemia, rheumatoid arthritis and other connective tissue disorders, monoclonal gammopathy of uncertain significance (MGUS), and other diseases.

II. MULTIPLE MYELOMA

A. Epidemiology. Myeloma accounts for 1% of all malignant disease and more than 10% of hematologic malignancies in the United States.

1. It is a disease of **older people;** the median age at diagnosis is 65–70 years.
2. The incidence in **African Americans** is twice that in Caucasians.

B. Clinical manifestations of multiple myeloma. The most common presenting symptoms are **related to anemia, bone pain,** and **infection.** The important clinical manifestations of multiple myeloma can be remembered using the mnemonic "PLASMA."

MNEMONIC **Important Clinical Manifestations of Multiple Myeloma ("PLASMA")**

Proteinuria/renal insufficiency
Lytic bone lesions and hypercalcemia
Anemia and **A**bnormal bleeding
Sepsis and infections
Marrow involvement
Amyloidosis

1. **Proteinuria/renal insufficiency** is multifactorial in etiology, with causes including light-chain proteinuria, hypercalcemia, hyperuricemia, amyloidosis, and pyelonephritis.
2. **Lytic bone lesions** and **hypercalcemia.** Bone pain occurs in 70% of patients, usually involving the back and ribs. Because the lesions are lytic, plain radiographs are better than bone scans.
3. **Anemia** and **abnormal bleeding.** Seventy percent of patients will have anemia (usually normocytic) at the time of diagnosis. Rouleaux formation is frequently seen due to the paraprotein. Paraproteinemias may cause qualitative platelet dysfunction, leading to abnormal bleeding, but patients with myeloma also frequently have thrombocytopenia.
4. **Sepsis** and **infections.** Because of the excess production of abnormal immunoglobulins, myeloma patients usually have decreased levels of normal immunoglobulins leading to increased susceptibility for infections. Seventy-five percent of patients will have a serious infection at some time.
5. **Marrow involvement.** The bone marrow is infiltrated by plasma cells, which initially causes anemia and thrombocytopenia, but may lead to bone marrow failure.
6. **Amyloidosis** develops in a minority of patients and occurs when light chains deposit in normal tissue. This may lead to carpal tunnel syndrome, congestive heart failure (CHF), or renal or liver disease.

C. Laboratory findings

1. **Proteinuria** may be evident on urinalysis, but the dipstick is often negative because it tests for albumin, not globulin.
2. **Anemia** is usually normocytic and normochromic, and **rouleaux formation** may be noted on the peripheral smear.

3. **Narrow anion gap.** Because globulin is cationic, the increased unmeasured cations decrease the anion gap.
4. **Low serum bicarbonate.** A type 2 renal tubular acidosis may result from proximal tubular damage as a result of filtered light chains.
5. **Elevated creatinine** signifying renal damage may be present.
6. **Pseudohyponatremia** may result from increased paraprotein, which can cause laboratory errors.
7. **Hypercalcemia** may occur from increased osteoclast activity leading to lytic bone lesions.
8. **Elevated erythrocyte sedimentation rate (ESR).** The ESR is frequently elevated, but this is a nonspecific finding.

D. Approach to the patient

1. **Protein electrophoresis** on serum and urine is usually ordered based on suspicious symptoms, signs, or laboratory test results.
   a. **Procedure.** Albumin and α-, β-, and γ-globulin are separated by differing mobilities through a gel in an electric field. In myeloma, an increased monoclonal paraprotein causes an abnormal spike (usually in the γ region). This spike may not be seen unless immunofixation is performed on the separated gel.
   b. **Results.** When used together, serum and urine protein electrophoresis will miss approximately 1% of myeloma patients (those who are minimal or nonsecretors). However, of patients who have a variant of myeloma (solitary bone plasmacytoma or extramedullary plasmacytoma), fewer than 30% will have a positive protein electrophoresis.
      (1) **Serum protein electrophoresis** will confirm the diagnosis of myeloma in 80%–90% of patients. Approximately two-thirds of patients with positive serum protein electrophoresis results will also test positive on urine protein electrophoresis.
      (2) **Urine protein electrophoresis.** In approximately 15% of patients, only the light chain is secreted. The light chain can be detected using urine protein electrophoresis with immunofixation or a spot urine Bence-Jones protein assessment.
      (3) Free light-chain proteins can also be quantified from the serum using an immunodiagnostic turbidity assay (serum free light chain).
2. **Immunoelectrophoresis** is performed to determine if the abnormal spike is polyclonal or monoclonal.
   a. A **polyclonal spike** is seen in reactive conditions (e.g., infection, malignancy, collagen vascular disease).

b. A **monoclonal (M component)** spike often signifies a plasma cell dyscrasia but may also be found in many other conditions (e.g., chronic lymphocytic leukemia, lymphoma, sarcoidosis). Therefore, this test should not be used to screen asymptomatic patients because the clinical setting is critical to interpreting the test correctly.

3. **Diagnostic criteria for multiple myeloma (Table 72-1)**
   a. Multiple criteria exist for establishing the diagnosis of multiple myeloma (vs. smoldering myeloma or MGUS).

TABLE 72-1

DIAGNOSIS OF MYELOMA

International Myeloma Working Group*	World Health Organization Criteria[†]
1. Presence of a serum or urinary monoclonal protein 2. Presence of clonal plasma cells in the bone marrow or a plasmacytoma 3. Presence of end-organ damage felt related to the plasma cell dyscrasia, including one of the following: a. Lytic bone lesions b. Increased calcium (>11.5 mg/dl) c. Anemia (hemoglobin <10 g/dl) d. Renal failure (creatinine >2 mg/dl) e. Others including symptomatic hyperviscosity, amyloidosis, recurrent bacterial infections (more than two episodes in 12 mo)	***Major Criteria*** 1. Plasmacytoma 2. Bone marrow plasmacytosis (>30% plasma cells) 3. Monoclonal immunoglobulin spike on serum or urine electrophoresis: • IgG >3.5 g/dl or IgA >2.0 g/dl • Urine κ or λ light chain excretion >1.0 gram per 24 hours ***Minor Criteria*** a. Bone marrow plasmacytosis (10%–30% plasma cells) b. Monoclonal immunoglobulin spike present but of lesser magnitude than given above c. Lytic bone lesions d. IgM <50 mg/dl, IgA <100 mg/dl, or IgG <600 mg/dl

*Must have each of three factors present for the diagnosis of symptomatic myeloma. Adapted from the International Myeloma Working Group. Criteria for the classification of monoclonal gammopathies, multiple myeloma, and related disorders: a report of the International Myeloma Working Group. Br J Haematol 2003;121(5):749–757.

[†]Myeloma may be diagnosed with any two major criteria, or one major criterion plus one minor criterion, or three minor criteria. Adapted from Jaffe ES, Harris NL, Stein H, et al. Tumors of Haematopoietic and Lymphoid Tissues. Pathology and Genetics. World Health Organisation Classification of Tumours. Lyon, France: IARC Press, 2001; as well as van Marion AMW, Lokhorst HM, van den Tweel JG. Pathology of multiple myeloma. Curr Diagn Pathol 2003;9(5):281–337.

b. The International Myeloma Working Group criteria have largely replaced the World Health Organization (WHO) criteria in the diagnosis.

An IgG spike greater than 3.5 g/dl or an IgA spike greater than 2 g/dl almost always represents myeloma (and will be seen as a monoclonal spike when tested by immunoelectrophoresis alone).

4. **Differential diagnosis.** The main disorder to distinguish from myeloma is **MGUS.** Characteristics of MGUS usually include:
   a. M component usually less than or equal to 3 g/dl
   b. Marrow plasmacytosis less than 10%
   c. Absence of anemia, renal disease, hypercalcemia, and bone lesions

For patients diagnosed with MGUS, approximately 1% of patients per year will progress to multiple myeloma.

E. Prognosis is influenced by multiple factors.
1. The serum **β_2 microglobulin** level is an important prognostic indicator and should be checked at diagnosis.
2. As with many hematopoietic malignancies, cytogenetic changes are prognostically significant for both the anticipated response to chemotherapy as well as overall survival. Translocations involving chromosomes 4 and 14 [t(4;14)], chromosomes 14 and 16 [t(14;16)], and deletion of chromosome 13 or the short arm of chromosome 17 (del17p) are associated with a poor prognosis.
3. Circulating plasma cells ($CD38^+/CD45^-$ cells) are also associated with a poorer prognosis.
4. A commonly used prognostic model is the **International Staging System** (Table 72-2).

F. Treatment. The only known curative option for multiple myeloma is an allogeneic bone marrow transplant. However, newer chemotherapies have drastically improved the overall survival in most patients.
1. **Chemotherapy** traditionally involved the use of an alkylating agent (i.e., melphalan) and prednisone, or combination cytotoxic chemotherapy (vincristine, doxorubicin, and dexamethasone). Melphalan and prednisone still provide a

TABLE 72-2

INTERNATIONAL STAGING SYSTEM FOR MULTIPLE MYELOMA*

Stage	Serum Markers
Stage 1	β_2 microglobulin <3.5 mg/L and serum albumin $\geq$3.5 g/dl
Stage 2	Neither stage I nor stage III
Stage 3	β_2 microglobulin $\geq$5.5 mg/L

*Derived from Greipp PR, San Miguel J, Durie BG. International staging system for multiple myeloma. J Clin Oncol 2005;23(15):3412–3420.

solid backbone for the treatment of patients who are not considered candidates for bone marrow transplantation.

2. **Targeted chemotherapies** have dramatically increased the response rate and overall survival. Targeted therapies are now being evaluated in combinations together with traditional chemotherapeutics.
   a. **The immunomodulatory drugs—thalidomide** and **lenalidomide—** are active agents against myeloma.
   b. The proteosomal inhibitor **bortezomib** also shows significant efficacy.
3. Autologous bone marrow transplant is frequently used as a consolidation treatment after initial chemotherapy. Allogeneic bone marrow transplant is frequently used in relapsed disease after failing an autologous transplant.
4. **Radiation** is also used for individual painful bone lesions or plasmacytomas.
5. **Bisphosphonates** are administered monthly to reduce skeletal complications.
6. **Pneumococcal vaccination** should be given to help prevent infectious complications.

III. WALDENSTRÖM'S MACROGLOBULINEMIA. Macroglobulinemia describes an elevated production of an IgM antibody. In Waldenström's macroglobulinemia, a clonal B cell proliferates and secretes a clonal IgM protein.

A. Clinical manifestations of Waldenström's macroglobulinemia. The secreted IgM protein accounts for most of the symptomatic manifestations. The clinical manifestations **are similar to those of myeloma;** however, there are some **important differences.**

1. **Hyperviscosity** is much more common in Waldenström's macroglobulinemia than in multiple myeloma. Symptoms may include headache, altered mental status, visual disturbances, stroke, and mucosal bleeding.

2. **Hepatomegaly, adenopathy,** and **splenomegaly** are commonly seen in Waldenström's macroglobulinemia but not in myeloma.
3. Hypercalcemia, bony lesions, and renal insufficiency are much less common in Waldenström's macroglobulinemia.
4. A simple way to remember the features that may distinguish Waldenström's macroglobulinemia from multiple myeloma is to use the mnemonic "Uncle Waldo loves HAMS."

MNEMONIC **Characteristics of Waldenström's Macroglobulinemia ("Uncle Waldo loves HAMS")**

Hyperviscosity
Adenopathy
Ig**M**
Splenomegaly

B. Treatment

1. Waldenström's macroglobulinemia is an indolent disease with a median survival of over 8 years but is largely incurable. Therefore, treatment is directed toward minimizing symptoms and complications from the macroglobulinemia. Asymptomatic patients may be only observed.
2. Alkylating agents (i.e., chlorambucil) are typically considered for patients who are not candidates for bone marrow transplantation.
3. Nucleoside analogs (i.e., fludarabine) can be used as initial therapy or after failing chlorambucil.
4. Rituximab (a monoclonal antibody to the cell surface B-cell antigen CD20) demonstrates significant activity in Waldenström's macroglobulinemia but may precipitate hyperviscosity symptoms.
5. Plasmapheresis may also be needed frequently to treat symptoms of hyperviscosity.

REFERENCES

Kyle RA, Rajkumar SV. Monoclonal gammopathy of undetermined significance. Clin Lymphoma Myeloma 2005;6(2):102–114.
Kyle RA, Rajkumar SV. Multiple myeloma. Blood 2008;111(6):2962–2972.
Vijay A, Gertz MA. Waldenström's macroglobulinemia. Blood 2007;109(12):5096–5103.

Metastatic Neoplasms

73

I. INTRODUCTION

A. Detection of malignancies. Malignancies are usually detected in one of three main ways:

1. **Screening** (e.g., as with breast, cervical, prostate, and colorectal cancer)
2. As a result of **local symptoms** or **findings** (e.g., pain, a change in bowel habits, hematuria, a lump)
3. As a result of **systemic symptoms** or **findings** (e.g., metastatic disease, paraneoplastic syndromes)

B. Common sites of metastasis. This chapter will help you remember the malignancies that commonly metastasize to the **bone, brain, liver,** and **lung.** If no primary source of metastasis is found, the term **carcinoma of unknown primary (CUP)** is used, and treatment is centered around the most likely cause.

C. Common malignancies capable of metastasis. Although there are many malignancies capable of metastasizing to different areas, there is a core group that can usually go anywhere—**thyroid cancer, lung cancer, breast cancer, gastrointestinal malignancies, renal cell carcinoma, sarcoma, prostate cancer,** and **melanoma.**

II. METASTASIS TO BONE

A. Common malignancies capable of metastasizing to bone are depicted in Figure 73-1.

1. **Melanoma** encircles the diagram denoting the typical skin origin of this malignancy. However, metastatic melanoma should be considered when a patient has a metastatic malignancy in any organ.
2. **Thyroid cancer**
3. **Lung cancer**
4. **Breast cancer**
5. **Gastrointestinal tract malignancies** (usually only the mucinous subtype goes to bone)
6. **Renal cell carcinoma**
7. **Sarcoma**
8. **Prostate cancer**

Multiple myeloma is not included in Figure 73-1 because it is a cancer that arises within the skeletal system rather than metastasizing to the skeletal system. Nevertheless, if you want to include myeloma on the "benzene ring" diagram, just place the sarcoma next to myeloma. **(Myeloma is a hematopoietic neoplasm.)**

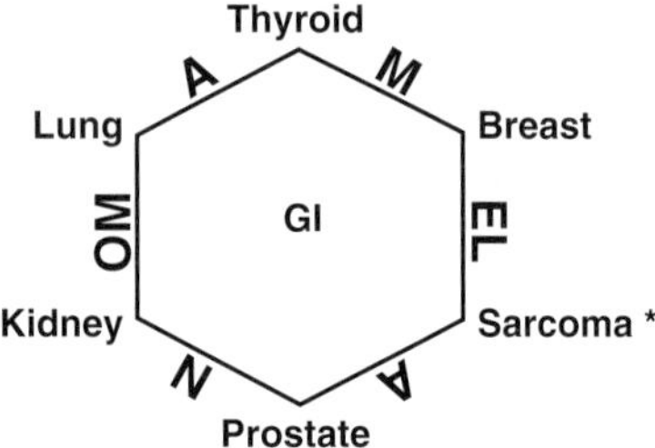

Figure 73-1 Despite the long lists of malignancies capable of metastasis contained in conventional textbooks, the most common cancers that involve the bone, brain, liver, and lungs can practically all be contained in an easy-to-remember, "benzene ring" diagram. The benzene ring represents the human body; the cancers are placed at their approximate anatomic position. (*Sarcoma can arise anywhere.) Even though this diagram is set up to help you remember those cancers that metastasize to bone, the same diagram (with some slight modifications) can be used to recall the cancers that go to the brain, liver, and lung.

B. **Sites of metastasis.** The bones most commonly involved are the **vertebrae, femur, pelvis, ribs,** and **sternum** (in that order).
   1. Cancers that cause lytic bone lesions (renal, thyroid, liver, myeloma) can be seen on plain radiographs (skeletal surveys) but will not show up on bone scans.
   2. Cancers that cause sclerotic bone lesions (prostate, breast, colon, melanoma, and sarcoma) can better be seen on bone scans.

C. **Symptoms and signs of bone cancer.** Cancers that involve the skeletal system can be asymptomatic or produce pain, deformity, pathologic fractures, and hypercalcemia.

D. **Treatment.** Along with malignancy-specific therapy, bone metastases can be treated palliatively with local radiation, surgical stabilization, and bisphosphonates depending on the histology.

III. METASTASIS TO THE BRAIN

A. **Common malignancies capable of metastasizing to the brain.** This list is the same as the one for cancers that metastasize to bone, with one exception: prostate cancer tends not to go to the brain (or lung).
   1. **Thyroid cancer**
   2. **Lung cancer** (most common)
   3. **Breast cancer**
   4. **Gastrointestinal tract malignancies**
   5. **Renal cell carcinoma**
   6. **Sarcoma**

B. Sites of metastasis. Most metastases are **supratentorial** and are often **multiple.**

C. Symptoms and signs of brain metastasis include evidence of **increased intracranial pressure** or **brain disturbances** (focal or diffuse).

D. Treatment. Steroids (usually **dexamethasone**) can be effective in acutely controlling symptoms of cerebral edema and should strongly be considered at the time of diagnosis. Whole brain irradiation is currently the mainstay of therapy for brain metastases, although in some cases focal irradiation to an individual lesion or systemic chemotherapy can be useful. Surgical resection or stereotactic radiosurgery can sometimes be used depending on the number and distribution of metastasis.

IV. METASTASIS TO THE LIVER. Metastatic involvement of the liver is very common and can involve virtually any cancer (except primary brain cancer). In the United States, the incidence of metastatic cancer to the liver is much more common than primary hepatocellular carcinoma. Only cirrhosis causes more cases of fatal liver disease.

A. Common malignancies capable of metastasizing to the liver. Again, this list is very similar to that for cancers that metastasize to the bone. The major difference is that pancreatic cancer commonly goes to the liver (which is not surprising, given the proximity of the two organs), whereas renal cell carcinoma, prostate cancer, and sarcomas involve the liver to a lesser extent (but still can).

1. **Thyroid cancer**
2. **Lung cancer**
3. **Breast cancer**
4. **Gastrointestinal tract malignancies**
5. **Pancreatic malignancy**
6. **Renal cell carcinoma**
7. **Sarcoma**
8. **Prostate cancer**

B. Symptoms and signs of liver metastasis. Often the first (and sometimes only) serum abnormality seen is an elevated alkaline phosphatase. Left upper quadrant pain can be a late sign. Palpable hepatomegaly can be a clue that leads to further radiographic confirmation of hepatic involvement. Finally, obstructive jaundice can occur but there must be an obstruction of the common hepatic duct or common bile duct to lead to jaundice.

C. Treatment. Surgical resection is the only curative option and should only be done if the primary site of disease is also surgically resectable. Systemic chemotherapy is commonly utilized but rarely curative. Other options include hepatic intra-arterial chemotherapy, percutaneous injection, cryosurgery, and hyperthermic coagulation depending on the size and distribution of lesions. External hepatic radiation therapy is limited by its effect on normal liver.

In patients with isolated elevations of alkaline phosphatase, always consider metastatic involvement of the liver as a cause.

V. METASTASIS TO THE LUNG

A. Common malignancies capable of metastasizing to the lung. Although almost any malignancy can involve the lung, the most common include:

1. **Thyroid cancer**
2. **Breast cancer**
3. **Gastrointestinal tract malignancies**
4. **Renal cell carcinoma**
5. **Testicular cancer** (instead of prostate cancer)

B. Sites of metastasis. Classically, lung metastases tend to be multiple and involve the peripheral areas of the lung parenchyma; lesions are most common in the lower lobes. Endobronchial metastases are very unusual.

C. Symptoms and signs of lung metastasis. Chest wall or pleuritic pain can occur depending on the sites of involvement. Shortness of breath and hemoptysis can also occur due to direct extension of the mass into the airway. Horner's syndrome can occur if a lesion involves the sympathetic chain. Incidental metastases to the lung are often detected by staging imaging studies.

D. Treatment. Chemotherapy, radiation, bronchial stenting, and surgery may all be viable options for therapy depending on a number of contributing factors.

REFERENCES

Coleman RE. Risks and benefits of bisphosphonates. Br J Cancer 2008; 98(11):1736–1740.

Herold CI, Blackwell KL. The impact of adjuvant endocrine therapy on reducing the risk of distant metastases in hormone-responsive breast cancer. Breast 2008;17(Suppl 1):S15–24.

Nordlinger B, Sorbye H, Glimelius B, et al. Perioperative chemotherapy with FOLFOX4 and surgery versus surgery alone for resectable liver metastases from colorectal cancer (EORTC Intergroup trial 40983): a randomised controlled trial. Lancet 2008;371(9617):1007–1016.

Patchell RA, Tibbs PA, Walsh JW, et al. A randomized trial of surgery in the treatment of single metastases to the brain. N Engl J Med 1990; 322(8):494–500 [Classic article].

Monoarticular Arthritis

74

I. INTRODUCTION. By addressing the following **three questions** in a patient with joint complaints, you will focus the differential diagnosis while dictating the pace and nature of the evaluation.

A. Does the patient have **true arthritis?** Joint pain (i.e., arthralgia) must be accompanied by signs of inflammation to be considered true arthritis.

B. Is the arthritis **monoarticular or polyarticular?** It is crucial to perform a complete musculoskeletal examination because a patient, distracted by knee pain for example, may overlook swelling and tenderness of other joints or soft tissues. The **number of joints involved** will change your differential diagnosis.

C. Are there any hints of **systemic involvement?** Historical points such as fevers, unintended weight loss, fatigue, or physical signs such as new skin lesions suggest multisystem disease.

II. CAUSES OF MONOARTICULAR ARTHRITIS. Once you have established true arthritis of one joint, **you must rule out an infectious etiology** because if left untreated this could lead to permanent joint damage and, in some cases, sepsis. With this caveat in mind, the mnemonic "If I Make The Diagnosis, No More Harm" will help you recall the common causes of monoarticular arthritis, with infection being first on the list.

MNEMONIC **Causes of Monoarticular Arthritis ("If I Make The Diagnosis, No More Harm")**

Infectious disease
Inflammatory disease
Metabolic disorders
Trauma
Degenerative joint disease
Neoplasm
Miscellaneous (foreign body synovitis, avascular necrosis)
Hemarthrosis

A. Infection

1. Common joint pathogens include **Staphylococcal** and **Streptococcal infection,** particularly in the setting of **skin breakdown.**

Gonorrheal infections should be considered when arthritis is accompanied by pustules and/or tendonitis.

B. **Inflammatory disorders** (e.g., **psoriatic arthritis, rheumatoid arthritis, reactive arthritis,** and other **collagen vascular diseases**). Although these diseases are usually polyarticular and often accompanied by hints of systemic involvement, they may begin as a monoarticular swelling and thus have to be considered in an acute setting when the other causes are ruled out.

C. **Metabolic disorders** [e.g., **gout, pseudogout** (calcium pyrophosphate dihydrate deposition disease (CPPDD)].
   1. **Acute gout can be indistinguishable from a septic joint.** Both give prominent systemic symptoms, and both may have very high white blood cell count in joint fluid. Polarized light microscopic examination of synovial fluid reveals urate crystals seen as ye**ll**ow crystals when para**ll**el to the condenser (i.e., negative birefringence) and of course, gout is treated by a**ll**opurinol (but not acutely). Gout can also be superinfected with a bacterial pathogen. Pseudogout usually has a less acute presentation and tends to be accompanied by chondrocalcinosis that may be visible radiographically. Examination of synovial fluid may reveal rhomboid-shaped **p**seudogout crystals with a **p**ositive birefringence pattern.

D. **Trauma** to a joint (e.g., torn ligament, bone fracture) can lead to hemarthrosis or internal joint derangement. The patient should always be asked specifically about a history of trauma to the affected joint.

E. **Degenerative joint disease (DJD),** a very common disorder, when present in the elderly often causes polyarthritis (see Chapter 75). Monoarticular DJD usually is posttraumatic (e.g., old football injury).

F. **Neoplasm** is a rare cause of monoarticular swelling but should be considered. Examples include **osteoid osteoma** and **pigmented villonodular synovitis.**

G. **Miscellaneous.** This category includes **foreign body synovitis** and **avascular necrosis** (e.g., due to trauma, steroid use, or alcohol).

H. **Hemarthrosis.** Bleeding into a joint, when not related to trauma, is usually seen in patients with clotting abnormalities or those receiving anticoagulants.

III. APPROACH TO THE PATIENT

A. Patient history

1. Determine if there are any hints of **systemic disease.**
2. Determine if arthritis has primarily an **inflammatory or mechanical component.**
   a. **Inflammatory.** Pain and stiffness worse at the day's beginning or with disuse, then "loosens up"; associated with swelling and redness that are often appreciated by others

b. **Mechanical.** Pain worse with use or at the end of the day; recent trauma or overuse; minimal swelling

B. Physical examination

1. Determine if the patient has true arthritis [i.e., look for periarticular processes that may mimic arthritis (e.g., cellulitis, bursitis, tendinitis)].
2. Determine the number of joints involved.
   a. **Monoarticular.** Infection and crystalline arthropathy are most common.
   b. **Oligoarticular** (i.e., two to five joints involved). Consider gonococcal infection, crystal deposition, or seronegative spondyloarthropathies.
   c. **Polyarticular** (i.e., more than three joints involved). See Chapter 75.
3. Look for signs of systemic disease (e.g., cardiac murmur, skin lesions, nail changes).

C. Other diagnostic modalities

1. **Plain radiographs** in the acute setting have a very low yield when there is no history of trauma or prominent bone pain on examination. Remember, infections require about 10 days before changes to the bone will be detectable by plain radiographs.
2. **Arthrocentesis** with **joint fluid analysis** is the **mainstay of diagnosis** and should be performed in all patients with a palpable effusion.
   a. Send fluid for white blood cell (WBC) count with differential, Gram stain and culture, and crystal examination.
   b. Based on the results of the joint fluid analysis, the disorder can be categorized as noninflammatory, inflammatory, or septic (Table 74-1).

Always consider infection, regardless of the joint fluid analysis results because a low cell count may represent early or partially treated infection.

IV. TREATMENT

A. A **septic joint,** once established as a diagnosis either definitively, with organisms detected in the joint fluid, or highly suspected based on risk factors for infection and a high WBC cell in the joint fluid, **is an urgent medical condition. Patients must be admitted to the hospital** with cultures of the joint fluid, blood, and any other relevant sites. Parenteral empiric antibiotics must be initiated to treat the most likely pathogens including skin flora such as *Staphylococcal aureus.* To achieve

TABLE 74-1

JOINT FLUID ANALYSIS*

	Normal	Noninflammatory	Inflammatory	Septic
WBCs/mm^3	<200	200–10,000	10,000–25,000	>25,000
% PMNs	<25%	<25%	50%–90%	50%–100%
Possible causes	—	DJD, trauma, aseptic necrosis	Collagen-vascular diseases, crystal-induced disease, TB, mycotic infections	Pyogenic bacterial infections

DJD = degenerative joint disease; *PMNs* = polymorphonuclear neutrophils; *TB* = tuberculosis; *WBCs* = white blood cells.
*Results in different diseases may be variable.

adequate drainage, all septic joints need to be lavaged in the operating room. Often the joint requires serial drainage either by arthrocentesis if possible or by surgical lavage. Antibiotics are continued for 4–6 weeks depending on the clinical circumstances.

B. Gout can best be treated with early intervention with oral **non-steroidal anti-inflammatory drugs (NSAIDs).** The time to symptom resolution roughly correlates with duration of symptoms once treatment is initiated. If patients have contraindications to NSAIDs (e.g., renal insufficiency, prior peptic ulcer disease), consider injection of corticosteroids into the affected joint. Alternatively, a 5-day course of oral prednisone is also effective. Allopurinol and colchicine have no role in the treatment of acute gout.

REFERENCES

Cassetta M, Gorevic PD. Crystal arthritis. Gout and pseudogout in the geriatric patient. Geriatrics 2004;59(9):25–30.

Mathews C, Coakley G. Septic arthritis: current diagnostic and therapeutic algorithm. Curr Opin Rheumatol 2008;20:457–462.

75

Polyarticular Arthritis

I. INTRODUCTION. Once you have established that a **polyarticular process (true arthritis of more than three joints)** is present, you must then address the following questions:

A. What is the **distribution of affected joints?**

1. **Symmetric processes** involve paired joints bilaterally (e.g., bilateral wrists, bilateral shoulders, bilateral small proximal joints of hands).
2. **Asymmetric processes** will involve nonpaired joints (e.g., left knee with right wrist).

B. Is there any evidence of **systemic involvement (e.g., fever, chills, weight loss)?**

II. CAUSES OF POLYARTICULAR ARTHRITIS. There are three main categories: symmetric, asymmetric, and miscellaneous (Table 75-1).

A. Symmetric seropositive arthritis. In addition to the characteristic joint distribution, a patient often will have accompanying **autoantibodies and frequently will also have systemic signs and symptoms.**

1. **Rheumatoid arthritis**
   a. **Epidemiology.** The disease affects women twice as often as men, and the usual age at onset is 20–40 years.
   b. **Clinical manifestations.** The onset is **insidious,** but 20% will have brisk progression. **Major symptoms** include malaise, fever, and morning stiffness relieved with hot bath and exercise. **Joints classically involved** include proximal interphalangeal joints (PIPs), metacarpal phalangeal joints (MCPs), wrists, shoulders, knees, ankles, and metatarsal phalangeal joints (MTPs). **Extra-articular manifestations,** most common in patients with high-titer rheumatoid factor (RF), may include subcutaneous nodules, pulmonary interstitial infiltrates, lymphadenopathy, and cutaneous ulcers. The classic bone **radiographic findings** include periarticular osteoporosis and erosions along the margin of the joint.

Eighty-five percent of patients with rheumatoid arthritis are RF positive. Eighty percent of patients with the autoantibody anticyclic citrullinated peptide have rheumatoid arthritis.

TABLE 75-1

COMMON CAUSES OF POLYARTICULAR ARTHRITIS

Symmetric seropositive polyarthritis
- Rheumatoid arthritis
- Systemic lupus erythematosus (SLE)
- Systemic sclerosis
- Polymyositis
- Overlap syndrome

Asymmetric seronegative spondyloarthropathy
- Ankylosing spondylitis
- Psoriatic arthritis
- Reactive arthritis (Reiter's syndrome when accompanied by conjunctivitis and urethritis)
- Arthritis related to enteric disorders (e.g., due to Crohn's disease or ulcerative colitis)

Miscellaneous
1. Gonorrheal—disseminated gonococcal infection
2. Spirochetal— early Lyme disease, secondary syphilis
3. Viral—human immunodeficiency virus (HIV), hepatitis B, parvovirus B19
4. Other—infiltrative diseases, Still's disease, rheumatic fever, vasculitis

2. **Systemic lupus erythematosus (SLE)** is a multisystem autoimmune disorder.
   a. **Epidemiology.** Eighty-five percent of all patients are women 20–40 years of age.
   b. **Clinical manifestations.** Because SLE can **affect most organ systems,** diagnosis can be based on the presence of 4 of 11 characteristics. To receive a passing grade in our medical school, we needed to know the 11 criteria for SLE; therefore, we were all in "P-MOAD"—7 Ps and

MNEMONIC **Criteria for the Diagnosis of SLE ("P-MOAD")**

Positive antinuclear antibody (ANA): seen in 99% of patients
Positive other immunologic test [antibody (Ab) to double-stranded DNA, Ab to Smith, LE cell preparation, or false-positive syphilis serology]
Psychosis, seizures, or other neurologic abnormalities
Photosensitivity rash
Polyserositis (pleuritis, pericarditis, or peritonitis)
Proteinuria or renal involvement

Pancytopenia or single-cell line "penia" (antibody-mediated anemia, thrombocytopenia, or leukopenia)
Malar rash
Oral ulcers (painful)
Arthritis
Discoid rash (heaped-up borders, almost cheloid in appearance)

M O A D. The first two Ps are positive lab tests; the next five Ps are arranged from head to toe (see mnemonic).

3. **Systemic sclerosis (scleroderma)** is characterized by the presence of a positive ANA, early Raynaud's phenomenon (90% of patients), and fibrosis of the skin and internal organs, which falls into two forms: diffuse and limited (CREST syndrome).
   a. **Clinical manifestations.** The diffuse form (affecting 20% of patients) has widespread skin thickening with frequent interstitial lung disease, an increased risk of suffering a renal crisis, and an association with anti-SCL-70 autoantibodies.
   b. The **limited** form (CREST syndrome) is characterized by **c**alcinosis, **R**aynaud's phenomenon, **e**sophageal motility dysfunction, **s**clerodactyly, and **t**elangiectasia. Those with CREST syndrome have a decreased risk of renal involvement, a higher risk of pulmonary hypertension, and correlation with serum anticentromere antibodies.
4. **Myositis-related arthritis,** when present, most commonly occurs in the hands and wrists.
   a. **Polymyositis** is arthritis associated with true weakness of proximal muscles (e.g., deltoids and quadriceps).
   b. **Dermatomyositis** is arthritis and weakness with an accompanying violaceous skin lesion most commonly located on the eyelids, on the forehead, and over the knuckles of the PIPs and DIPs (Gottron's papules).

B. Asymmetric seronegative arthritis. The classic seronegative spondyloarthropathies are characterized by **asymmetric involvement of the spine and peripheral joints, early onset of disease** (usually before age 40), an **absence of RF or ANA** (hence, the term "seronegative"), and a strong association with **human leukocyte antigen (HLA)-B27.** Consider pelvic films to assess the sacroiliac joint involvement that characterizes this group of disorders.

1. **Ankylosing spondylitis.** This chronic inflammatory disease leads to pain and stiffening of the spine, affects men more than women, and usually occurs in the second or third decades of life.

2. **Psoriatic arthritis.** Look for subtle skin changes at the umbilicus, gluteal crease, and hairline.
3. **Reactive arthritis.** Usually follows an episode of invasive infectious diarrhea or venereal infection with chlamydia. **Reiter's syndrome** is classically characterized by the clinical triad of **conjunctivitis, urethritis,** and **arthritis**—the patient cannot "see, pee, or bend at the knees."
4. **Arthritis related to enteric disorders** [e.g., inflammatory bowel disease (IBD), Whipple's disease, enteric infection]

C. Miscellaneous causes. There are many other causes of polyarthritis. Most can easily be remembered in the following manner: one gonorrheal, two spirochetal, three viral, and four others.

1. **Gonorrheal. Disseminated gonococcal infection** (as a result of *Neisseria gonorrhoeae* infection) may result in migratory polyarthralgias of the ankles, knees, and fingers; tenosynovitis; fever; and/or a pustular rash often on the dorsum of the hands.
2. **Spirochetal**
   a. **Lyme disease** (caused by *Borrelia burgdorferi* infection) is characterized by flu-like symptoms, erythema migrans, and unilateral knee arthritis. Late stages include neurologic problems (e.g., seventh nerve palsy, meningitis), cardiac conduction abnormalities, and/or chronic large joint arthritis.
   b. **Secondary syphilis** can involve almost any part of the body, including the joints.
3. **Viral.** The three common viral etiologies include **human immunodeficiency virus (HIV), hepatitis B virus,** and **parvovirus B19.**
4. **Other**
   a. **Infiltrative diseases** include **sarcoidosis, amyloidosis,** and polyarticular **tophaceous gout;** biopsy is usually necessary to make the diagnosis.
   b. **Still's disease** is a form of juvenile rheumatoid arthritis that affects adults. It is characterized by spiking fevers, arthritis, and an evanescent, salmon-colored rash.

Degenerative joint disease, the most common cause of polyarticular arthritis, is a slowly progressive noninflammatory process that destroys articular cartilage. (It is a mechanical arthritis.) Its natural history, distribution of involved joints (i.e., primarily distal interphalangeal joints, shoulders, knees, and hips), and characteristic radiologic findings (i.e., joint space narrowing, bone spurs, and sclerosis) make this a relatively straightforward diagnosis.

c. **Rheumatic fever** is discussed in Chapter 53.
d. **Vasculitis** is discussed in Chapter 76.

REFERENCES

Braun J, Sieper J. Ankylosing spondylitis. Lancet 2007:369(9570):1379–1390.

Conaghan PG, Dickson J, Grant RL. Care and management of osteoarthritis in adults. BMJ 2008; 336(7642):502–503.

D'Cruz DP, Khamshta MA, Hughes GR. Systemic lupus erythematosus. Lancet 2007;369(9561):587–596.

Donahue KE, Gartlehner G, Jonas DE, et al. Systemic review: comparative effectiveness and harms of disease-modifying medications for rheumatoid arthritis. Ann Intern Med 2008;148(2):124–134.

Lee DM, Weinblatt ME. Rheumatoid arthritis. Lancet 2001;358(9285):903–911 [Classic article].

76 Vasculitis

I. **INTRODUCTION.** The vasculitides are characterized by inflammation of the blood vessels disrupting blood flow with resultant ischemic damage. Because of the broad distribution and varied nature of blood vessels, the clinical manifestations of vasculitis similarly are quite varied and often subtle.

II. **CLINICAL MANIFESTATIONS OF VASCULITIS.** The vasculitides can present with any combination of the following (although disease presentation is primarily influenced by specific vessel involvement):

A. **Constitutional symptoms** (e.g., fever, fatigue, anorexia, weight loss)

B. **Arthralgias**

C. **Symptoms of organ ischemia** referable to affected viscera (e.g., pulmonary hemorrhage, glomerulonephritis)

D. **Peripheral neuropathy** from small vessel involvement

E. **Skin findings** (e.g., palpable purpura, livedo reticularis, necrotic lesions, infarcts of the tips of digits)

Palpable purpura is pathognomonic of a cutaneous, small vessel vasculitis of any etiology. Inflammation of the vessel allows extravasation of blood and fluid, resulting in palpable edema. Because the blood is no longer intravascular, the lesion is purpuric (nonblanchable) rather than erythematous (blanchable).

III. **CAUSES OF VASCULITIS.** To help organize your approach, consider the vasculitides affecting large, medium, and small blood vessels. Because there are a large number of entities that can cause small vessel vasculitis, a mnemonic to make it easier to remember the different causes will be provided.

A. **Large vessel vasculitides.** These diseases affect vessels that have elastic lamina.

1. **Giant cell (temporal) arteritis**

   a. **Epidemiology.** Giant cell arteritis is rare in patients younger than 50 years. Women are affected more often than men.

b. **Clinical manifestations.** A new headache or change in character of ongoing headaches is the most common clinical finding, whereas jaw claudication is the most specific symptom. Sudden blindness, due to retinal ischemia, is the most dreaded complication. Since treatment with corticosteroids can prevent retinal ischemia, early diagnosis is crucial. There is a close association with polymyalgia rheumatica, which is characterized by proximal muscle pain and stiffness.

c. **Diagnosis.** Suspect in an elderly patient who complains of a headache and has an erythrocyte sedimentation rate (ESR) greater than 50 mm/hr. A temporal artery biopsy of at least 2 cm in length, to account for skip lesions, is needed for definitive diagnosis. If your pretest probability is high enough to merit a biopsy, empiric treatment with steroids needs to be strongly considered.

2. **Takayasu's aortitis**

a. **Epidemiology.** Takayasu's aortitis is rare. Young Asian women are most commonly affected.

b. **Clinical manifestations.** Patients have findings resulting from involvement of the aortic arch and its primary branches; thus, transient ischemic attacks and absent radial pulses yielding the moniker "pulseless disease" are most common.

c. **Diagnosis.** Clinical suspicion must be supported by diagnostic angiography.

B. Medium vessel vasculitis

1. **Polyarteritis nodosa (PAN)**

a. **Epidemiology.** The average age at onset is approximately 45 years. Men are affected more often than women. In 30% of patients, PAN is associated with hepatitis B antigenemia.

b. **Clinical manifestations.** Virtually any organ system can be involved, making description of a "classic" case of PAN difficult. Due to the significant inflammation, fever and weight loss are common. Diffuse vessel involvement can cause new-onset hypertension, whereas involvement of specific medium arteries supplying the kidneys yields renal failure with a bland urinary sediment; mesenteric vessel involvement yields abdominal pain; disruption of blood to muscles causes myalgia and weakness; and neuropathies occur secondary to nerve ischemia.

c. **Diagnosis.** Definitive diagnosis is made by biopsy of involved organs or by visceral angiography, which may reveal aneurysms, areas of stenosis, or obliteration of vessels.

C. Small vessel vasculitides. The mnemonic "VAASCULITIS" can help you remember the diverse and large number of causes of this group.

MNEMONIC **Causes of Small Vessel Vasculitis ("VAASCULITIS")**

Various drugs
ANCA (antineutrophilic cytoplasmic antibody) associated
Autoimmune disorders
Serum sickness
Cryoglobulinemia
Ulcerative colitis
Low complement (hypocomplementemic urticarial vasculitis)
Infections
Tumors
IgA nephropathy (Henoch-Schönlein purpura)
Smoking related (thromboangiitis obliterans)

1. **Various drugs.** Penicillins, sulfa drugs, and propylthiouracil are just a few of the many drugs that can cause hypersensitivity vasculitis.
2. **ANCA associated**
   a. **Wegener's granulomatosis**
      (1) **Clinical manifestations.** Pulmonary involvement with cough, dyspnea, hemoptysis, or asymptomatic infiltrates occurs in approximately 95% of patients. The upper and lower respiratory tract are involved, resulting in ulcerations of the nasal mucosa, saddle nose deformity (secondary to perforation of the nasal septum), chronic sinusitis, serous otitis, or pulmonary infiltrates or cavities. The kidney is involved in approximately 85% of patients, leading to hematuria, proteinuria, and/or glomerulonephritis with rapidly progressive renal failure if treatment is delayed.
      (2) **Diagnosis.** Biopsy, preferably lung or kidney, reveals necrotizing granulomas in small arteries and veins. Serum antibodies yield a circulating ANCA (C-ANCA) pattern with enzyme-linked immunosorbent assay (ELISA) positive for proteinase-3.
   b. **Churg-Strauss syndrome** (allergic angiitis and granulomatosis)
      (1) **Epidemiology.** Churg-Strauss syndrome is associated with adult-onset reactive airway disease that is not related to smoking.

(2) **Clinical manifestations.** Pulmonary involvement (with asthma and, occasionally, fleeting pulmonary infiltrates) is most common. Mononeuritis multiplex is also well described. Peripheral eosinophilia can be significant.

(3) **Diagnosis.** Biopsy (usually of lung tissue) shows small vessel vasculitis, extravascular granulomas, and eosinophil infiltration. Perinuclear ANCA (P-ANCA) pattern is associated with positive ELISA for myeloperoxidase molecules.

c. **Microscopic polyangiitis (MPAN)**

(1) **Clinical manifestations.** Most important distinctions from classic PAN are rapidly progressive glomerulonephritis and small vessel involvement of the lung yielding alveolitis and hemorrhage.

(2) **Diagnosis.** Biopsy shows necrotizing inflammation of capillaries, venules, and arterioles with no granulomas. P-ANCA pattern is characteristic with serum antibodies positive for myeloperoxidase.

d. **Pauci-immune necrotizing glomerulonephritis**

(1) Identical to MPAN except no lung involvement

3. **Autoimmune disorders.** Systemic lupus erythematosus (SLE) and rheumatoid arthritis may cause a vasculitis.
4. **Serum sickness** occurs 7–10 days after a primary exposure to an antigen (e.g., penicillin) or 2–4 days after a secondary exposure.
5. **Cryoglobulinemia** is characterized by immunoglobulins that precipitate in cold temperatures. The condition is correlated with hepatitis C infection, acute or chronic.

   a. **Type I cryoglobulins** are monoclonal and usually associated with multiple myeloma, Waldenström's macroglobulinemia, or other lymphoproliferative disorders.

   b. **Type II cryoglobulins,** which have one monoclonal component and one polyclonal component, and **type III cryoglobulins,** which have two polyclonal components, are both considered mixed cryoglobulins. They are often associated with infections (e.g., hepatitis), connective tissue diseases, or lymphoproliferative disorders; patients are rheumatoid factor positive. **Essential mixed cryoglobulinemia** is diagnosed when no precipitating condition can be elicited.

6. **Ulcerative colitis** is occasionally associated with a secondary vasculitis.
7. **Low complement. Hypocomplementemic urticarial vasculitis** occurs predominantly in young women. Recurrent bouts of urticarial lesions, most commonly found on the trunk and extremities, are the most notable feature; lesions

often become confluent. All serum complement levels are low.

8. **Infections** should always be considered as a cause of small vessel vasculitis because they may be life-threatening.
   a. **Bacterial.** *Neisseria* spp., *Staphylococcus aureus, Streptococcus* spp, and *Pseudomonas aeruginosa* infections are most commonly associated with vasculitis. Syphilis and Lyme disease should also be considered.
   b. **Viral.** The most commonly implicated viruses are hepatitis B and C virus, Epstein-Barr virus, and cytomegalovirus (CMV).
   c. **Rickettsial.** Rocky Mountain spotted fever may be associated with vasculitis. The characteristic rash usually appears on the extremities 2–6 days after the onset of fever.
9. **Tumors. Lymphoma** and **multiple myeloma** are the malignancies most often associated with vasculitis.
10. **IgA nephropathy (Henoch-Schönlein purpura)** usually occurs in children or young adults. Classically, palpable purpura appears over the lower extremities, followed by abdominal pain, arthritis, and renal involvement. IgA deposits can be found in the skin and kidney.

IgA deposits may be found on skin biopsy in patients with Henoch-Schönlein purpura, making this the only vasculitis that can be diagnosed by simple skin biopsy.

11. **Smoking related. Thromboangiitis obliterans (Buerger's disease)** was first described in men but also is seen in women who are younger than 40 years and heavy smokers. It is likely that a significant vasospastic component causes vessel wall damage and inflammation leading to impaired arterial blood supply, Raynaud's phenomenon, thrombophlebitis, or deep venous thrombosis. Smoking cessation is the mainstay of therapy.

There are several additional types of vasculitis of which you may be aware. These involve either small vessels (e.g., Goodpasture's syndrome, Behçet's disease) or medium vessels (e.g., Kawasaki's disease, primary granulomatous central nervous system vasculitis).

IV. APPROACH TO THE PATIENT

A. Patient history. A travel history and medication history may provide insight into the cause of the vasculitis (e.g., infection, drug therapy).

B. Laboratory studies. With the exception of the SLE-, rheumatoid arthritis (RA)-, and ANCA-associated vasculitides, no specific tests will focus the diagnosis. Notably, an elevated ESR only suggests that inflammation of any cause is present in the patient. Use lab tests to characterize the distribution and magnitude of end-organ involvement.

1. **Complete blood count (CBC).** Look for leukocytosis, anemia, or thrombocytosis.
2. **Renal panel.** Look for elevated creatinine levels.
3. **Urinalysis.** Look for hematuria or proteinuria. If blood is present, you must examine the urine sediment for casts or dysmorphic red blood cells (RBCs) since these findings indicate glomerulonephritis.
4. **ESR** (usually elevated)
5. **Antinuclear antibody (ANA)** and **rheumatoid factor (RF) levels**
6. **ANCA and if available specific ELISA for myeloperoxidase and proteinase-3**
7. **Cryoglobulins**
8. **Complement levels (C3, C4)**
9. **Blood cultures** (especially to rule out endocarditis)
10. **Cultures for gonococcal infection** (e.g., oral, anal, cervical, urethral)
11. **Serologies for hepatitis B** and **C virus, Epstein-Barr virus, CMV,** ***Treponema pallidum,*** or ***Borrelia burgdorferi***

C. Diagnosis is very difficult to make conclusively without tissue biopsy. Use the history and physical examination to guide you to tissues most likely to be affected (e.g., skin, lung, peripheral nervous system).

V. TREATMENT.

A rheumatology consult is often useful when treating a patient with vasculitis. These diseases are uncommon; therefore, it is crucial to recognize that many infections, neoplasms, metabolic disorders, and drug reactions can serve as mimickers.

Because therapy involves immunosuppression, always ask yourself, "Am I about to start treating an infection with steroids?"

A. Large vessel vasculitides are often treated initially with **glucocorticoids** (e.g., prednisone, 1 mg/kg/day). In general, temporal arteritis responds to steroids alone, and its timely administration can be vision saving. After the first 4 weeks with high-dose steroids, if the patient is clinically responding consider a slow taper of the steroids. Patients usually require 1–2 years to successfully taper off the treatment.

B. **Medium vessel and ANCA-associated small vessel vasculitides**
   1. Evidence of **generalized organ-threatening disease** requires immunosuppression with a combination of corticosteroids and cyclophosphamide, either intravenous pulses or daily oral dosing, to induce remission. Maintenance of the remission can be achieved by substituting azathioprine or mycophenolate mofetil at 3–6 months of treatment while continuing the corticosteroid taper.
   2. If you suspect a **mimic of vasculitis,** the underlying condition must be treated. Empiric antibiotics may be given if an infection (e.g., meningococcemia, endocarditis, Rocky Mountain spotted fever) is suspected. Stop the use of any possible offending drugs (e.g., propylthiouracil).

REFERENCES

Bosch X, Guilabert A, Espinosa G, et al. Treatment of antineutrophilic cytoplasmic antibody associated vasculitis: a systematic review. JAMA 2007;298(6):655–669.

Molloy ES, Langford CA. Vasculitis mimics. Curr Opin Rheumatol 2008;20(1):29–34.

Salvarani C, Cantini F, Hunder GG. Polymyalgia rheumatica and giant cell arteritis. Lancet 2008;372:234–245.

Seo P, Stone JH. Small-vessel and medium-vessel vasculitis. Arthritis Rheum 2007;57(8):1552–1559.

Suresh E. Diagnostic approach to patients with suspected vasculitis. Postgrad Med J 2006;82(970):483–488.

77 Hypercalcemia

I. INTRODUCTION

A. Definition. Hypercalcemia is an elevated level of ionized calcium in the blood. Hypercalcemia is a common problem in both inpatients and outpatients. In the former, hypercalcemia is usually secondary to malignancy; in the latter, hyperparathyroidism is more common.

B. Because **albumin binds calcium,** it is important to make sure that hypercalcemia is real and not just a reflection of hyperalbuminemia.

For every 1-mg increase in albumin (the normal albumin level is 4 mg/dl), you must decrease the calcium level by 0.8 mg/dl. The converse is true for hypoalbuminemia. For example, if the serum calcium is 10.5 mg/dl and the albumin is 5 mg/dl, the corrected calcium is 9.7 mg/dl (and the patient is not hypercalcemic).

II. CLINICAL MANIFESTATIONS OF HYPERCALCEMIA

A. Symptoms are usually nonspecific and tend to be more obvious when the serum calcium level exceeds 12 mg/dl. The severity of symptoms is also dependent on the acuity of the calcium elevation. "**Abdominal moan, psychiatric groan, kidney stone,** and **urination zone** (i.e., the bathroom)" is a way to recall common symptoms.

1. **Gastrointestinal** symptoms include constipation, nausea, vomiting, and anorexia. Patients may develop acute pancreatitis.
2. **Central nervous system (CNS) symptoms** may range from depression and fatigue to confusion, lethargy, and weakness. Progression to coma and death may occur with severe hypercalcemia.
3. **Renal** symptoms include nephrolithiasis, renal failure, and polyuria leading to dehydration. Hypercalcemia impairs urinary concentrating ability, leading to frequent urination and worsening dehydration.

B. Signs of hypercalcemia include hypertension, hypotonia, decreased deep tendon reflexes, and a shortened QT interval on the electrocardiogram (ECG).

III. CAUSES OF HYPERCALCEMIA. There are many causes of hypercalcemia. The mnemonic "MISHAP + F" will help you remember the most important ones.

MNEMONIC **Causes of Hypercalcemia ("MISHAP + F")**

Malignancy
Intoxication (vitamin D)
Sarcoidosis (and other granulomatous diseases)
Hospitalization and **H**ydrochlorothiazide
Adrenal disease and milk-**A**lkali syndrome
Primary hyperparathyroidism and **P**aget's disease
+
Familial hypocalciuric hypercalcemia (FHH)

A. Malignancy. Hypercalcemia occurs secondary to **local osteolysis** (seen with extensive bone involvement by the tumor) or **humoral influences** [induced by parathyroid hormone (PTH)-related peptide]. **Lymphomas** may produce excess 1,25-dihydroxyvitamin D.

B. Intoxication with vitamin D. Some patients take large amounts of vitamin D for unclear reasons; serum 25-hydroxyvitamin D or 1,25-dihydroxyvitamin D levels (depending on what form of vitamin D was ingested) will confirm this diagnosis.

C. Sarcoid and **other granulomatous diseases** (e.g., **tuberculosis, berylliosis**). Hypercalcemia results from increased formation of 1,25-dihydroxyvitamin D in granulomatous tissues.

D. Hospitalization. Hypercalcemia occurs in the setting of **prolonged immobilization.** It is most commonly seen in patients with active bone turnover, such as younger patients with maturing bone or older patients with Paget's disease.

E. Hydrochlorothiazide. Patients receiving thiazide diuretics may have elevated serum calcium levels.

F. Adrenal disease. Addison's disease and **pheochromocytoma** are uncommon causes of hypercalcemia.

G. Alkali ingestion. Hypercalcemia can occur as a result of excess calcium carbonate ingestion (e.g., patients with peptic ulcer disease taking large amounts of calcium-containing antacids).

H. Primary hyperparathyroidism. Primary hyperparathyroidism is caused by solitary adenomas (85% of patients), four-gland hyperplasia (10% of patients), or carcinoma (<5% of patients).

Patients are usually asymptomatic at the time of diagnosis. Serum phosphate levels are often low.

I. Paget's disease, a metabolic bone disease of unknown etiology, is characterized by excessive bone destruction and disorganized repair leading to skeletal deformities (e.g., kyphosis, tibial bowing, and skull enlargement).

J. Familial hypocalciuric hypercalcemia (FHH) is a benign, autosomal dominant genetic disease characterized by hypercalcemia, hypocalciuria (<50 mg/24 hours), and occasionally hypermagnesemia. The serum PTH level is often slightly increased, which can lead to a mistaken diagnosis of hyperparathyroidism. In primary hyperparathyroidism, however, urinary calcium is typically normal or elevated.

IV. TREATMENT is warranted if symptoms are present or if serum calcium exceeds 12 mg/dl.

A. Initial therapy entails fluids, fluids, and more fluids, **followed** by loop diuretics primarily to prevent fluid overload. Other therapies include **bisphosphonates, calcitonin, corticosteroids,** and **plicamycin.**

B. Definitive treatment will, of course, depend on the underlying cause.

REFERENCES

Bushinsky DA, Monk RD. Calcium. Lancet 1998;352(9124):306–311 [Classic article].

LeGrand SB, Leskuski D, Zama I. Narrative review: furosemide for hypercalcemia: an unproven yet common practice. Ann Intern Med 2008; 149(4):259–263.

78

■ Hypocalcemia

I. INTRODUCTION

A. Definition. Hypocalcemia is a decreased ionized calcium level. Hypocalcemia is a common occurrence in very ill, hospitalized patients.

B. Because **albumin binds calcium,** it is important to make sure that hypocalcemia is real and not just a reflection of hypoalbuminemia.

For every 1-mg decrease in albumin (the normal albumin level is 4 mg/dl), you must increase the calcium by 0.8 mg/dl. For example, if the serum calcium is 7.5 mg/dl and the albumin is 2 mg/dl, then the corrected serum calcium is 9.1 mg/dl (and the patient is not hypocalcemic).

C. In patients with respiratory alkalosis (such as hyperventilation), the total serum calcium is normal but the ionized calcium is low. This may result in signs and symptoms of hypocalcemia.

II. CLINICAL MANIFESTATIONS OF HYPOCALCEMIA. Because hypocalcemia leads to enhanced excitation of the nervous system and muscle cells, the symptoms and signs primarily involve the **neuromuscular** and **cardiovascular** systems.

A. Symptoms include paresthesias of the lips and extremities, muscle cramps (which can progress to tetany), and laryngospasm with wheezing or life-threatening stridor (in severe cases).

B. Signs include **hypotension, Chvostek's sign** (tapping the facial nerve leads to contraction of the facial muscles), and **Trousseau's sign** (occlusion of the brachial artery with a blood pressure cuff leads to carpal spasm). The **electrocardiogram** (ECG) may show a prolonged QT interval or atrioventricular (AV) block.

III. CAUSES OF HYPOCALCEMIA. There are many causes of hypocalcemia; the mnemonic "HIPOCAL" will help you remember the most important ones.

MNEMONIC **Causes of Hypocalcemia ("HIPOCAL")**

Hypoparathyroidism
Infection
Pancreatitis
Overload states
Chronic renal failure
Absorption abnormalities
Loop diuretics

A. **Hypoparathyroidism.** The major causes of hypoparathyroidism are **thyroidectomy** with damage to the parathyroid glands and **autoimmune parathyroid destruction**. Rare causes include DiGeorge's syndrome and parathyroid injury as a result of infection or irradiation. Functional hypoparathyroidism [i.e., decreased secretion of parathyroid hormone (PTH)] may result from magnesium deficiency.
B. **Infection.** Up to 20% of patients with **gram-negative sepsis** are hypocalcemic due to acquired defects in the parathyroid–vitamin D axis. This hypocalcemia may cause hypotension that is responsive to calcium replacement.
C. **Pancreatitis.** Serum calcium less than 8 mg/dl is one of Ranson's criteria; the calcium level may correlate with the severity of acute pancreatitis.
D. **Overload states.** Occasionally, hypocalcemia may be seen in cases of rapid intravascular **volume expansion.**
E. **Chronic renal failure.** Vitamin D is metabolized in the normal kidney to 1,25-dihydroxyvitamin D, which promotes intestinal calcium absorption. With renal failure, intestinal calcium absorption decreases and patients become hypocalcemic.
F. **Absorption abnormalities.** Patients with malabsorption (due to any cause) of calcium, magnesium, or vitamin D will often have hypocalcemia.
G. **Loop diuretics.** Unlike thiazide diuretics (which can cause hypercalcemia), furosemide and other loop diuretics lead to enhanced renal excretion of calcium.

IV. TREATMENT

A. If the patient has tetany, arrhythmias, laryngospasm, or seizures, immediate therapy with **intravenous calcium gluconate** is indicated. This is in addition to any other acute interventions necessary to treat a life-threatening complication.
B. If the patient has asymptomatic hypocalcemia, **oral calcium** and **vitamin D** are usually sufficient.
C. If the patient has hypomagnesemia, replacement of magnesium is usually required to correct hypocalcemia.

REFERENCES

Bushinsky DA, Monk RD. Calcium. Lancet 1998;352(9124):306–311 [Classic article].

Shoback, D. Hypoparathyroidism. N Engl J Med 2008;359(4):391–403.

79 Diabetic Ketoacidosis

I. INTRODUCTION

A. Definition. Diabetic ketoacidosis (DKA) is a life-threatening complication of diabetes mellitus caused by a relative or absolute deficiency of insulin along with an excess of "stress hormones" (i.e., glucagon, epinephrine, and cortisol). This imbalance results in impaired cellular uptake of glucose, along with increased gluconeogenesis, lipolysis, and ketogenesis. Patients present with hyperglycemia, hyperosmolarity, significant dehydration from a glucose-induced osmotic diuresis, and acidosis from ketone production. DKA can be seen in both type 1 and type 2 diabetes, and initial management is the same for both disorders.

B. Causes. Infection, surgery, myocardial infarction (MI), or noncompliance with insulin therapy may all lead to DKA in patients with diabetes.

II. CLINICAL MANIFESTATIONS OF DKA

A. Signs and symptoms. DKA may present with any of the following signs and symptoms:

1. **Hypotension** and **tachycardia** often reflect volume depletion, but sepsis should always be considered, especially if fever is present.
2. **Tachypnea** is common and often reflects the hyperventilation needed to compensate for the metabolic acidosis.
3. **Mild hypothermia** is usually present. Even a mild temperature elevation is a strong indicator of an underlying infection.
4. **Neurologic abnormalities,** including **seizures** and **altered mental status,** may be present. (Stroke may also precipitate DKA.)
5. **Abdominal pain** associated with **nausea** or **vomiting** may occur as a result of the ketoacidosis itself or as a result of intra-abdominal pathology (e.g., cholecystitis).
6. **Polyuria** and **polydipsia** often precede other symptoms by 1–2 days and reflect the osmotic diuresis generated by glycosuria. The **differential diagnosis for polyuria** can be remembered as the **"6 Ds":**

MNEMONIC **Differential Diagnosis for Polyuria ("6 Ds")**

Diabetes mellitus
Diabetes insipidus
Diuretics
Diuretic phase of acute tubular necrosis (ATN)
Drinking too much
Darn! Too much calcium

B. Laboratory findings

1. **Blood glucose levels greater than 300 mg/dl** are usually found in conjunction with **4+ glycosuria.**
2. **Ketonemia** and **ketonuria** are present.
3. **Anion gap acidosis** with a pH less than 7.3 is typical.
4. **Hyponatremia** usually results from the hyperglycemia, which exerts an osmotic pull of water into the intravascular space, thereby decreasing sodium concentration. Vomiting with fluid losses accompanied by free water replacement may also contribute to hyponatremia. Significant hyperlipidemia may accompany DKA, resulting in pseudohyponatremia (see Chapter 43).
5. **Profound potassium, magnesium,** and **phosphate depletion** are typically present. The acidosis of DKA results in a compensatory movement of hydrogen ions intracellularly pushing potassium ions into the extracellular (i.e., intravascular) space; this may normalize or even elevate the serum potassium despite significant total body depletion.
6. An **elevated blood urea nitrogen (BUN)** and **creatinine level** usually result from **prerenal azotemia.**
7. An **elevated white blood cell (WBC) count** with a **left shift** can occur even without infection.
8. An **increased amylase level** is common but reflects both salivary and pancreatic sources; therefore, it is not a good marker for pancreatitis.

III. APPROACH TO THE PATIENT

A. Diagnose DKA. The diagnosis of DKA is made by the association of **acidosis, hyperglycemia,** and **serum ketonemia.**

B. Identify treatable underlying causes.

1. The possibility of an underlying infection should be investigated, even if the patient does not have a fever. A chest radiograph, urinalysis, and urine and blood cultures are usually obtained; other evaluation depends on the clinical presentation.
2. Whether to image the abdomen in patients with DKA and abdominal pain is an extremely difficult decision that

Because immediate serum ketone determinations are not always available, understanding the implications of urine ketone and serum electrolyte determinations is extremely useful:

- **Urine ketones.** Ketones are concentrated in the urine, so the **absence of ketonuria usually rules out DKA.** Urine ketones are, however, nonspecific; therefore, a diagnosis of DKA requires other clinical criteria (i.e., acidosis, hyperglycemia).
- **Serum electrolytes.** The **absence of an anion gap acidosis usually rules out DKA**.

must be based on associated findings (e.g., fever, significant leukocytosis, liver test abnormalities) and clinical judgment.

3. Patients with diabetes are at increased risk for myocardial infarction (with or without chest pain). This may be the cause, or the result, of DKA, and should always be considered early in the evaluation of a patient with DKA.

IV. TREATMENT

A. Fluid replacement. Aggressive intravenous fluid replacement is the first line of action to help correct both volume depletion (5–6 L on average) and hyperglycemia.

1. **How much?** The most common mistake is not giving enough fluids. At least 1 L should be given in the first hour, often followed by 0.5–1 L/hr intravenously. Patients with cardiac dysfunction should have frequent lung examinations and oxygen saturation measurements to assess the possibility of pulmonary edema.
2. **What kind?** A useful way of deciding between normal saline and half-normal saline is to determine the **corrected sodium concentration,** which corrects for the dilution caused by hyperglycemia. For every extra 100 mg/dl of glucose over normal (e.g., 100 mg/dl), the serum sodium concentration needs to be increased by approximately 1.6–2.0 mg/dl:

$$\text{Corrected sodium} = \frac{(\text{Serum glucose} - 100)}{100} \times 1.6 + \text{Serum sodium}$$

   a. **Normal saline** is often used if the corrected sodium is less than or equal to 142 mg/dl or if hypotension is present.
   b. **Half-normal saline** may be a better choice for patients with a corrected serum sodium that is greater than 142 mg/dl. In these patients, normal saline (with a sodium concen-

tration of 150 mg/dl) would keep the sodium high and contribute to persistent hyperosmolarity, which is correlated with poor outcome.

B. Insulin. Because patients with DKA are significantly volume depleted, insulin is best given following or during fluid replacement. Giving insulin first may precipitate significant hypotension by moving glucose and water from the already depleted intravascular space to the intracellular space.

1. **Insulin bolus.** Regular insulin in a dose of 0.1–0.3 units/kg should be administered intravenously. An initial dose of 10 units avoids overdosage and is usually adequate until an insulin drip can be started.
2. **Insulin drip**
   a. **Initiation.** A starting dose of 0.1 unit/kg/hr is effective and can be titrated to keep the glucose level at 200–300 mg/dl.
   b. **Continuation.** The insulin drip needs to be continued until the anion gap is back to normal, even if the glucose level has fallen to near-normal levels. Once the glucose level is below 250 mg/dl, change the fluids to 5% dextrose in normal saline solution or 5% dextrose in half-normal saline solution and continue the insulin drip (adjusting the drip rate to keep the glucose level at 200–300 mg/dl).
   c. **Termination.** The half-life of intravenous insulin is only 8 minutes, so subcutaneous insulin should be administered well before the insulin drip is stopped.

Changing to subcutaneous insulin prematurely will result in a rebound of ketoacidosis.

3. **Subcutaneous insulin.** Both long-acting (e.g., NPH, glargine, detemir) and short-acting insulins should be used during the transition from intravenous to subcutaneous insulin therapy. A rapidly acting insulin analog, such as lispro, aspart, or glulisine, is generally preferred over regular insulin. The patient's glucose level is checked every 4 hours initially. Once the patient is clinically stable and is eating meals, monitoring should be done before meals, before bed, and at 3:00 a.m. Short-acting subcutaneous insulin may initially be administered on a sliding scale; approximate doses are given in Table 79-1. However, optimal glucose control requires a combination of basal long-acting insulin combined with meal-specific dosing of rapidly acting insulin.

TABLE 79-1

SUBCUTANEOUS INSULIN DOSES IN THE TREATMENT OF DIABETIC KETOACIDOSIS

Glucose Level (mg/dl)*	Dose (Regular Insulin)
<150	0 units
>150 but <250	3 units
>250 but <350	5 units
>350 but <450	7 units
>450	9 units; call house officer

*If the glucose level is less than 70 mg/dl, the patient may be given 1 cup of orange juice. If the glucose level is less than 70 mg/dl and the patient cannot take fluids orally, administer 0.5 ampule of 50% dextrose and call the house officer.

C. Electrolyte replacement

1. **Potassium repletion** is essential to prevent hypokalemia and potentially life-threatening arrhythmias. The potassium level universally falls during the treatment of DKA as a result of fluid replacement and correction of acidosis. Patients with renal insufficiency, hypotension, or significant volume depletion require careful potassium repletion to avoid causing hyperkalemia. Hypotensive or significantly volume-depleted patients should not have a standing potassium dose given in their intravenous fluids, because they may inadvertently receive an excessive amount of potassium with large volume replacement.
   a. A potassium level **below 4.5 mEq/L** is usually **the trigger for initiating replacement therapy.** A potassium level **below 4 mEq/L** should alert you to aggressively replete potassium, because the level is likely to continue falling with therapy.
   b. A potassium level of **4–5 mEq/L** is the **goal.** Often 20–40 mEq of potassium is given in each liter of intravenous fluid, depending on the rate of intravenous fluid administration. Extra potassium can be given to keep the potassium level in the desired range.
2. **Magnesium replacement** is frequently necessary and will also help correct hypokalemia associated with hypomagnesemia. If the magnesium level is **less than 1.6 mEq/L,** intravenous magnesium sulfate may be given and repeated as needed. Magnesium repletion also needs to be titrated carefully in the presence of renal failure.

Generally, each 10 mEq of potassium given will raise the potassium level approximately 0.1 mEq/L (assuming normal renal function and no major change in volume or acid-base status).

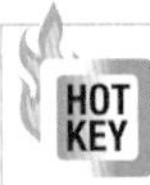

Always confirm that the patient has adequate urine output before administering potassium.

3. **Phosphate replacement** is often not required, but a level **less than 1 mg/dl** may be an indication for replacement with potassium phosphate (usually 9–15 mmol given at a maximal rate of 3 mmol/hr, repeated as needed). If the patient is able to take fluids orally, milk is very high in phosphate and an effective treatment of hypophosphatemia.

D. pH regulation. Patients with a symptomatic acidosis (e.g., cardiac pump dysfunction) or severe asymptomatic acidosis (pH <7.0) are sometimes given sodium bicarbonate to keep the pH greater than 7.0. In general, routine therapy with sodium bicarbonate is not indicated as it increases hypokalemia, shifts the hemoglobin–oxygen dissociation curve to the left (increasing tissue hypoxia), increases intracellular acidosis, and is not associated with any survival advantage.

E. Frequent monitoring is the key to treating patients with DKA.

1. An arterial line is often useful because frequent arterial blood gas and electrolyte measurements are needed.
   a. **pH.** If the pH is less than 7.2, it should be followed closely until a steady upward trend is noted. Once it reaches 7.2, less frequent evaluation can be instituted.
   b. **Electrolytes** (including glucose) are usually checked each hour initially and may be followed by checks every 2–4 hours after improvement is noted.
2. Following the electrolytes and the anion gap is more useful than following the serum ketones, because serum ketone measurements may not include β-hydroxybutyrate.
   a. In patients with DKA and concomitant tissue hypoxia or circulatory collapse (e.g., sepsis), β-hydroxybutyrate is produced preferentially, so serum ketones may appear falsely low when the patient is very sick.
   b. With therapy, β-hydroxybutyrate (which is not measured) may be converted to acetoacetate (which is measured). Thus, serum ketone measurements may appear to increase despite clinical and biochemical improvement.

REFERENCES

Kitabchi AE, Umpierrez GE, Fisher JN et al. Thirty years of personal experience in hyperglycemic crises: diabetic ketoacidosis and hyperglycemic hyperosmolar state. J Clin Endocrinol Metab 2008;93(5):1541–1552.

Trence DL, Hirsch IB. Hyperglycemic crises in diabetes mellitus type 2. Endocrinol Metab Clin North Am 2001;30(4):817–831 [Classic article].

Thyroid Disease

I. APPROACH TO THE PATIENT. Because thyroid hormone affects virtually all systems, abnormal thyroid function has **protean manifestations.** The simplest approach is to:

A. Decide whether the patient is hypothyroid or thyrotoxic based on both **clinical manifestations** and the results of **thyroid function tests.**

B. List the possible causes of the abnormal thyroid function and begin the process of elimination, using the clinical scenario and laboratory data. Determining the etiology of thyrotoxicosis may also require a radioactive iodine uptake study.

II. HYPOTHYROIDISM

A. Causes

1. **Primary hypothyroidism** results from a thyroid abnormality. Common causes include:
   a. **Hashimoto's disease** (the most common cause and a chronic process)
   b. **Thyroiditis** (subacute, postpartum)
   c. **Drugs** (thionamides, lithium, amiodarone, or iodide. Note: amiodarone and iodide may cause either hypothyroidism or thyrotoxicosis.)
   d. **Surgical resection** or **radiation** of the thyroid gland
2. **Secondary hypothyroidism** results from pituitary disorders.
3. **Tertiary hypothyroidism** has a hypothalamic basis.

B. Clinical manifestations of hypothyroidism

1. **Symptoms**
   a. Weakness, fatigue, and lethargy
   b. Arthralgias or myalgias
   c. Cold intolerance

Remember:
Hyp**o**thyroidism produces c**o**ld intolerance.

   d. Skin dryness or edema
   e. Slow speech or hoarseness
   f. Menstrual irregularities, galactorrhea, or both

g. Weight gain (usually no more than 10 pounds)
h. Constipation
i. Decreased sense of taste, smell, and hearing
j. Peripheral neuropathy and carpal tunnel syndrome

2. **Signs**
   a. Thin, brittle nails or thin, coarse hair
   b. Delayed return phase of deep tendon reflexes
   c. Puffiness of the face and eyelids or thickened tongue
   d. Pitting edema
   e. Effusions (anywhere)
   f. Hypothermia, bradycardia, or hypotension in severe cases. (However, diastolic blood pressure may be mildly elevated with moderate hypothyroidism.)
   g. Goiter is variably present

Goiter refers only to thyroid enlargement, not to the etiology. It may be present in either hypothyroidism or thyrotoxicosis.

3. **Laboratory studies**
   a. Elevated levels of thyroid-stimulating hormone (TSH) and decreased levels of free thyroxine (T_4) are diagnostic of primary hypothyroidism. Both tests are low in secondary and tertiary hypothyroidism.
   b. Serum levels of cholesterol, creatine kinase, prolactin, and liver enzymes may be increased.
   c. Anemia, usually normocytic or macrocytic
   d. Hypoglycemia and hyponatremia
   e. Positive antithyroid antibodies (i.e., anti-TPO or anti-microsomal antibodies and antithyroglobulin antibodies) in patients with Hashimoto's disease. However, antithyroid antibodies may also be present in a variety of other thyroid disorders.
   f. Sinus bradycardia, low-voltage QRS complexes, and nonspecific T-wave abnormalities

C. Treatment

1. **Primary hypothyroidism.** Replacement therapy with **L-thyroxine** is the treatment of choice in almost all cases of primary hypothyroidism. Consider the (unusual) possibility of concomitant adrenal insufficiency before initiating thyroid hormone replacement.
   a. If the free T_4 is normal and the patient has only mild symptoms, start therapy at just below the expected final replacement dose (1.5 μg/kg of lean body mass per day of L-thyroxine).

b. If the free T_4 is low or the patient is significantly symptomatic, start with a low dose of thyroxine and increase by 25–50 μg every 2–4 weeks until a maintenance dose level is achieved.

c. **TSH levels should be monitored** every 5–6 weeks until the patient is biochemically euthyroid. Thereafter, monitoring can take place on an as-needed basis.

2. **Secondary** or **tertiary hypothyroidism.** L-Thyroxine should be administered only after adrenal insufficiency has been excluded or treated.

D. Myxedema coma is a **life-threatening manifestation of hypothyroidism;** usually patients are stuporous, hypothermic, bradycardic, hypotensive, hypoxemic, and hypercapnic.

1. **Approach to the patient.** Since the hypothyroidism is almost always longstanding, make sure to search for, and treat, the precipitating cause of the acute decompensation (e.g., infection, ischemia, stroke, acute abdomen, pulmonary embolus).
2. **Treatment.** Patients often require ventilatory support and should be admitted to the intensive care unit (ICU). Intravenous L-thyroxine may be administered after adrenal insufficiency has been excluded or treated.

III. THYROTOXICOSIS

A. There are many causes of **"thyrotoxicosis"** (a term that simply implies **symptoms and signs attributed to increased levels of thyroid hormones**). The causes can be subdivided into those that are attributable to thyroid hyperfunction (hyperthyroidism) and those that are not. A **radioactive iodine uptake** will reveal the functional status of the gland, expressed as the percentage of radioactive iodine captured by the thyroid.

1. **Hyperfunctioning thyroid (hyperthyroidism).** The scan will reveal **high radioactive iodine uptake.**

   a. **TSH-secreting tumor.** This pituitary tumor is rare and should be considered in thyrotoxic patients with normal (or moderately elevated) TSH levels.

   b. **Autonomous toxic adenoma(s).** Hyperthyroidism may be caused by a single adenoma or by a toxic multinodular goiter. There are no associated Graves'-specific findings, such as infiltrative ophthalmopathy, antithyroid antibodies, or thyroid-stimulating immunoglobulins (TSIs).

   c. **Graves' disease,** an autoimmune disorder that causes diffuse thyroid enlargement, is the most common cause of hyperthyroidism. Women 20–40 years of age are most commonly affected. Graves' disease may be associated with an infiltrative ophthalmopathy, dermopathy, or systemic autoimmune disorders and is usually associated with elevated TSI (and other antithyroid antibody) levels.

MNEMONIC **Causes of Thyrotoxicosis—Hyperfunctioning Gland ("TAG")**

TSH-secreting tumor
Autonomous toxic adenoma (younger patients) or multinodular goiter (older patients)
Graves' disease

All causes of thyrotoxicosis may be associated with "stare" (i.e., being able to see sclera above the iris on direct gaze). Only Graves' disease causes infiltrative ophthalmopathy with periorbital swelling, erythema, true proptosis, and the sensation of grittiness in the eyes. More severe Graves' ophthalmopathy may lead to diplopia and decreased visual acuity. The latter is a medical emergency.

2. **Damaged or nonfunctioning thyroid.** The thyroid uptake will reveal **low radioactive iodine uptake** (think of a "fist" obscuring the view—see below).
   a. **Factitious thyrotoxicosis** results from the ingestion of large amounts of exogenous thyroid hormone.
   b. **Iodine-induced thyrotoxicosis (Jod-Basedow disease)** occurs when a patient with a multinodular goiter receives a large iodine load (e.g., following radiographic contrast studies or amiodarone therapy).
   c. **Struma ovarii** An exceedingly small percentage of ovarian dermoid tumors and teratomas contain thyroid tissue, which may autonomously secrete thyroid hormone.
   d. **Thyroiditis** is an autoimmune disease resulting in thyroid destruction. In the early phase, thyrotoxicosis may result from leakage of thyroid hormone. Hypothyroidism typically follows and may be transient or permanent.

MNEMONIC **Causes of Thyrotoxicosis—Decreased or Absent Thyroid Function ("FIST")**

Factitious thyrotoxicosis
Iodine-induced thyrotoxicosis
Struma ovarii
Thyroiditis

B. Clinical manifestations of thyrotoxicosis

1. **Symptoms**
   a. Nervousness, emotional lability, and restlessness
   b. Heat intolerance and increased sweating
   c. Fatigue, weakness, and muscle cramps
   d. Palpitations and angina
   e. Weight loss (despite hyperphagia) and hyperdefecation (not diarrhea)
2. **Signs**
   a. Agitation and anxiety
   b. Warm, moist palms
   c. Stare and lid lag
   d. Fine tremor and hyperreflexia
   e. Irregularly irregular pulse (a sign of atrial fibrillation), widened pulse pressure, and, occasionally, evidence of high-output heart failure
3. **Laboratory studies**
   a. Serum free T_4 and free triiodothyrinone (T_3) are usually increased, and serum TSH is decreased (except with a TSH-secreting tumor).
   b. Hypercalcemia, anemia, and increased alkaline phosphatase levels may be seen in thyrotoxicosis.

C. Treatment. There are many ways to treat thyrotoxic patients—with the choice depending on the cause and clinical setting.

1. Symptomatic relief is provided by **β-blockers** (e.g., propranolol). β-blockers do not decrease thyroid hormone secretion but reduce adrenergic stimulation.
2. **Reduction of thyroid hormone secretion (in true hyperthryoidism)** can be accomplished using **thionamide drugs** (methimazole, propylthiouracil), **radioactive iodine, iodinated agents,** or **thyroid surgery.**
3. **Thyroiditis.** Patients with thyrotoxicosis secondary to thyroiditis are best treated symptomatically (typically with β-blockers) until the condition resolves spontaneously. These patients will then usually require treatment for **hypo**thyroidism, either transiently (if thyroid function returns) or permanently.

D. Thyroid storm is a **life-threatening exacerbation of thyrotoxicosis.**

1. **Approach to the patient.** Always look for a precipitating cause of clinical decompensation as well as the etiology of thyrotoxicosis (e.g., myocardial infarction, infection, surgery).
2. Clinical manifestations include the usual features of thyrotoxicosis and the precipitating event, plus **fever** and **psychosis** (hallmarks of **thyroid storm**), nausea, vomiting, and seizures.
3. **Treatment** goals include suppression of the effects of thyroid hormone and rapid reduction of circulating thyroid hormone levels.

a. These goals are usually accomplished by β-blockade, thionamide therapy, corticosteroids, and iodide (**following** thionamide administration). Aspirin should be avoided, as it displaces thyroid hormone from its binding protein.
b. Definitive treatment occurs once the patient is rendered euthyroid.

REFERENCES

Brent GA. Graves' disease. N Engl J Med 2008;358(24):2594–2605.
Dayan CM. Interpretation of thyroid function tests. Lancet 2001;357(9256): 619–624 [Classic article].
Pearce EN. Diagnosis and management of thyrotoxicosis. BMJ 2006; 332(7554):1369–1373.

81

Adrenal Insufficiency

I. INTRODUCTION

A. Definitions. Adrenal insufficiency is defined as the inadequate production of glucocorticoids, mineralocorticoids, or both. However, glucocorticoid deficiency has the greater clinical manifestations and is therefore the focus of this chapter

1. **Glucocorticoid insufficiency** occurs when **glucocorticoid production** by the adrenal gland **is deficient.** This may be due to adrenal gland dysfunction (primary adrenal insufficiency) or inadequate secretion of adrenocorticotropic hormone (ACTH) (secondary adrenal insufficiency).
2. **Hypoaldosteronism** occurs when **mineralocorticoid production is impaired.** It can occur with adrenal insufficiency (as in Addison's disease) or as an isolated finding; when hypoaldosteronism occurs as an isolated finding, it is usually the result of defective renin secretion.

II. CAUSES OF ADRENAL INSUFFICIENCY

A. Primary adrenal insufficiency (Addison's disease) results from destruction of the adrenal glands and is therefore accompanied by hypoaldosteronism. One way to remember the common causes of primary adrenal insufficiency is to use the mnemonic "ADDISON'S":

MNEMONIC **Causes of Addison's Disease ("ADDISON'S")**

Amyloidosis
Destruction (autoimmune or hemorrhage following trauma)
Drugs (anticoagulants leading to bilateral adrenal hemorrhage)
Infections [bacterial sepsis (especially meningococcus), tuberculosis, disseminated fungal infections, cytomegalovirus (CMV) in acquired immunodeficiency syndrome (AIDS) patients, syphilitic gummas]
Sarcoidosis
Overload of iron (hemochromatosis)

Neoplasm (bilateral metastatic disease, usually from the lung)
Surgical (hemorrhage during open-heart surgery or following bilateral adrenalectomy)

B. **Secondary adrenal insufficiency** is caused by pituitary dysfunction. There are many causes of secondary adrenal insufficiency, but the most important are summarized in Table 81-1. All these causes affect the pituitary gland and lead to **hypopituitarism;** the most common disorders are ACTH suppression due to **chronic exogenous corticosteroids** and **ACTH deficiency due to pituitary tumors.**

C. **Tertiary adrenocortical insufficiency** occurs with **hypothalamic disorders, pituitary stalk destruction,** and certain **central nervous system (CNS) diseases.**

III. CLINICAL MANIFESTATIONS OF ADRENAL INSUFFICIENCY

A. **Primary adrenal insufficiency.** The clinical manifestations vary depending on the time course of adrenal destruction.

1. **Chronic insufficiency.** Most patients (75%) present with chronic insufficiency due to gradual destruction of the adrenal gland. More than 90% of the gland must be destroyed before symptoms occur; therefore, symptoms occur over many months and, in some cases, years. Table 81-2 can be used to determine "WWHHOOO" may have chronic insufficiency.

TABLE 81-1

CAUSES OF SECONDARY ADRENAL INSUFFICIENCY

Category	Specific Cause
Congenital	Familial hypopituitarism
Hematologic	Pituitary apoplexy (hemorrhage)
Pregnancy related	Sheehan's syndrome
Drugs	Withdrawal of chronic exogenous corticosteroids
Metabolic/endocrine	Chronic renal failure, diabetes mellitus, hemochromatosis
Infectious	Tuberculosis, syphilis, fungal disease
Iatrogenic	Irradiation of the pituitary gland
Idiopathic	Empty sella syndrome, sarcoidosis
Neoplasm	Pituitary tumors
Surgical	Pituitary surgery

TABLE 81-2

CLINICAL MANIFESTATIONS OF CHRONIC ADRENAL INSUFFICIENCY ("WWHHOOO")

Clinical Manifestation	Incidence
Weakness	Common
Weight loss	Common
Hyperpigmentation	Common
Hypotension	Variable
Obstipation and other gastrointestinal symptoms (nausea, vomiting, diarrhea, pain)	Variable
Orthostasis	Variable
Other (hyponatremia, hyperkalemia, nonanion gap metabolic acidosis, fever, hypoglycemia, eosinophilia)	Variable

Hyperpigmentation may precede other manifestations. It tends to be generalized but is accentuated in sun-exposed areas; on pressure points (e.g., knees and knuckles); and on the nail beds, nipples, and palmar creases. In dark-skinned patients, the only signs of hyperpigmentation may be on the tongue and in the perilimbal region of the eyes.

2. **Acute insufficiency (adrenal crisis).** Only 25% of patients with adrenal insufficiency will present acutely, but when it occurs, it can be **life-threatening.** Adrenal crisis is usually seen in a patient with adrenal insufficiency (known or not) who experiences a significant stress (e.g., infection, cardiac ischemia, surgery). It may also be seen in a previously healthy patient if acute adrenal destruction occurs (e.g., adrenal hemorrhage due to sepsis or anticoagulation therapy).
   a. **Signs and symptoms**
      (1) **Profound anorexia, nausea,** and **vomiting** may be seen.
      (2) **Abdominal pain** may be mistaken for a "surgical abdomen."
      (3) **Hypotension** may be severe and is typically unresponsive to saline hydration.
      (4) **Fever** may occur, even in the absence of an initiating infection.
      (5) **Hypoglycemia.** Remember, *gluco*corticoids stimulate *gluco*neogenesis.
      (6) **Hyperpigmentation** may occur but is not as common as in chronic insufficiency.

b. **Laboratory findings** are similar to the findings in chronic insufficiency (see Table 81-2).

B. Secondary adrenal insufficiency. The development of signs and symptoms can be chronic or acute. The clinical manifestations are the same as in primary adrenal insufficiency, with the following exceptions:

1. Patients may have **other evidence of pituitary dysfunction** (e.g., hypothyroidism, hyperprolactinemia, diabetes insipidus, gonadotropin deficiency).
2. **Hyperkalemia** and a **nonanion gap metabolic acidosis** are usually **not present** (because aldosterone is sill secreted **appropriately**).
3. **Hyperpigmentation** usually **does not occur.**

IV. APPROACH TO THE PATIENT

A. The most difficult aspect of diagnosing adrenal insufficiency is **considering the diagnosis.** The pattern of clinical manifestations and lab findings should alert you to the possibility of adrenal insufficiency. When a patient presents with hypotension, weakness, abdominal pain, unexplained fever, hypoglycemia, or nonspecific findings, consider Addison's disease.

B. Confirmation of the diagnosis is straightforward.

1. **Plasma cortisol assay.** If the plasma cortisol level is greater than 18 μg/dl, adrenal insufficiency is very unlikely.
2. **Cosyntropin (ACTH) stimulation test.** If the plasma cortisol level is less than 18 μg/dl, perform a 1-hour cosyntropin stimulation test. A normal response rules out primary (but not secondary) adrenal insufficiency.
3. **Plasma ACTH level.** ACTH levels are elevated in primary adrenal insufficiency. A low ACTH level in the setting of cortisol deficiency usually confirms the diagnosis of secondary adrenal insufficiency.

V. TREATMENT

A. Acute insufficiency (adrenal crisis). If there is strong clinical suspicion for adrenal crisis, appropriate treatment should not be delayed until diagnostic testing is completed.

Dexamethasone does not interfere with the plasma cortisol assay and can be used initially.

1. **Intravenous glucocorticoids.** High doses of glucocorticoids (e.g., hydrocortisone, 100 mg every 8 hours) are administered

initially; mineralocorticoids may also be used but are not routinely given until the cortisol dose has been tapered to lower levels. (High doses of hydrocortisone have sufficient mineralocorticoid activity.)

2. **Supportive treatment** (e.g., intravenous fluids, oxygen) should also be instituted in a monitored setting.
3. **Precipitating causes should be treated.**

B. Chronic insufficiency

1. **Primary adrenal insufficiency.** Both glucocorticoids and mineralocorticoids are administered.
   a. Doses vary, but a rough estimate for a maintenance dose is 20–25 mg of cortisol daily and 0.1–0.2 mg of fludrocortisone daily.
   b. Patients should be counseled that treatment is **lifelong** and that doses should be increased during times of stress. Patients should also carry a wallet card or wear a bracelet with their diagnosis.
2. **Secondary** or **tertiary insufficiency.** Usually, only glucocorticoid therapy is needed.

REFERENCES

Annare D, Maxime V, Ibrahim F, et al. Diagnosis of adrenal insufficiency in severe sepsis and septic shock. Am J Respir Crit Care Med 2006;174(12):1319–1326.

Bouillon R. Acute adrenal insufficiency. Endocrinol Metab Clin N Am 2006;35(4):767–775.

Lamberts SW, de Herder WW, van der Lely AJ. Pituitary insufficiency. Lancet 1998;352(9122):127–134 [Classic article].

PART X
NEUROLOGY

Altered Mental Status

I. **INTRODUCTION.** Altered mental status has myriad causes, ranging from acute focal brain lesions (e.g., stroke) to metabolic derangements (e.g., alcohol withdrawal) to chronic neurodegenerative diseases (e.g., Alzheimer's dementia). A key to diagnosis is to distinguish between a focal deficit, delirium, and dementia.

A. **A focal lesion** that results in aphasia can mimic delirium. Some brain lesions can cause both a focal deficit and delirium through mass effect (e.g., a subdural hematoma causing hemiparesis and somnolence).

B. **Delirium** is an alteration in mental status that is characterized by **acute onset, fluctuating course, impaired attention,** and either a disturbance in the **level of consciousness** or **disorganized thinking**.

1. The history of **acute onset** and **fluctuating course** is usually obtained from family members or care providers.
2. Patients with **impaired attention** have difficulty keeping track of a conversation and are easily distractible.
3. A disturbance in the **level of consciousness** may span the spectrum from vigilant and hyperalert through drowsy, difficult to arouse, and finally coma.
4. **Disorganized thinking** is manifested by rambling or irrelevant speech, or an illogical flow of ideas. Other cognitive deficits in delirium may involve orientation, memory, judgment, abstract thinking, recognition, language skills, or personality.

C. **Dementia.** If the change in mental status presents as **a slow deterioration in cognition and appears chronic,** it is classified as dementia rather than delirium.

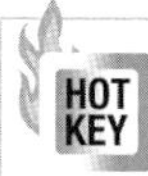

Patients with dementia are at especially high risk for developing delirium.

II. **CAUSES OF ALTERED MENTAL STATUS.** The mnemonic "MIST-P" is a useful way to help remember a long list of differential diagnoses and roughly divides the causes into three broad classes:

A. **M**etabolic disorders;

B. **I**nfectious, **I**nflammatory, and **I**nherited disorders (which is a very broad category);

C. **S**eizures and **S**tructural problems (stroke/vascular disorders, **T**umor, **T**rauma); and

D. **P**sychiatric disorders.

Although a single cause of altered mental status is sought, a combination of factors is often responsible (e.g., a urinary tract infection in an elderly person who has Alzheimer's disease and is receiving multiple medications).

III. APPROACH TO THE PATIENT. Given the overlap in the differential diagnoses for delirium, coma, and dementia as well as the potential consequences of an incorrect or delayed diagnosis, all patients with altered mental status should be evaluated in a thorough and systematic manner.

MNEMONIC

Causes of Altered Mental Status (MIST-P)

Metabolic

- **M**edicines: medications that either are directly psychoactive (e.g., benzodiazepines) or have significant cognitive side effects (e.g., anticholinergics)
- **E**lectrolyte derangements (e.g., disorders of sodium, magnesium, or calcium) or **E**ndocrine disorders (increased or decreased levels of glucose, cortisol, thyroid hormone)
- **T**emperature derangements (i.e., hypothermia or hyperthermia)
- **A**lcohol and other drugs, either in toxicity or causing a withdrawal syndrome
- $\mathbf{B}_{12}$ and other vitamin deficiencies, [e.g., niacin deficiency (pellagra) or thiamine deficiency (Wernicke-Korsakoff syndrome)]
- **O**xygen deficiency or hypercarbia [oxygen deficiency may result from insufficient oxygen in the blood (i.e., hypoxemia), an inadequate number of red blood cells (RBCs) to carry the oxygen (i.e., anemia), or insufficient forward flow (i.e., decreased cardiac output)]
- **L**iver or kidney disease causing encephalopathy

Infectious disorders either affecting the central nervous system (CNS) directly (e.g., encephalitis, brain abscess) or due to a systemic infection (e.g., urosepsis)

Inflammatory (e.g., collagen vascular diseases, sarcoidosis)
Inherited or degenerative diseases (e.g., Huntington's disease, Alzheimer's disease)
Seizures (actively seizing or due to a postictal state)
Strokes and other vascular disorders
- Ischemic infarcts (from emboli, thromboses, or vasculitis)
- Bleeds (epidural, subdural, subarachnoid, or intracerebral)
- Hypertensive encephalopathy
- Thrombotic thrombocytopenic purpura (TTP) or disseminated intravascular coagulation (DIC)
- Hyperviscosity syndrome (seen with plasma cell dyscrasias or significantly elevated RBC counts)

Tumors: malignant processes may lead to altered mental status either because of an intracranial lesion or because of a paraneoplastic process
Trauma (e.g., concussion)
Psychiatric disorders
Porphyria

A. Perform the ABCs.
1. **Airway.** Consider intubation, especially if the Glasgow Coma Scale score is less than 8.
2. **Breathing.** Consider intubation.
3. **Circulation.** Check vital signs.

B. Assess the need for intravenous access and fluids, oxygen, and electrocardiographic monitoring.

C. Rule out easily reversible conditions.
1. **Thiamine** (100 mg intravenously) is usually given.
2. **Fifty percent dextrose (D50)** is usually given empirically when a fingerstick test for glucose is not readily available. Always give thiamine before dextrose to avoid precipitating Wernicke-Korsakoff syndrome.
3. **Naloxone hydrochloride** should be administered if an opiate overdose is suspected.

Remember to always carefully consider all the medications a patient has been receiving as a potential cause of altered mental status.

D. Rule out common, immediately life-threatening conditions. Check the pupils, corneal reflexes, oculocephalic reflex, gag, motor response, meningeal signs, and vital signs, looking for evidence of any of the following disorders:

1. **Mass effect** (e.g., tumor, infarct, bleed, or abscess). If mass effect is suspected, make arrangements for emergent neuroimaging and an emergent neurosurgical consult. Mannitol, steroids, or intubation with hyperventilation may be indicated.
2. **Meningitis.** Initial measures include blood cultures and early empiric antibacterial therapy followed by a lumbar puncture (see Chapter 88).
3. **Status epilepticus.** Lorazepam, fosphenytoin, and, if necessary, phenobarbital are administered (see Chapter 86).
4. **Hypertensive encephalopathy.** Nitroprusside is often administered.
5. **Hyperthermia.** Cooling measures should be initiated.

E. Continue the work-up if the cause of altered mental status is still not apparent.

1. **Patient history** and **physical examination.** Perform a thorough examination, with particular focus on the neurologic examination and a search for occult infection.
2. **Laboratory studies.** The following studies are often useful:
    a. **Complete blood count (CBC)**
    b. **Electrolyte panel** (including glucose and calcium)
    c. **Blood urea nitrogen (BUN)** and **creatinine levels**
    d. **Liver tests**
    e. **Prothrombin time (PT)** and **partial thromboplastin time (PTT)**
    f. **Arterial blood gases** (possibly including carboxyhemoglobin)
    g. **Toxicology screen**
    h. **Urinalysis**
3. **Other studies.** An electrocardiogram (ECG), chest radiograph, lumbar puncture (with an opening pressure), head computed tomography (CT) or magnetic resonance imaging (MRI) scan, and electroencephalogram (EEG) may be appropriate.
4. **Neurology consult.** Consultation with a neurologist may be necessary if the diagnosis still cannot be made.

F. Treatment of delirium involves a three-tiered approach:

1. Treat the **underlying cause.**
2. **Nonpharmacologic measures.** Frequently reorient patients, use sitters and family members, provide eyeglasses and hearing aids, avoid restraints and Foley catheters, and maintain normal sleep–wake cycles.
3. **Pharmacologic measures.** Use only if delirium is disrupting necessary medical care or compromising patient safety.

Low doses of antipsychotics (e.g., haloperidol) are preferred. Benzodiazepines should be reserved for cases of alcohol withdrawal.

REFERENCES

Blennow K, de Leon MJ, Zetterberg H. Alzheimer's disease. Lancet 2006;368(9533):387–403.

Joshi S, Morley JE. Cognitive impairment. Med Clin North Am 2006;90(5):769–787.

Young J, Inouye SK. Delirium in older people. BMJ 2007;334(7598):842–846.

Peripheral Neuropathy

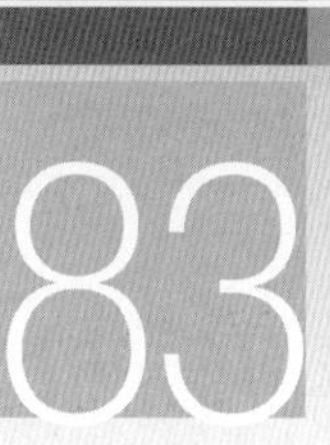

I. INTRODUCTION

A. Clinical syndromes. Peripheral neuropathies can be divided into three clinical syndromes:

1. **Polyneuropathies** present with **symmetric** abnormalities in sensation, strength, or both.
2. **Mononeuritis multiplex** is an **initially asymmetric** abnormality in more than one nerve occurring either simultaneously or over days to years.
3. **Mononeuropathies** imply **focal** involvement of a single nerve (e.g., carpal tunnel syndrome) and usually result from local nerve compression or stretch.

B. Because **polyneuropathy** is the most common peripheral neuropathy and poses the greatest difficulty in differential diagnosis, it is the **focus of this chapter.**

II. CLINICAL MANIFESTATIONS OF POLYNEUROPATHY

A. Sensory abnormalities in the feet are usually the first symptom of polyneuropathy.

1. **Hypesthesia** (decreased sensation), **anesthesia** (absent sensation), **paresthesia** ("pins and needles" sensation without any stimuli), **dysesthesia** (burning sensation with or without stimuli), and **hyperpathia** (exaggerated pain perception) may all be noted. Initially, subjective complaints may be unaccompanied by objective findings.
2. Later, a pansensory loss in the feet may occur and progress centrally. Finger involvement often occurs once the shins are affected; eventually, the classic **"stocking-glove"** pattern may be seen.

B. Motor abnormalities may also occur. The extensors are usually more involved than the flexors (i.e., weakness of dorsiflexion of the toes is a common finding). The ankle reflex is often diminished early in the course of the disease, and a diminished knee reflex and foot drop are seen with progression.

III. CAUSES OF POLYNEUROPATHY.

Polyneuropathies may result from a variety of disorders. The mnemonic "MOVE, STUPID" can be used.

MNEMONIC **Causes of Polyneuropathy ("MOVE, STUPID")**

Metabolic disorders (diabetes mellitus)
Other (including heredofamilial disorders such as Charcot-Marie-Tooth)
Vasculitis or **V**itamin deficiency (vitamin B_{12}, thiamine, pyridoxine, folate)
Endocrine disorders (hypothyroidism)

Syphilis or **S**arcoid
Tumor related (i.e., paraneoplastic syndrome)
Uremia or liver disease (chronic liver disease, hepatitis B and C)
Paraproteinemia/amyloidosis,[1] **P**orphyria, **P**rimary biliary cirrhosis, or **P**olycythemia vera
Infections,[2] **I**nflammatory [e.g., Guillain-Barré syndrome, chronic inflammatory demyelinating polyneuropathy (CIDP)], or **I**diopathic causes
Drugs or toxins (including alcohol, antiretroviral nucleoside analogs)

IV. APPROACH TO THE PATIENT. Many of the disorders that can cause polyneuropathies are potentially life-threatening if not appropriately diagnosed and treated. Because the differential diagnosis is extensive and the etiology may or may not be obvious, the evaluation needs to be tailored to the situation. If the diagnosis is not initially apparent, a four-step process may be used to cover most of the possibilities.

A. Take a thorough patient history.

1. Make sure to ask about **recent events** that may provide a clue to the diagnosis. Specifically, inquire about recent viral illnesses (which may suggest Guillain-Barré syndrome), the presence of similar symptoms in family members or co-workers (which may suggest a toxic exposure or hereditary disease), and systemic symptoms (e.g., weight loss, which may raise suspicion for an occult malignancy).
2. Obtain a **medication history.** Some drugs that may be responsible for polyneuropathy include amiodarone, dapsone, hydralazine, isoniazid, metronidazole, nitrofurantoin,

[1]Amyloidosis may cause peripheral neuropathy without an accompanying paraproteinemia but is listed with paraproteinemia because these disorders are often thought of together.

[2]Peripheral neuropathy can be associated with infection [e.g., Lyme disease, leprosy, or acquired immunodeficiency syndrome (AIDS)]. Patients with AIDS may develop polyradiculopathy with abnormalities on cerebrospinal fluid analysis that may be secondary to cytomegalovirus infection.

phenytoin, vincristine, nucleoside reverse transcriptase inhibitors, and high doses of pyridoxine.

3. Inquire about **toxin exposures.** The most common toxins include heavy metals (e.g., arsenic, lead, mercury, thallium); industrial agents; and pesticides (e.g., organophosphates); diphtheria toxin should also be considered but is quite rare.

Remember, common things are common. If diabetes or uremia is present or if the patient is a long-time alcoholic, you may not need to look any further.

B. Assess the time course. Only a few disorders commonly result in an **acute polyneuropathy** (i.e., one that occurs over a few days). Furthermore, unlike subacute or chronic polyneuropathies, acute disorders usually produce predictable patterns on **electrodiagnostic evaluation** (i.e., **electromyography, nerve conduction studies**).

1. **Acute axonal polyneuropathies** have relatively preserved nerve conduction and are usually caused by **porphyria** or **intoxications** (e.g., arsenic).
2. **Acute demyelinating polyneuropathies** display a significant decrease in nerve conduction and are essentially synonymous with **Guillain-Barré syndrome,** although **diphtheria** and **toxic berry** (buckthorn) **ingestion** may rarely produce the same clinical picture.

C. Perform appropriate laboratory studies if the diagnosis is still not evident. Review the list of possible causes and obtain the laboratory tests that will help shorten the list. Tests that may be requested include:

1. Complete blood count (CBC)
2. Erythrocyte sedimentation rate (ESR)
3. Renal panel with electrolytes
4. Fasting glucose level
5. Vitamin B_{12} level
6. Thyroid function tests
7. Liver tests
8. Fluorescent treponemal antibody absorbed (FTA-ABS) test for syphilis
9. Serum and urine protein electrophoresis and serum immunofixation

D. Consider occult disorders. The simple laboratory tests outlined in IV C may not rule out some of the more occult processes (e.g., tumor, vasculitis, sarcoidosis), but they may provide evidence for or against a possible diagnosis (e.g., a normal ESR makes vasculitis less likely). The following tests may be useful in certain clinical settings:

1. **Antinuclear antibody (ANA), rheumatoid factor (RF),** and **serum cryoglobulin** assessments may be used in the evaluation of suspected vasculitis (see Chapter 76).
2. **Radiography**
   a. **Chest radiographs** may show evidence of sarcoidosis or an occult tumor.
   b. A **computed tomography (CT) scan** may be performed if an intra-abdominal malignancy is suspected.
3. **Urinary heavy metal** and **porphobilinogen levels** can be used to evaluate the possibility of toxic metal exposures and acute intermittent porphyria, respectively.
4. **Lyme titers** are only useful in the appropriate clinical setting because they lack specificity.
5. **Cerebrospinal fluid evaluation**
   a. Findings include high protein levels and a normal cell count in patients with Guillain-Barré syndrome or CIDP.
   b. In AIDS patients with cytomegalovirus polyradiculopathy, findings include neutrophilic pleocytosis, high protein levels, and low glucose levels.
6. **Electrodiagnostic studies** may be performed (if they have not been already) to help categorize whether there is primarily axonal degeneration or demyelination. These studies may be especially helpful in diagnosing CIDP.
7. **Sural nerve biopsy.** The ankle is the easiest place to obtain a cutaneous nerve biopsy.
   a. Nerve biopsy is of low yield in symmetric polyneuropathies but should be considered in patients with suspected **mononeuritis multiplex** because a vasculitis may be more likely. The yield of biopsy is also increased in patients with suspected **vasculitis, amyloidosis, sarcoidosis,** or **leprosy** and in those with palpably thickened nerves.
   b. Because **heredofamilial disorders** often present at an early age and have a characteristic histopathology, a sural nerve biopsy should also be considered in **children.**

V. TREATMENT is generally aimed at the underlying disorder. Some general measures and specific therapies are discussed here.

A. General measures

1. **Relief of neuropathic pain** can be challenging. **Tricyclic antidepressants** (e.g., desipramine, amitriptyline), the serotonin-norepinephrine reuptake inhibitors **duloxetine** or **venlafaxine**, or the **anticonvulsants gabapentin or pregabalin** are often tried. Other anticonvulsants (e.g., carbamazepine) and **topical capsaicin or lidocaine** may also be helpful in some cases.

2. **Ankle–foot orthotics** can help prevent Achilles tendon contractures and relieve foot-drop.

B. Specific therapies

1. **Guillain-Barré syndrome**
   a. Most patients require hospitalization for observation and **supportive care** (e.g., intubation for respiratory failure).
   b. **Plasmapheresis** or **intravenous immunoglobulin (IVIG)** is beneficial (especially within the first 2 weeks of illness). Steroids are not effective.
   c. Approximately 85% of patients will recover completely or have only mild residual defects. The mortality rate is approximately 3%–4%.
2. **CIDP** may be treated with **steroids, immunosuppressants,** and **IVIG** or **plasmapheresis** if ambulation is threatened.
3. **Isoniazid overdose** can be treated with **intravenous pyridoxine** (1 g for each gram of isoniazid ingested).
4. **Acute intermittent porphyria**
   a. **Acute treatment.** Intravenous **glucose** and **hematin** may be needed for acute attacks.
   b. **Chronic treatment** entails **avoiding precipitating factors** (e.g., sulfa drugs) and **adhering to a high-carbohydrate diet.**

REFERENCES

Dworkin RH, O'Connor AB, Backonja M, et al. Pharmacologic management of neuropathic pain: evidence-based recommendations. Pain 2007;132(3):237–251.

England JD, Asbury AK. Peripheral neuropathy. Lancet 2004;363(9427):2151–2161.

Hughes RA. Peripheral neuropathy. BMJ 2002;324(7335):466–469 [Classic article].

Hughes RA, Swan AV, Raphael JC, et al. Immunotherapy for Guillain-Barre syndrome: a systematic review. Brain 2007;130(Pt 9):2245–2257.

■ Vertigo

84

I. INTRODUCTION

A. Definitions

1. **Dizziness** is a term used to describe an unusual head sensation or gait unsteadiness. Faintness and vertigo are forms of dizziness.
2. **Faintness** is usually described as a sense of light-headedness and is usually caused by an insufficient supply of oxygen, blood, or glucose to the brain. Faintness often occurs with hyperventilation, with hypoglycemia, or just before a syncopal event.
3. **Vertigo,** the topic of this chapter, is the illusion of movement (usually spinning). The patient may describe the environment as moving while he or she remains stationary, or vice versa.

B. Clinical manifestations of vertigo

1. **Nausea** and **vomiting** usually accompany vertigo.
2. **Gait unsteadiness** and **ataxia** are common.
3. Vertigo **worsens with head movement.**

C. Etiology. Vertigo most commonly results from a defect in the vestibular system, but defects in the visual system or the somatosensory system can cause vertigo as well.

II. TYPES OF VERTIGO.
Prognostically, it is important to distinguish **central** vertigo from **peripheral** vertigo.

A. Central vertigo often has a **poorer prognosis** than peripheral vertigo.

1. **Clinical manifestations of central vertigo**
   a. Central vertigo is usually accompanied by other **brain stem** or **cerebellar** (occasionally even **cerebral hemispheric**) **signs** (e.g., headache, limb ataxia, true weakness, paresthesias, dysarthria, diplopia, dysphagia). **Nystagmus** may be present and can take any form: horizontal, vertical, or multidirectional.

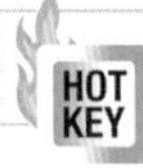

Vertical nystagmus is almost always due to a central cause.

b. Central vertigo is usually not accompanied by tinnitus or hearing loss.

2. **Causes of central vertigo.** The most common causes of central vertigo can be remembered with the mnemonic "MAIM." (Often patients with central vertigo are "maimed" because of their poor prognosis.)

MNEMONIC **Causes of Central Vertigo ("MAIM")**

Multiple sclerosis
Acoustic neuroma or other cerebellopontine angle tumor
Ischemia or central nervous system (CNS) lesions [especially basilar transient ischemic attack (TIA)]
Migraine (especially basilar)

B. Peripheral vertigo

1. **Clinical manifestations of peripheral vertigo** tend to cause more patient distress than those of central vertigo and are more often associated with nausea and vomiting; however, the episodes are briefer because the CNS tends to adapt.
   a. **Tinnitus** and **hearing loss** are common.
   b. **Nystagmus,** which is usually present, occurs unidirectionally, is horizontal, and is worse when looking toward the unaffected ear. The fast component is toward the side of the unaffected ear. Unlike the nystagmus of central vertigo, the nystagmus of peripheral vertigo is inhibited by visual fixation. **Otherwise, the neurologic examination is completely normal.**
2. **Causes of peripheral vertigo.** Peripheral vertigo is usually a result of processes that involve the **labyrinth** (inner ear) or **eighth cranial nerve.** Causes can be remembered by the mnemonic "AMPLITUDE":

MNEMONIC **Common Causes of Peripheral Vertigo ("AMPLITUDE")**

Acoustic neuroma (also causes central vertigo)
Ménière's disease (vertigo, hearing loss, and tinnitus)
Positional [benign paroxysmal positional vertigo (BPPV)]: very brief (e.g., <1 minute) episodes of vertigo, usually brought on by head movement and often following ear trauma or infection
Labyrinthitis and vestibular neuritis lead to acute, severe vertigo, nausea, and vomiting in patients who have had a recent viral syndrome.
Infection of the inner ear

Trauma (head)
ψchogenic causes (considered in patients with a normal neurologic examination and lacking nystagmus during an episode of vertigo)
Drugs (especially aminoglycoside antibiotics, vincristine)
Endocrine disorders (e.g., hypothyroidism, diabetes)

III. APPROACH TO THE PATIENT

A. Patient history. In many patients, the cause of vertigo can be determined from the history alone. Key elements on which to focus include the onset and duration of vertigo (episodic vs. continuous); associated symptoms (nausea, vomiting, neurologic symptoms, headache); recent illness or trauma; medications; and presence of tinnitus or hearing loss.

B. Physical examination. The examination should focus on the ears, eyes, and nervous system.

1. The presence or absence of an **ear infection, nystagmus,** and **neurologic deficits** should be ascertained.
2. The **Nylen-Bárány maneuver** is important in the assessment of BPPV. The seated patient turns his or her head to one side while quickly lying down so that the head hangs over the edge of the table. If the vertigo that is reproduced (along with nystagmus) has a delayed onset of 1–2 seconds, lasts 10–20 seconds, and fatigues with repeated testing, the patient is likely to have BPPV.

C. Special tests should be ordered in the following situations:

1. If hearing loss or tinnitus is a major component, an audiogram is useful to evaluate for Ménière's disease or acoustic neuroma.
2. If thyroid disease or diabetes mellitus is suspected, **blood work** is useful.
   a. **Thyroid-stimulating hormone (TSH) levels** may be useful if thyroid disease is suspected.
   b. **Serum glucose values** may prove useful if diabetes is suspected.
3. If peripheral causes seem unlikely or if the patient has neurologic abnormalities, brain **magnetic resonance imaging (MRI)** and **magnetic resonance angiography (MRA)** are indicated. The decision to forego imaging must be made carefully in a patient with vascular risk factors (e.g., advanced age, hypertension, diabetes, smoking).

IV. TREATMENT

A. Central vertigo. Treatment depends on the cause. For patients suspected of having vertebrobasilar TIAs, see Chapter 87.

B. Peripheral vertigo. For acute peripheral vertigo of almost any cause, the patient should be prescribed antihistamines, anticholinergics, and/or benzodiazepines. The patient should be cautioned regarding falls.

1. Medications may prevent CNS adaptation to peripheral vertigo and, therefore, should not be used for an extended period.
2. A mild vestibular exercise program can expedite the adaptation process.
3. For BPPV, the Epley maneuver can be performed in the office and is curative in 60%–80% of cases. Sometimes the maneuver needs to be repeated at a subsequent visit or by the patient at home. (See Fife et al. 2008 in the References for instructions on how to properly perform the Epley maneuver.)
4. For acute vestibular neuritis, methylprednisolone has been shown to improve extent of recovery at 12 months and is a treatment option.

REFERENCES

Fife TD, Iverson DJ, Lempert T, et al. Practice parameter: therapies for benign paroxysmal positional vertigo (an evidence-based review). Neurology 2008;70:2067–2074.

Strupp M, Zingler VC, Arbusow V, et al. Methylprednisolone, valacyclovir, or the combination for vestibular neuritis. N Engl J Med 2004;351(4): 354–361.

Tusa RJ. Vertigo. Neurol Clin 2001;19(1):23–55 [Classic review article].

Singultus

I. INTRODUCTION. A hiccough is an inspiratory sound caused by the abrupt closure of the glottis in the setting of rhythmic spasm of the diaphragm and respiratory muscles. Hiccoughs can occur at any age and can last for years (but usually only last for a few minutes). There is a strong male predominance.

II. CAUSES OF SINGULTUS. Singultus may be caused by a wide variety of conditions that have one thing in common—they involve the reflex arc shown in Figure 85-1. Causes can be classified as **peripheral** (i.e., involving the vagus or phrenic nerves or structures adjacent to the diaphragm) or central.

MNEMONIC **Common Causes of Singultus ("SINGULTUS")**

Surgery (following abdominal, thoracic, or neck surgery)
Infection of structures adjacent to the diaphragm (e.g., lower lobe pneumonia, subphrenic abscess, peritonitis)
Nervous system disorders (e.g., stroke, meningitis, brain tumor, multiple sclerosis)
Gastric distention (very common cause)
Uremia
Low serum calcium, sodium, or potassium
Tumor of the pancreas
ψchiatric disorders
Steroids and other drugs (e.g., alcohol, benzodiazepines, barbiturates)

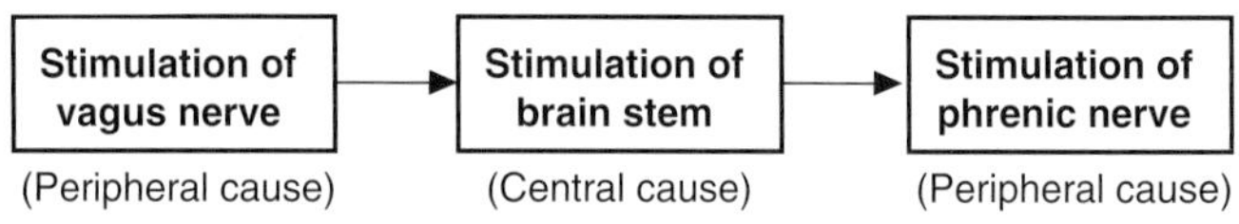

Figure 85-1. The many causes of singultus involve this reflex arc in some way.

III. TREATMENT. Treating the underlying disorder is the best course of action.

A. Several benign strategies to relieve hiccoughs have been anecdotally successful. These include (in no particular order):

1. Having the patient swallow a tablespoon of granulated sugar
2. Massaging the soft palate or applying traction to the tongue
3. Placing a nasogastric tube or a nasopharyngeal catheter
4. The age-old scare tactic

B. Pharmacologic therapy (e.g., with chlorpromazine, metoclopramide, or baclofen) may be instituted if the benign strategies fail.

REFERENCES

Goldstein R. Practice tips. Simple method for curing hiccups. Can Fam Physician 1999;45:1459.

Smith HS, Busracamwongs A. Management of hiccups in the palliative care population. Am J Hosp Palliat Care 2003;20(2):149–154.

86 Seizure Disorders

I. INTRODUCTION

A. Definitions

1. A **seizure** is a paroxysmal abnormality of cerebral function caused by uncontrolled, excessive discharges from a group of neurons.
2. **Epilepsy** is the tendency to have recurrent (unprovoked) seizures.
3. **Status epilepticus** is continuous seizure activity. Practically, any seizure lasting more than 5 minutes or occurrence of more than two subsequent seizures without returning to baseline between seizures may be considered status epilepticus. (Most seizures last 30 seconds to 2 minutes.)

A prolonged seizure is a medical emergency.

4. An **aura** is a subjective sensation experienced before a seizure. In fact, auras represent simple partial seizures (see III A).
5. **Automatisms** are repetitive movements such as lip smacking, chewing, and scratching that often accompany complex partial seizures.
6. **Postictal** refers to "after the ictus (or event)." Patients are often tired and disoriented after a seizure and may have a transient focal paralysis secondary to seizure activity, called Todd's paralysis. Typically, all symptoms improve over the course of minutes to hours.

B. Epidemiology.

Epilepsy is a relatively common neurologic problem, affecting about 0.5% of the population.

II. DIFFERENTIAL DIAGNOSIS

A. Syncope.

This condition is most often confused with seizures because it involves loss of consciousness and is accompanied by brief "seizure-like" movements that may occur with the loss of consciousness. Some factors that help distinguish syncope from seizures include the following:

1. **Precipitating factors. Seizures** usually have **no immediate precipitating factors** and **no premonitory symptoms except for an aura.** In contrast, syncope is often associated with emotional stress, Valsalva maneuvers, or cardiac conditions and it may be preceded by tiredness, nausea, diaphoresis, and "graying out" of vision. Syncope usually begins with an erect posture, whereas seizures are variable.
2. **Course. Seizures** usually lead to **immediate unconsciousness, lasting for several minutes,** with a **period of sleepiness or disorientation for minutes to hours after the event.** Syncope usually leads to unconsciousness, lasting for several seconds, with a rapid return (seconds to several minutes) to full consciousness and alertness (if the patient has been allowed to assume a recumbent position).

B. Other conditions. Migraine, transient ischemic attack, stroke, movement disorders, pseudoseizures and other psychiatric disorders are also diagnostic possibilities.

III. TYPES OF SEIZURES The most important distinction to make when evaluating a patient who has had a seizure is deciding if the event is a partial or a generalized seizure. This distinction helps determine etiology, location of brain abnormality, prognosis, and subsequent treatment.

A. Partial seizures. Partial seizures are those that **begin in one "part" of the brain** and are the **most common type of seizure.** In adults, they most often **occur following brain injury** (e.g., tumor, trauma, stroke). Partial seizures are also known as "localization-related seizures."

1. **Simple partial seizures** result in a **focal neurologic deficit without alteration of awareness.** These seizures may include shaking of a limb, numbness on one side, rising epigastric sensation, odd smell or taste, auditory or visual phenomena, a sense of familiarity (déjà vu), or a sense of strangeness (jamais vu).
2. **Complex partial seizures** result in a **loss of awareness. Complex partial seizures with secondary generalization** refer to a seizure that begins focally and then spreads to involve the brain diffusely, leading to a generalized seizure.

Most generalized seizures occurring in adults are secondarily generalized.

B. Generalized seizures. Generalized seizures **begin with a diffusely abnormal discharge of neurons leading to widespread cortical involvement.** These seizures occur in the **inherited epilepsies** or **secondary to diffuse brain injury.**

1. **Tonic-clonic seizures** are one of the **most widely recognized generalized seizures.**
   a. They usually begin with **alteration of consciousness.**
   b. Then **bilateral stiffening** (tonic phase) of limbs, often with a clenched jaw, occurs, followed by **rhythmic shaking of limbs** (clonic phase), followed by **complete loss of tone.**
   c. **Afterward, patients may be difficult to arouse** and it may take minutes to hours to return to baseline.
2. **Tonic seizures** involve **tonic stiffening,** usually for about 10 seconds, often causing individuals to fall.
3. **Clonic seizures** involve **rhythmic shaking,** with no tonic phase.
4. **Atonic seizures** involve **sudden and sometimes complete loss of body tone.** They often lead to a fall.
5. **Absence seizures** involve **"staring spells,"** which last for several seconds.
   a. Onset is abrupt and cause individuals to stop what they are doing. Absence seizures often occur **many times per day** and **more frequently in children** compared with adults.
   b. Although individuals are not responsive during an episode, they **often return to baseline level of consciousness immediately.**
   c. **Associated symptoms** may include **eye blinking, lip smacking,** or **swallowing.**
6. **Myoclonic seizures** are myoclonic jerks, which are brief, lightning-fast jerks of a group of muscles. These movements are associated with a generalized electrical discharge. Myoclonic seizures may be associated with an inherited epilepsy syndrome, progressive epilepsy syndromes, or neurodegenerative disorders.

It is important to distinguish myoclonic seizures from the more common medical causes of myoclonic jerks, such as transitions in and out of sleep, severe hypoxic injury, and metabolic derangements.

IV. APPROACH TO THE PATIENT

A. Assess and protect the airway. Both during and after a seizure, patients should be positioned on their side to avoid aspiration.

B. Always consider whether the patient may still be seizing. If the patient is seizing for more than 5 minutes, acute intervention to stop the seizure should be taken (see V B). A patient often does not return to baseline mental status immediately after a seizure, but the typical course is that of constant improvement.

C. Do not forcefully restrict limbs, but make sure that obstacles such as beds or chairs are cleared out of the way to avoid injury. All hospitalized patients with a recent history of seizures should have padded bed rails to help decrease injury.

D. Obtain a detailed history and perform a detailed physical examination, which most often help distinguish between seizure and other disorders with transient neurologic deficits. The evaluation of a patient with a known seizure disorder who has a seizure typical of that condition obviously differs from the evaluation of a patient with a first-time seizure.

E. Obtain several laboratory studies, because metabolic derangements (e.g., hyponatremia) may provoke seizures. A **glucose level** should be obtained immediately. It may often be appropriate to treat a patient with intravenous glucose (and thiamine) presumptively. **Other laboratory studies** should include complete blood count, electrolyte panel, blood urea nitrogen, creatinine, calcium, magnesium, phosphorous, liver panel, anticonvulsant medication levels (if appropriate), and toxicology screen (including ethanol level).

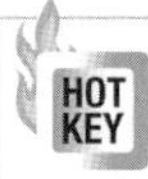

Almost all patients briefly stop breathing during a generalized seizure and therefore become acidemic.

F. Consider performing an infectious work-up in all patients with a seizure. In patients with a known seizure disorder, an intercurrent infection is a common cause of worsening of seizures.

G. Consider performing cerebrospinal fluid (CSF) studies. Although not every patient with a seizure needs a lumbar puncture, the likelihood of a causal central nervous system (CNS) infection should always be strongly considered.

CNS infections commonly present with seizures and may be especially difficult to recognize without CSF studies in immunosuppressed or elderly patients.

H. Obtain brain imaging if the episode is a new-onset seizure or represents a change in the type of seizure for a patient with epilepsy. A **magnetic resonance imaging (MRI) scan of the brain is**

the imaging modality of choice. The acuity of the presentation and rapidity with which an MRI can be obtained often determine if computed tomography (CT) is obtained before the MRI. Immediate CT is indicated if the patient is at high risk for an acute intracranial process (e.g., hemorrhage, infection, stroke, hydrocephalus).

I. Consider obtaining an electroencephalogram (EEG). An EEG should be obtained if a patient's exam is not improving after a generalized seizure to rule out ongoing nonconvulsive status. EEG is also used to monitor patients with status epilepticus treated with drug-induced coma. For an outpatient, the EEG may help distinguish between types of epilepsy or direct attention to a given area.

V. TREATMENT

A. Non–medication-related management

1. **Seizure precautions** should be instituted for all inpatients.
2. Patients should be told to use common sense and to **avoid activities that would be dangerous if they were to have another seizure** (e.g., swimming alone, working on ladders, driving a motorized vehicle). In many states, a seizure must be reported to state public health agencies, who will in turn notify the department of motor vehicles. All patients with seizures should be told specifically not to drive until the seizure disorder is under adequate control, as determined by the treating physician and, in many states, the department of motor vehicles.

B. Medications

1. **Status epilepticus.** Patients should be in a monitored setting and may require intubation for airway protection.
   a. Give **intravenous thiamine** (100 mg) and **glucose** (50 ml of 50% dextrose).
   b. Give 0.1 mg/kg **lorazepam** (Ativan), the first-line acute anticonvulsant medication, at 2 mg/min via intravenous push. Note that lorazepam only temporarily (for about 15–20 minutes) halts status epilepticus, but this often allows enough time to begin determining the etiology.
   c. If the seizure does not stop immediately, give 20 mg/kg **fosphenytoin** at 150 mg/min. Watch for hypotension.
   d. If the seizure continues, repeat the intravenous fosphenytoin load with 10 mg/kg at 150 mg/min.
   e. If the seizure has not stopped, consider **phenobarbital** 20 mg/kg intravenously at 75 mg/min or proceed to general anesthesia with propofol, midazolam, or pentobarbital if the seizures have already lasted 60 minutes.
2. **Epilepsy.** Almost all anticonvulsant drugs treat partial seizures (and the generalized seizures that begin in a partial

TABLE 86-1

PHARMACOLOGIC AGENTS COMMONLY USED FOR SEIZURES

Agent	Seizure Type	Adverse Effects
Phenytoin (fosphenytoin, Dilantin)	Partial, tonic-clonic	Dizziness, diplopia, ataxia, neuropathy, confusion, slurred speech, rash, gingival hyperplasia, hirsutism, blood dyscrasias, toxic hepatitis, facial coarsening
Carbamazepine (Tegretol)	Partial, tonic-clonic	Ataxia, dizziness, diplopia, vertigo, nausea, aplastic anemia, hyponatremia, blood dyscrasias, toxic hepatitis
Oxcarbazepine (Trileptal)	Partial, tonic-clonic	Similar to carbamazepine, hyponatremia
Valproic acid (Depakote, Depacon, Depakene)	All	Ataxia, sedation, tremor, toxic hepatitis, thrombocytopenia, hair loss, weight gain, nausea
Phenobarbital	Partial, tonic-clonic	Somnolence, cognitive and behavioral changes, rash, blood dyscrasias
Topiramate (Topamax)	Partial, tonic-clonic, others	Psychomotor slowing, sedation, fatigue, paresthesias, speech or language problems, weight loss, kidney stones
Lamotrigine (Lamictal)	All	Dizziness, diplopia, sedation, headache, ataxia, rash
Levetiracetam (Keppra)	Partial, tonic-clonic	Irritability, disinhibition
Gabapentin (Neurontin)	Partial	Sedation, dizziness, ataxia
Pregabalin (Lyrica)	Partial	Sedation
Zonisamide (Zonegran)	Partial	Kidney stones, impaired sweating, rash, blood dyscrasias
Ethosuximide	Absence	Nausea, anorexia, rash, blood dyscrasias, somnolence

manner). A subset of anticonvulsant drugs specifically treats generalized seizures (e.g., valproic acid). Side effect profile and ease of administration are most important in the treatment of partial seizures. Table 86-1 lists some medications commonly used to control seizures, along with their potential side effects.

a. **Monitor for side effects**

(1) Almost all anticonvulsant drugs have **potential serious side effects,** including an allergic reaction,

hematologic and liver toxicity, and hyponatremia. Rash, fever, or other reactions should be evaluated immediately. A complete blood count, liver enzymes, and an electrolyte panel are followed frequently when starting a new anticonvulsant drug.

(2) Almost all anticonvulsant drugs have some **non–life-threatening CNS side effects** (e.g., sedation, nausea, nystagmus, ataxia), drug interactions, and potential teratogenicity.

b. **Build dose gradually.** To minimize side effects, most anticonvulsant drugs are started at a low dose and are gradually increased to either maximum tolerated dose or control of seizures.

c. **Try other medications if needed.** Approximately 65% of patients achieve full seizure control with the first medication tried. If the first medication fails, generally monotherapy with a second agent is attempted before treating with two antiepileptics.

C. Other therapies. In specialized cases in which medications fail to provide adequate control, the following may be considered: undergoing surgery to remove a seizure focus, implanting a device that delivers recurrent low-dose electrical stimuli to the vagus nerve (vagus nerve stimulator), or following a restrictive (i.e., ketogenic) diet.

REFERENCES

Ahmed S, Chadwick D, Walker RJ. The management of alcohol-related seizures: an overview. Hosp Med (London) 2000;61(11):793–796 [Classic review article].

French JA, Pedley TA. Clinical practice. Initial management of epilepsy. N Engl J Med 2008;359(2):166–176.

Lowenstein DH. Treatment options for status epilepticus. Curr Opin Pharmacol 2005;5(3):334–339.

Perucca E. An introduction to antiepileptic drugs. Epilepsia 2005;46(Suppl 4): 31–37.

87 Stroke

I. INTRODUCTION

A. Definitions. A stroke is an acute focal neurologic deficit produced by a disturbance in cerebral circulation that results in ischemic infarction, hemorrhage, or both. If the deficit resolves within 24 hours, the incident is a **transient ischemic attack (TIA).**

B. Epidemiology. Stroke is the third leading cause of death and a leading cause of disability in the United States. Mortality rates from stroke have fallen by more than 50% in the past 30 years, probably due to better control of hypertension and other risk factors.

II. CAUSES OF STROKE

A. Ischemic infarction

1. **Distribution.** Cerebral infarcts can be classified according to the type of vessel involved.
   a. **Small vessel.** Chronic stress to vessels produces lipohyalinosis, leading to stenosis and occlusion.
   b. **Large vessel.** Embolism from a vessel, valve, or cardiac chamber or thrombosis (often caused by a ruptured atherosclerotic plaque) leads to stenosis and inadequate perfusion. Affected arteries include the:
      (1) **Middle cerebral artery**
      (2) **Anterior cerebral artery**
      (3) **Carotid artery**
      (4) **Posterior cerebral artery**
      (5) **Vertebrobasilar circulation**
   c. **Watershed** infarctions may occur at the junction of the anterior and middle cerebral arteries or the junction of the posterior and middle cerebral arteries during systemic hypotension.
   d. **Venous.** Thrombosis occurring in the superior sagittal sinus or other large cerebral veins may also result in cerebral infarction.
2. **Source.** Small vessel, large vessel, watershed, and venous infarctions may be produced by local processes or disease in the systemic circulation. It is helpful to remember the sources of infarcts by beginning in the arterioles of the

brain, working backward to the heart, and then through the venous system to the brain again (Table 87-1).

B. **Hemorrhage**

1. **Intraparenchymal hemorrhage** is usually caused by hypertension; an underlying vascular malformation, cerebral amyloid angiopathy, or tumor may also result in intraparenchymal hemorrhage.
2. **Subarachnoid hemorrhage** is usually caused by ruptured cerebral aneurysms. A sudden onset of headache and neck stiffness is characteristic.
3. **Subdural hematoma** can occur with or without a history of preceding trauma.
4. **Epidural hematoma** is almost always sudden and posttraumatic.
5. **Hemorrhagic transformation.** Bleeding occurs into an ischemic infarct.

III. APPROACH TO THE PATIENT

A. **Consider differential diagnoses**

1. **Migraine**
2. **Postictal state**
3. **Hypoglycemia**
4. **Hypertensive encephalopathy**

B. **Brain imaging**

1. **Infarction.** In the first 6 hours after ischemic infarction, head computed tomography (CT) and magnetic resonance imaging (MRI) may be unrevealing; therefore, the patient's history and physical examination findings are particularly important. Localization of the lesion helps to identify the infarction as large vessel, small vessel, watershed, or venous, thereby limiting the differential diagnosis and directing treatment. Table 87-2 summarizes the clinical manifestations and findings on imaging studies for each type of cerebral infarct.
2. **Hemorrhages** will usually be apparent immediately using CT or MRI, although lumbar puncture is required to rule out subarachnoid hemorrhage, which may not be seen on imaging.

C. **Search for an underlying cause**

1. Almost all patients should undergo the studies summarized in Table 87-3. Local practice varies greatly regarding whether patients with TIA need to be admitted to the hospital for evaluation and/or observation. Risk for stroke after TIA can be determined using the ABCD2 score: **a**ge older

---

[1]Focal weakness following a seizure (i.e., Todd's paralysis) is occasionally seen.

TABLE 87-1

SOURCES OF CEREBRAL INFARCTS

Source	Distribution	Risk Factors	Useful Data
Small arteries	Small vessel	Hypertension, diabetes mellitus	Glucose, Hg-A1C
Large and medium arteries	Large vessel	Diabetes mellitus, elevated cholesterol, vasculitis, Asian decent, syphilis, dissection	Glucose, Hg-A1C, cholesterol panel, ESR, toxicology screen, MHA-TP, MRA, CTA or angiography
Carotid stenosis	Large vessel	Diabetes mellitus, elevated cholesterol	Glucose, Hg-A1C, cholesterol panel; MRA, CTA, Doppler ultrasound, or angiography
Aortic arch	Large vessel	Elevated cholesterol, coronary artery disease	Transesophageal echocardiogram
Left ventricle	Large vessel	History of anterior myocardial infarction, ejection fraction <30%	ECG, cardiac monitoring, echocardiogram
Heart valves	Large vessel	Abnormal or prosthetic valves, endocarditis	Echocardiogram, ESR, blood cultures
Left atrium	Large vessel	Atrial fibrillation, left atrial enlargement	ECG, cardiac monitoring, echocardiogram
Hypotension	Watershed	Coronary artery disease, arrhythmia, shock	ECG, cardiac monitoring, CBC
Hematologic	Venous; large or small vessel	Polycythemia, thrombocytosis, leukocytosis, hypercoagulable states, sickle cell anemia	CBC, PT, PTT, anticardiolipin antibody, Russell viper venom test, hexagonal antiphospholipid antibodies, protein C and S, antithrombin III, IgM, factor V Leiden and prothrombin 20210 mutations, viscosity studies
Systemic veins	Large vessel	Deep venous thrombosis with patent foramen ovale or atrial septal defect	Echocardiogram with contrast, lower extremity Doppler ultrasound
Cerebral veins or sinuses	Venous	Dehydration, hypercoagulable state, otitis, sinusitis	Magnetic resonance venogram, conventional venogram

CBC = complete blood count; *CTA* = computed tomographic angiogram; *ECG* = electrocardiogram; *ESR* = erythrocyte sedimentation rate; *Hg-A1C* = glycosylated hemoglobin; *MHA-TP* = microhemagglutination-*Treponema pallidum*; *MRA* = magnetic resonance angiogram; *PT* = prothrombin time; *PTT* = partial thromboplastin time.

TABLE 87-2

CLINICAL MANIFESTATIONS OF CEREBRAL INFARCTS*

Type	Clinical Manifestations	Imaging Study Findings
Small vessel	Lacunar syndrome (e.g., pure motor hemiparesis, ataxic hemiparesis, pure sensory deficit, clumsy hand dysarthria)	Small, often round, lesions in the white matter, deep gray matter, and brain stem
Large vessel		
Middle cerebral artery	Hemiparesis and hemisensory deficit (face = arm > leg), visual field cut, gaze preference, aphasia (left hemisphere) or neglect (right hemisphere)	Infarction in wedge of cortex and underlying white matter
Anterior cerebral artery	Hemiparesis and hemisensory deficit (leg > arm, sparing face), gaze preference	
Carotid artery	Signs of middle cerebral artery infarct plus or minus signs of anterior cerebral artery infarct or amaurosis fugax	
Posterior cerebral artery	Visual field cut	
Vertebrobasilar circulation	Cranial nerve palsies, ataxia, coma	
Watershed	"Man in the barrel" with proximal arm and leg weakness and numbness	Infarction in cortex and underlying white matter in a line from eyes to occiput
Venous	Variable; headache often present; legs often affected	Infarction and hemorrhage near the superior sagittal sinus or in the temporal lobe

*Specific neurologic deficits in a given patient are often more complex and depend on the exact location of the infarct.

than 60 years (1 point); systolic **b**lood pressure greater than 140 (1 point); **c**linical features including speech impairment without weakness (1 point) or unilateral weakness (2 points); **d**uration 10–59 minutes (1 point) or longer than 60 minutes (2 points); and **d**iabetes mellitus (1 point). The

TABLE 87-3

INITIAL WORK-UP FOR THE EVALUATION OF STROKE PATIENTS

Tests	Purpose
CBC, PT, PTT	Rule out hematologic problem
ESR, MHA-TP	Rule out vasculitis, syphilis
ECG	Rule out arrhythmia, myocardial infarction
Head CT or MRI scan	Rule out nonstroke, differentiate ischemic infarction from hemorrhage*

CBC = complete blood count; *CT* = computed tomography; *ECG* = electrocardiogram; *ESR* = erythrocyte sedimentation rate; *MHA-TP* = microhemagglutination-*Treponema pallidum*; *MRI* = magnetic resonance imaging; *PT* = prothrombin time; *PTT* = partial thromboplastin time.

*Head CT may not show evidence of ischemic infarction until 6 hours postinfarction but is relatively sensitive for hemorrhage immediately. Contrast is rarely helpful. MRI is more sensitive for ischemic infarct, especially in the brain stem and cerebellum where bone obscures the CT view but is more expensive and time consuming.

total score predicts the 2-day risk of stroke as follows: 0–3 points, 1%; 4–5 points, 4%; 6–7 points, 8%. Urgent evaluation is warranted in patients at high risk.

2. The following studies are indicated in certain circumstances:
   a. **Carotid Doppler ultrasound** is indicated following a large vessel TIA or stroke when endarterectomy or stent is being considered.
   b. **Cardiac echocardiography** is indicated following a large vessel TIA or stroke.
   c. **CT angiography** is often considered in the setting of an acute stroke when knowledge of intracranial vasculature may affect treatment.
   d. **Magnetic resonance angiography.** A magnetic resonance angiogram (MRA) of the head is indicated for patients with possible intracranial large vessel disease or suspected arterial dissection. MRA of the neck can also confirm abnormal carotid Doppler ultrasound findings.
   e. **Conventional angiography** may be appropriate if carotid endarterectomy is being considered or when vasculitis, aortic dissection, or subarachnoid hemorrhage is suspected.
   f. **Transcranial Doppler** ultrasound is often indicated for patients with possible intracranial large vessel disease or vasospasm following subarachnoid hemorrhage.
   g. **Lumbar puncture** is indicated if subarachnoid hemorrhage is a possibility and not visualized on CT scan.
   h. **Hypercoagulability** studies (see Chapter 67) are appropriate in young patients (i.e., those younger than 45 years) with no other risk factors for stroke.

i. **Toxicology screen.** A toxicology screen is often performed in young patients with stroke to rule out cocaine or amphetamine use.

IV. TREATMENT

A. Ischemic infarction. Treatment has been primarily supportive and focused on secondary prevention, but therapies directed at dissolving clots and protecting the patient from cerebral ischemia have been evolving rapidly.

1. **Generally accepted therapies**

a. **Pharmacologic therapy**

(1) **Warfarin** reduces the risk of a recurrent event by approximately 65% for patients with a known cardiac source of embolus (e.g., atrial fibrillation, mechanical heart valve, mural thrombus). There is no evidence supporting the use of heparin in the setting of acute stroke.

(2) **Aspirin** or another antiplatelet agent (e.g., clopidogrel) is usually indicated for stroke prophylaxis in patients who do not meet one of the above indications for warfarin.

(3) **Tissue plasminogen activator (t-PA).** Intravenous administration of t-PA may be beneficial for patients with a cerebral infarct who can be **treated** within 3 hours of symptom onset (defined as the time the patient can be last **confirmed** to be **normal**). Although this treatment does not currently appear to decrease mortality rates, t-PA may lead to a 50% relative increase in patients who are neurologically normal at 3 months. Importantly, t-PA may be associated with a 6% risk of serious intracranial hemorrhage (50% of which were fatal).

b. **Supportive measures**

(1) Hold or decrease antihypertensive agents and consider intravenous hydration to increase blood flow to the ischemic area around the infarct.

(2) Aspiration should be prevented by having a swallow therapist evaluate patients with dysarthria or poor cough; urinary tract infections should be prevented by removing urinary catheters as early as possible; deep vein thrombosis should be prevented with prophylactic doses of unfractionated or low-molecular-weight heparin.

c. **Secondary prevention**

(1) **Atorvastatin** 80 mg started acutely after ischemic stroke in patients with a low-density lipoprotein

(LDL) cholesterol level greater than 100 appears to reduce the risk of recurrent stroke.

(2) **Smoking cessation** counseling is mandatory in all stroke patients.

(3) After the acute period, treatment of **hypertension** reduces recurrent stroke risk.

(4) **Diabetes mellitus** should be tested for and if present, treated.

d. **Specific treatment** that addresses the cause of the stroke (e.g., carotid endarterectomy) should be carried out if indicated.

e. **Physical, occupational,** and **speech therapy** are necessary.

2. **Evolving therapies**

a. **Anticoagulation.** Antiplatelet versus warfarin therapy continues to be reevaluated in a variety of clinical settings (e.g., aortic arch disease and cardiomyopathy with low ejection fraction).

b. **Intra-arterial thrombolysis and thrombectomy.** Intra-arterial thrombolytic agents and mechanical thrombectomy may be beneficial if administered during cerebral angiogram within 6 hours or 8 hours of infarct onset, respectively.

c. **Neuroprotection.** A variety of neuroprotectant therapies are being investigated as a way of minimizing ischemic damage.

B. Hemorrhage

1. **Hemorrhagic transformation.** The treatment is the same as that for ischemic infarction, except heparin and aspirin are withheld briefly.

2. **Intraparenchymal hemorrhage**

a. Blood pressure is usually lowered acutely to minimize risk of hematoma expansion.

b. Coagulopathy (e.g., warfarin therapy) should be reversed with fresh frozen plasma or recombinant factor IX in addition to vitamin K.

c. Consultation with a neurosurgeon is warranted as surgical evacuation may be possible, depending on the size and location of the hemorrhage. In addition, placement of an external ventricular drain (EVD) or other intracranial pressure monitor may be necessary.

3. **Subarachnoid hemorrhage**

a. Consultation with a neurosurgeon or interventional radiologist is indicated to explore the possibility of early aneurysm clipping or coiling. In addition, placement of an EVD may be necessary if there is acute hydrocephalus.

b. Prior to securing the aneurysm, blood pressure is usually lowered to minimize risk of rerupture. After the aneurysm is secured, blood pressure is often raised to prevent vasospasm.

c. Nimodipine therapy and hydration are indicated.

4. Subdural and **epidural hemorrhages.** Consultation with a neurosurgeon to investigate the possibility of evacuation is appropriate.

REFERENCES

Adams HP Jr, del Zoppo G, Alberts MJ, et al. Guidelines for the early management of adults with ischemic stroke: a guideline from the American Heart Association/American Stroke Association Stroke Council, Clinical Cardiology Council, Cardiovascular Radiology and Intervention Council, and the Atherosclerotic Peripheral Vascular Disease and Quality of Care Outcomes in Research Interdisciplinary Working Groups: the American Academy of Neurology affirms the value of this guideline as an educational tool for neurologists. Circulation 2007;115:e478–534.

Gage BF, Fihn SD, White RH. Warfarin therapy for an octogenarian who has atrial fibrillation. Ann Intern Med 2001;134:465–474 [Classic article].

Johnston SC, Rothwell PM, Nguyen-Huynh MN, et al. Validation and refinement of scores to predict very early stroke risk after transient ischaemic attack. Lancet 2007;369:283–292.

Sacco RL, Adams R, Albers G, et al. Guidelines for prevention of stroke in patients with ischemic stroke or transient ischemic attack: a statement for healthcare professionals from the American Heart Association/American Stroke Association Council on Stroke: co-sponsored by the Council on Cardiovascular Radiology and Intervention: the American Academy of Neurology affirms the value of this guideline. Circulation 2006;113:e409–449.

Tissue plasminogen activator for acute ischemic stroke. The National Institute of Neurological Disorders and Stroke rt-PA Stroke Study Group. N Engl J Med 1995;333:1581–1587 [Classic article].

Meningitis

I. INTRODUCTION. Meningitis may result from infection, malignancy (i.e., carcinomatous meningitis), or systemic illness (e.g., lupus, sarcoidosis). Infectious etiologies (particularly acute bacterial meningitis) are common, life-threatening causes of meningitis and are the major focus of this chapter. Infectious meningitis can be classified as easy as "A, B, C."

MNEMONIC **Classification of Infectious Meningitis ("A, B, C")**

Aseptic meningitis
Bacterial meningitis (acute)
Chronic meningitis

II. CAUSES OF INFECTIOUS MENINGITIS

A. Aseptic meningitis [inflammatory cerebrospinal fluid (CSF) with negative cultures]

1. **Viral infections,** including enterovirus, mumps, herpes simplex virus 1, coxsackievirus, Epstein-Barr virus, and cytomegalovirus (CMV), are common causes of aseptic meningitis.
2. **Spirochetal infections.** Secondary syphilis, Lyme disease, and leptospirosis may also cause aseptic meningitis.
3. **Parameningeal focus.** An infection near the arachnoid layer—but not invading it—may produce inflammation in the CSF (e.g., spinal epidural abscess or intracranial abscess) despite persistently negative CSF cultures.

B. Acute bacterial meningitis

1. ***Streptococcus pneumoniae*** is the most common cause of meningitis in adults.
2. ***Neisseria meningitidis*** infection may be epidemic or sporadic and is rare in adults older than 50 years.
3. ***Haemophilus influenzae*** infection, previously common in children younger than 6 years, has been significantly reduced by the *H. influenzae* vaccine.
4. ***Listeria monocytogenes*** infection is most often seen in infants, the elderly, the debilitated, alcoholics, and patients who are immunosuppressed, including during pregnancy.

5. ***Staphylococcus aureus, Staphylococcus epidermidis,*** and **gram-negative bacilli.** Infections with these organisms may occur following neurosurgical procedures, head trauma, or shunt infections. Left-sided endocarditis should always be considered when the infecting organism is *S. aureus*.

C. Chronic meningitis

1. **Fungal infections,** including *Coccidioides immitis* and *Cryptococcus neoformans* infections, are especially common causes of chronic meningitis. More virulent fungi and acute presentations may be seen in immunocompromised patients.
2. **Mycobacterial infections.** *Mycobacterium tuberculosis* is the most common mycobacterial cause of chronic meningitis.
3. **Spirochetal infections.** *Treponema pallidum* and *Borrelia burgdorferi,* the causes of syphilis and Lyme disease, respectively, may cause aseptic or chronic meningitis.

III. CLINICAL MANIFESTATIONS OF INFECTIOUS MENINGITIS

A. Fever and **headache** should always raise the suspicion of meningitis.

B. Neck stiffness, positive **Kernig's** and **Brudzinski's signs,** and **photosensitivity** are also common findings but are less likely with certain infections (e.g., cryptococcal meningitis).

C. Altered mental status (rare in aseptic meningitis), **focal neurologic abnormalities, seizures,** and **evidence of increased intracranial pressure** (e.g., papilledema) may all be seen.

D. Signs related to the causative organism may be present. For example, a petechial or purpuric rash caused by meningococcus infection is present in approximately 50% of patients with meningococcal meningitis.

Infants, the elderly, and immunosuppressed patients may not generate a high fever or signs of meningismus. The sensitivities of neck stiffness and the other findings are not high enough to rule out meningitis clinically; therefore, all patients with a fever and altered mental status, and many patients with a fever and a headache, require further evaluation.

IV. APPROACH TO THE PATIENT

A. Patient history. The time course of the patient's illness may provide a clue as to the type of meningitis; however, a lumbar puncture is always necessary.

1. **Aseptic meningitis** often presents acutely after a "flu-like" prodrome. More than 90% of patients are younger than 30 years.

2. **Acute bacterial meningitis** presents acutely (usually within hours to days) and typically with symptoms that are more severe than in **patients with aseptic meningitis.**
3. **Chronic** meningitis usually is more indolent; symptoms may not appear for days to weeks.

B. Blood cultures and **empiric therapy.** If acute meningitis is suspected, draw two sets of blood cultures and start empiric therapy with antibiotics (and possibly steroids) immediately (see V); the yield on Gram stain and culture of the CSF will probably not change within 4 hours of starting therapy. Blood cultures are positive in approximately 50% of patients with bacterial meningitis and should always be obtained because they may be diagnostic in patients with a negative CSF culture.

C. Lumbar puncture and **CSF fluid analysis.** Acute bacterial meningitis often cannot be distinguished from more benign processes (e.g., aseptic meningitis, common viral syndromes) on the basis of clinical criteria alone; therefore, a lumbar puncture should be performed whenever meningitis is a consideration.

1. **Lumbar puncture**
   a. **Contraindications.** A lumbar puncture can usually be done safely in the presence of normal mental status and a nonfocal neurologic exam with no evidence of increased intracerebral pressure (e.g., papilledema). If there is evidence of altered mental status, a focal neurologic examination, papilledema, an immunocompromised state, a history of CNS disease, or a new seizure, empiric therapy should be initiated and a computed tomography (CT) scan obtained before lumbar puncture.
   b. **Procedure**
      (1) **Premedicate the patient.** Premedicating with low doses of a benzodiazepine (e.g., lorazepam; 0.5–2 mg intravenously) and morphine sulfate (e.g., 2–4 mg) often lessens the pain and anxiety associated with lumbar puncture. These agents should be avoided in patients with altered mental status.
      (2) **Measure the opening pressure.** Opening pressure elevations are nonspecific, but significant elevations are common with acute bacterial meningitis. Normal or minimal elevations predominate in aseptic meningitis. The legs must be straightened to obtain an accurate opening pressure.
      (3) **Draw four samples.** You will usually have four tubes.
         (a) A **cell count** is usually performed on the CSF sample in tubes 1 and 4. If the last tube has a significantly decreased number of red blood cells (RBCs) in comparison to the first tube, a traumatic tap may be more likely than a true

disease process (e.g., subarachnoid hemorrhage, herpes encephalitis).

(b) **Protein** and **glucose levels** are often obtained from the sample sent in tube 1 or tube 4.

(c) **Gram staining** and **culture.** The CSF sample in tube 2 is usually used for Gram staining and culture. Only a small amount of CSF (e.g., 1 ml) is required.

(d) **Cryptococcal antigen (CRAG) titer,** an **India ink preparation,** and **fungal culture** can also be performed on the tube 2 sample in human immunodeficiency virus (HIV)-positive or immunocompromised patients; however, a serum CRAG is more sensitive than a CSF CRAG.

(e) **Other studies** may be needed. Tube 3 is often filled and refrigerated pending the results of the standard tests.

2. **CSF analysis**

a. **Cell count.** The normal cell count is 0–5 lymphocytes/μl. If pleocytosis is found, the predominant cell type helps to prioritize the differential diagnoses.

(1) **Neutrophilic [polymorphonuclear neutrophil (PMN)] pleocytosis**

(a) The patient should be considered to have **acute bacterial meningitis** until proven otherwise.

(b) **Early viral infections** can also be neutrophil predominant, but the worst should always be assumed first.

(c) PMN counts greater than 50,000 cells/μl should alert you to a possible **brain abscess with rupture into a ventricle.**

(2) **Lymphocytic pleocytosis.** An elevated lymphocyte count can occur with **all three categories of infectious meningitis** (i.e., the ABCs) as well as with **other processes.**

(a) **ABCs.** Aseptic and chronic meningitis typically have a lymphocytic predominance. Certain types of bacterial infections (e.g., early or partially treated bacterial meningitis, brain abscesses, parameningeal infections) may also cause lymphocytic pleocytosis.

(b) **Other causes.** These patients will probably need "2 ICE" cubes to help their headaches (see mnemonic next page).

b. **Protein level.** The normal protein level in adults is 15–45 mg/dl. Approximately 90% of patients with acute

MNEMONIC **Other Causes of Lymphocytic Meningitis ("2 ICE")**

Infections (malaria, toxoplasmosis, fresh water amebiasis, cysticercosis, Rocky Mountain spotted fever)
Intoxications [salicylates, barbiturates, heavy metals, nonsteroidal anti-inflammatory drugs (NSAIDs)]
Cancer (carcinomatous meningitis)
Collagen vascular disease [systemic lupus erythematosus (SLE)]
Endocrine disorder (pheochromocytoma)
Endocarditis

bacterial meningitis have an elevated CSF protein level, whereas patients with aseptic meningitis often have a normal or minimally elevated protein level.

c. **Glucose level.** The normal glucose level is 45–85 mg/dl. The CSF glucose may vary with the serum glucose.
   (1) The ratio of CSF to serum glucose is less than 0.4 (assuming that the serum glucose level is <250 mg/dl) in most patients with acute bacterial meningitis, but is normal (>0.4) in patients with aseptic meningitis.
   (2) Carcinomatous, fungal, and tuberculous meningitis are other common causes of depressed CSF glucose.

d. **Gram stain** and **culture**
   (1) **Gram stain.** The Gram stain is positive in the majority of cases of untreated acute bacterial meningitis. (*L. monocytogenes,* however, is notorious for not being identified.)
   (2) **Culture.** The CSF culture is positive in most cases of bacterial meningitis.

D. Ancillary tests

1. **Patients with neutrophilic pleocytosis** (i.e., a high probability of bacterial meningitis)
   a. **Latex agglutination tests** for bacterial antigen can be done on patients who may have a partially treated culture-negative bacterial meningitis.
   b. **Head CT scan** or **magnetic resonance imaging (MRI).** Acute bacterial meningitis may be caused by direct extension from sinusitis, otitis, or mastoiditis. An imaging study is necessary if extension is suspected.
2. **Patients with lymphocytic pleocytosis.** By considering the possible causes of a lymphocytic pleocytosis (i.e., the ABCs and the 2 ICE cubes) and the clinical setting, you can determine which diagnostic tests may be useful.

a. **ABCs**

(1) **Aseptic meningitis.** Mumps virus, herpes simplex virus (HSV), varicella-zoster virus, and CMV can be recovered from the CSF, and a Monospot test can be done for Epstein-Barr virus, but in most cases, the viral agent is not recovered. A **Venereal Disease Research Laboratory (VDRL) test** should always be sent and **Lyme titers and polymerase chain reaction (PCR) for HSV** are also a consideration in cases of suspected aseptic meningitis.

(2) **Bacterial meningitis.** Acute bacterial infection resulting from a parameningeal focus is a possibility and, depending on the presentation, a **CT scan** or **MRI** may be considered.

(3) **Chronic meningitis.** *M. tuberculosis* infection or fungal infection are possible etiologies. Commonly ordered tests include a **purified protein derivative (PPD) test,** a **CSF acid-fast bacillus stain** and **culture, CSF** and **serum CRAG titers,** and ***Coccidioides* serology** (other fungal serologies and cultures may also be ordered).

(a) Multiple CSF samples of up to 20 ml of CSF increase the yield on acid-fast bacillus staining and culture, but the culture may still be negative in up to 25% of patients with tuberculous meningitis. A PCR-based test for tuberculosis (TB) is under investigation.

(b) A history of TB, active TB, or basilar meningitis on MRI may support the diagnosis of tuberculous meningitis.

b. **Other causes. CSF cytology** is frequently sent when carcinomatous meningitis is a consideration. Multiple (often three) CSF samples and performing CSF flow cytometry can increase the yield.

V. TREATMENT. Medication doses are given for **adults** with **normal renal** function.

A. Empiric antibacterial therapy for acute bacterial meningitis is critical.

1. **No penicillin allergy**

a. **Ceftriaxone** (often 2 g intravenously every 12 hours) or cefotaxime (2 g intravenously every 4 hours) is the best choice because these drugs cover gram-negative organisms (including *H. influenzae*) as well as the emerging penicillin-resistant ***S. pneumoniae.***

b. **Vancomycin** (30–45 mg/kg/day divided every 8–12 hours) is usually recommended given the high prevalence of drug-resistant *S. pneumoniae*. Vancomycin should be added to cover *S. aureus* in cases involving head trauma, recent neurosurgery, or manipulation of a CSF shunt.

c. **Ampicillin** (12–18 g/day in divided doses every 4 hours) or **penicillin G** (18–24 million units intravenously per day divided or with continuous therapy) should be **added** in patients with epidemiologic risk factors for ***L. monocytogenes*** (immunocompromised, older than 50 years).

d. **Acyclovir** should be added for cases suspicious for HSV (while awaiting results of HSV PCR).

e. **Fungal coverage** should be considered in any immunocompromised patient.

2. **Penicillin allergy**
   a. In patients who are allergic to penicillin and have a history of anaphylaxis, **chloramphenicol** may be used. Chloramphenicol is also effective against *Listeria*.
   b. If the patient is allergic to penicillin but has no history of anaphylaxis, ceftriaxone or cefotaxime may be tried. **Trimethoprim-sulfamethoxazole (TMP/SMX)** can be added if *Listeria* infection is a possibility.

B. Steroids may be given in the following situations:
1. To decrease the incidence of deafness in children with *H. influenzae* infection.
2. In most cases of adult bacterial meningitis (usually dexamethasone 0.15 mg/kg intravenously every 6 hours for 4 days) if administered prior to or concomitant to the start of antibiotics. Steroids are probably only beneficial in pneumococcal meningitis and should only be continued if this diagnosis is confirmed by gram stain or culture; steroids may be harmful in patients with HIV.
3. In some cases of tuberculous meningitis of moderate severity

VI. PREVENTION. Rifampin prophylaxis (600 mg orally twice daily for 2 days for adults) is appropriate for close contacts of a patient with meningococcal meningitis. Household and daycare center contacts and hospital workers with intense exposure should all be given prophylaxis.

REFERENCES

Tunkel AR, Glaser CA, Bloch KC, et al. The management of encephalitis: clinical practice guidelines by the Infectious Diseases Society of America. Clin Infect Dis 2008;47(3):303–327.

Tunkel AR, Hartman BJ, Kaplan SL, et al. Practice guidelines for the management of bacterial meningitis. Clin Infect Dis 2004;39(9):1267–1284.

van de Beek D, de Gans J, Tunkel AR, et al. Community-acquired bacterial meningitis in adults. N Engl J Med 2006;354(1):44–53.

Weisfelt M, van de Beek D, Spanjaard L, et al. A risk score for unfavorable outcome in adults with bacterial meningitis. Ann Neurol 2008;63(1):90–97.

■ Spinal Cord Compression

I. INTRODUCTION. Spinal cord compression is a true medical emergency that requires prompt intervention. The clinical diagnosis of cord compression may be difficult because early symptoms are often attributed to more common processes. Furthermore, the characteristic symptoms often occur too late to prevent irreversible damage. Clinical suspicion is therefore paramount.

II. CAUSES OF SPINAL CORD COMPRESSION

A. Malignancy, most often from **metastatic disease,** is by far the most common cause of spinal cord compression. Consistent with the number of each type of vertebrae, the thoracic vertebrae are most often involved, followed by approximately equal involvement of the cervical and lumbosacral vertebrae.

1. If you remember the cancers that involve the bone—breast, lung, thyroid, kidney, prostate, and multiple myeloma—you will remember the most common causes of spinal cord compression (see also Chapter 73). **Breast, lung,** and **prostate cancer** account for most cases of cord compression.
2. Lymphomas, primary spinal tumors (i.e., meningiomas, neurofibromas), and many other malignancies can also cause spinal cord compression.

B. Infections. Epidural abscesses and osteomyelitis (e.g., from bacteria or tuberculosis) occasionally lead to cord compression.

C. Herniated discs that are large and central in location occasionally result in cord compression.

D. Epidural hemorrhage may occur spontaneously or result from arteriovenous malformations, trauma, anticoagulation therapy, or underlying tumors, resulting in cord compression.

E. Rheumatologic disorders. Arthritis (especially rheumatoid arthritis) with cervical involvement can result in cord compression from relatively minor trauma (e.g., whiplash or intubation). Ankylosing spondylitis may result in lumbar cord compression.

F. Trauma. Motor vehicle accidents, falls, and assault can cause spine fracture and cord compression. Injuries causing concussion (e.g., loss of consciousness) are frequently accompanied by spine injury.

III. CLINICAL MANIFESTATIONS OF SPINAL CORD COMPRESSION

A. Back pain is the most common symptom and is present in at least 80% of patients. The quality of the pain is variable and nonspecific and does not usually allow spinal cord compression to be distinguished from more benign disorders. **Point tenderness** over the involved vertebrae is common in spinal cord compression and should raise a red flag.

B. Neurologic findings are infrequent initially but become more prominent with time.

1. If the lesion is in the **cervical or thoracic spine**, upper motor neuron weakness will be seen (e.g., increased tone, hyperreflexia, and extensor > flexor weakness in the arms and flexor > extensor weakness in the legs). There may also be a sensory level, dissociated sensory signs (e.g., preserved pain/temperature but diminished vibration/joint position sense), constipation, and urge incontinence.
2. If the lesion affects the **lumbar spine** and thus the **cauda equina,** lower motor neuron weakness will be seen (e.g., decreased tone, hyporeflexia, and weakness in the pattern of the nerve roots affected). Saddle anesthesia, numbness in the distribution of a nerve root, constipation, and urinary retention with overflow incontinence are also seen.
3. Lesions in the **conus medullaris** (located at the level of vertebrae L1–2) can cause both upper and lower motor neuron weakness and often affect bladder function.

IV. APPROACH TO THE PATIENT.

Diagnosis depends on imaging studies.

A. Modalities

1. **Magnetic resonance imaging (MRI)** is extremely sensitive and noninvasive and is therefore the first choice. The entire cord needs to be evaluated because multiple skip lesions are often present.
2. **Computed tomography (CT)** with a **myelogram** can be used when MRI is not available or contraindicated.
3. **Radiographs** and **bone scans** are of little value in the diagnosis of cord compression (although they may be a useful initial screen in patients presenting only with back pain). Radiographs are not sensitive enough to detect vertebral metastases, and neither test evaluates the spinal cord itself.

B. Indications

1. **Absolute indications.** The following patients usually require testing:
   a. **All patients with a known cancer** accompanied by symptoms or signs of possible cord compression (e.g., back pain)
   b. **Patients with focal neurologic symptoms or signs** (e.g., gait difficulty, bowel/bladder incontinence, saddle anesthesia, bilateral weakness or numbness)

2. **Risk stratification.** In the remaining patients who present with back pain, you can perform a simple risk stratification to assess the likelihood of possible cord compression and the appropriateness of imaging studies.
   a. **Simple back pain.** Patients with back pain who are younger than 50 years, without a history of cancer or weight loss, and with no evidence of sciatica or neurologic deficit have musculoskeletal pain approximately 99% of the time. Usually, no tests are performed, and conservative therapy is recommended.
   b. **Back pain with risk factors.** Risk factors include pain worse at rest, history of or suspected malignancy, history of chronic infection, history of trauma, age older than 50, pain lasting for more than 1 month, history of intravenous drug use, steroid use, unexplained fever or weight loss, or spine percussion tenderness. These patients have a higher incidence of an underlying malignancy or infectious process and are often initially evaluated with plain radiographs, complete blood count (CBC), and an erythrocyte sedimentation rate (ESR). If these test results are abnormal or if conservative therapy has failed, additional diagnostic testing to rule out serious causes of back pain is usually indicated.

If spinal cord compression is a possibility, then imaging studies need to be performed immediately. Patients with stable symptoms may be evaluated on a less acute basis.

V. TREATMENT

A. Malignancy

1. **Steroids.** High-dose **dexamethasone** (often 10–100 mg via an intravenous bolus) followed by 4–24 mg every 6 hours (intravenously or orally) is often administered.

If cord compression is suspected, do not wait for the MRI results before initiating treatment. There is usually little harm in one dose of steroids if your clinical diagnosis proves incorrect.

2. **Radiation therapy** should be initiated once the diagnosis is made. The combination of steroid treatment plus radiation therapy is more beneficial than radiation alone presumably

because steroids decrease the swelling associated with radiation.

3. **Ketoconazole** administered intravenously can reduce malignant prostatic metastases acutely; therefore, it is sometimes used in patients who have known prostate cancer associated with cord compression.
4. **Chemotherapy** alone is sometimes effective in patients with extremely chemosensitive tumors (e.g., small cell lung cancer, lymphoma).
5. **Emergency surgery.** Early consultation with a neurosurgeon is very helpful. **Surgery** for cord compression is usually indicated:
   a. With rapidly progressive neurologic deficits
   b. When radiation therapy is failing or for spinal instability
   c. For radio-insensitive tumors
   d. When the etiology is unclear (i.e., for diagnostic and therapeutic purposes)

B. Infection. Whenever possible, a microbiologic diagnosis should be made. Treatment with **antibiotics** is tailored to the pathogen. **Surgery** may be indicated if the spine is unstable.

C. Herniated disc. Surgery is usually indicated if there is a myelopathy (e.g., spinal cord involvement), progressive motor deficit, bowel or bladder incontinence, or radicular pain unrelieved by conservative therapy for 6 months.

D. Traumatic spinal cord injury

1. **Hemodynamic support.** Maintenance of perfusion is critical in traumatic spinal cord injury. Thus, **hypotension** and **hypoxia** should be prevented.
2. **Steroids.** High-dose intravenous methylprednisolone is an option if the patient presents within 8 hours of the injury (30 mg/kg over 1 hour, then 5.4 mg/kg/hr for 24 hours if started within 3 hours of injury and 48 hours if started within 8 hours of injury).
3. **Surgery** may be indicated if there is an unstable spine fracture, and neurosurgical consultation is always indicated.

REFERENCES

Deyo RA, Weinstein JN. Low back pain. N Engl J Med 2001;344(5):363–370 [Classic article].

Kaplin AI, Krishnan C, Deshpande DM, et al. Diagnosis and management of acute myelopathies. Neurologist 2005;11(1):2–18.

Loblaw DA, Perry J, Chambers A, Laperriere NJ. Systematic review of the diagnosis and management of malignant extradural spinal cord compression: the Cancer Care Ontario Practice Guidelines Initiative's Neuro-Oncology Disease Site Group. J Clin Oncol 2005;23(9):2028–2037.

PART XI
DERMATOLOGY

Exanthems

I. INTRODUCTION

A. A vascular lesion is caused by congestion within the blood vessel and therefore usually blanches with pressure. The term **erythematous** implies that the lesion **blanches.**

The best way to determine blanchability is to place a glass microscope slide (or another transparent object) onto the lesion while applying pressure. You will be able to tell quickly whether the lesion blanches.

B. A **purpuric lesion,** on the other hand, is caused by the escape of blood into the perivascular tissue. Purpuric lesions **do not blanch with pressure.** Purpuric lesions may be more worrisome than erythematous ones because the diseases that can cause purpura are occasionally life-threatening (e.g., meningococcemia).

1. There are two types of purpuric lesions:
   a. **Petechiae** are small purpuric lesions.
   b. **Ecchymoses** are large purpuric lesions.
2. When purpuric lesions become raised, they are considered **"palpable purpura"** and represent a vasculitis (see Chapter 76).

C. An **exanthem** is an **acute, generalized rash.** Exanthemas are common in hospitalized patients and in those visiting the emergency department. Most of these eruptions are benign; however, life-threatening disorders can also cause exanthemas and must be considered. Exanthemas can be **morbilliform** or **scarlatiniform** eruptions. Both morbilliform and scarlatiniform eruptions blanch.

II. MORBILLIFORM RASH.

A morbilliform rash is an erythematous macular/papular, **nonconfluent** eruption that usually involves the torso. Morbilliform eruptions are much more common than scarlatiniform ones.

A. Causes

1. **Drug reactions.** Any drug can cause a morbilliform rash; however, **penicillins** and **sulfa-containing compounds** are the most common culprits. The skin reaction is usually symmetric

and involves the torso more than the appendages. In previously exposed patients, the rash appears within 3 days; in previously unexposed patients, the eruption appears 7–9 days into the course of treatment. Fever, pruritus, lymphadenopathy, and eosinophilia are sometimes present.

2. **Infections**
   a. **Viral infections** [e.g., **rubeola (measles), rubella, parvovirus, Epstein-Barr virus, echovirus, coxsackievirus, adenovirus,** and **early human immunodeficiency virus (HIV)**] are the most common infectious causes of morbilliform rashes.

Viral exanthemas are usually preceded by fever and constitutional symptoms.

   b. **Bacterial** causes include **typhoid fever** and **secondary syphilis.** Early **rickettsial** and **meningococcal** disease—diseases usually associated with purpuric lesions—can initially present as morbilliform reactions and must be considered, given the mortality associated with each. **If you suspect rickettsial or meningococcal disease, begin empiric antibiotics while awaiting the definitive diagnosis** (see Chapter 50).
3. **Acute graft versus host disease (GVHD)** is seen in allogeneic bone marrow transplant recipients when immunocompetent donor lymphocytes and macrophages are transplanted and attack the new host.

B. Diagnosis. If the diagnosis is unclear, skin biopsy (a safe, easy procedure) should be considered.

III. SCARLATINIFORM RASH. A scarlatiniform eruption is a generalized, confluent, blanching erythema. It may be difficult to distinguish a scarlatiniform rash from a morbilliform rash, which can begin to coalesce; however, scarlatiniform eruptions are **usually confluent at the outset.**

A. Scarlet fever. Patients with a β-hemolytic streptococcal (group A) pharyngitis or tonsillitis can develop a characteristic rash caused by an erythrogenic toxin. The rash, which is confluent, papular, and sandpaper-like in texture, begins on the neck and upper chest and then spreads over the extremities and abdomen. Circumoral pallor and a strawberry tongue are characteristic; desquamation of most of the involved areas occurs in 5 days.

B. Kawasaki disease is a multisystemic disorder of unknown etiology that mainly affects children.

1. **Clinical manifestations.** Kawasaki disease is characterized by fever, conjunctivitis, mucous membrane involvement, edema, cervical lymphadenopathy, and a scarlatiniform

(or sometimes a morbilliform) rash that is most prominent on the trunk.

2. **Treatment** is usually with intravenous immune globulin (IVIG) and aspirin.
3. **Complications.** Patients are at risk for coronary artery aneurysms and myocardial infarction.

Kawasaki disease rarely affects adults but may occasionally occur in epidemic fashion. One theory of pathogenesis proposes that staphylococcal toxin acts as a "superantigen" that interacts with T cells.

C. Toxic shock syndrome is a life-threatening disorder caused by toxins elaborated by ***Staphylococcus aureus*** or group A streptococci.

1. Toxic shock syndrome is most commonly seen in tampon-using menstruating women, postsurgical patients, and those with a site of toxin-producing staphylococcal or streptococcal infection (e.g., an abscess). **Whenever a patient has a scarlatiniform rash, always consider toxic shock syndrome.**
2. **Clinical manifestations.** Toxic shock syndrome is characterized by **fever, hypotension,** and **multiorgan involvement.**
   a. **Gastrointestinal.** Nausea, vomiting, diarrhea, elevated liver enzymes
   b. **Musculoskeletal.** Myalgias, arthralgias, myositis
   c. **Renal.** Acute renal failure
   d. **Mucous membranes.** Nonexudative conjunctivitis, strawberry tongue
   e. **Pulmonary.** Acute respiratory distress syndrome (ARDS)
   f. **Cutaneous.** Diffuse erythematous rash that blanches very easily; desquamation occurs after 1–2 weeks

The rash of toxic shock syndrome is often accentuated in the flexural folds.

REFERENCES

Issa NC, Thompson RL. Staphylococcal toxic shock syndrome. Suspicion and prevention are keys to control. Postgrad Med 2001;110(4):55–56 [Classic article].

Newburger JW, Takahashi M, Gerber MA, et al. Diagnosis, treatment and long-term management of Kawasaki disease. Circulation 2004:2747–2771.

Segal A, Doherty KM, Leggott J, et al. Cutaneous reactions to drugs in children. Pediatrics 2007;120:e1082–1096.

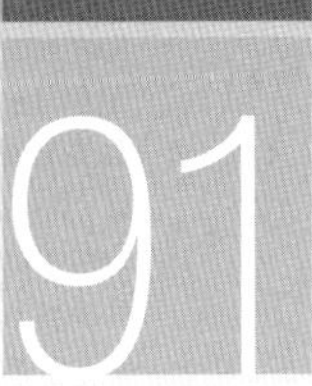

Pruritus

I. INTRODUCTION. Itching can be caused by a variety of dermatologic and nondermatologic disorders.

A. Dermatologic disorders. Itching is a very common symptom of dermatologic disorders. Skin lesions are usually present when a dermatologic disorder is the cause of the itching.

B. Systemic disorders. When no skin lesions are present, the itching is often caused by a systemic disorder. Approximately 15% of patients with itching but without skin lesions have a systemic disorder diagnosed at initial presentation.

II. CAUSES OF PRURITUS

A. Dermatologic disorders

1. **Xerosis (dry skin)** is a very common cause.
2. **Parasitic infestation** (e.g., scabies, pediculosis) and **insect bites** cause pruritus.
3. Other causes include **urticaria, atopic** or **contact dermatitis, superficial fungal infections, drug reactions, sunburn, dermatitis herpetiformis, fiberglass dermatitis, lichen planus,** and **folliculitis.**

B. Systemic disorders

1. **Uremia** is the most common cause of pruritus when lesions are not present.
2. **Primary biliary cirrhosis, extrahepatic biliary obstruction,** and **cholestatic drugs** cause **total bilirubin elevation,** bile salt retention, and pruritus.
3. **Cancer.** Neoplasms that can cause pruritus include lymphoma (especially **Hodgkin's disease**) and **breast, lung,** and **stomach cancer.**
4. **Hematologic disorders. Polycythemia vera** (and the other myeloproliferative disorders) and **iron deficiency anemia** can cause pruritus.
5. **Endocrine disorders** (e.g., diabetes mellitus, hyperthyroidism and hypothyroidism, carcinoid syndrome) can cause pruritus.

III. APPROACH TO THE PATIENT

A. Patient history. A detailed history focusing on medications; other medical conditions; travel; hobbies; occupation; and

MNEMONIC **Most Common Causes of Pruritus ("ITCHED")**

Infestation (e.g., scabies)
Total bilirubin elevation (e.g., primary biliary cirrhosis)
Chronic renal failure (uremia) or **C**ancer
Hematologic disorders
Endocrine disorders
Dermatologic disorders

the presence of constitutional symptoms (e.g., weight loss, fever) is very useful.

1. The itching associated with **Hodgkin's disease** is often described as a "burning" sensation, especially on the lower extremities.
2. Patients with **scabies** usually describe worsening of their pruritus at night.
3. **Polycythemia vera** is often associated with a "prickly" itch that usually occurs as the patient cools off after bathing.
4. **Xerosis** is common in the elderly, especially when the heater is turned on during the winter months.

B. Physical examination

1. A thorough dermatologic examination, focusing on the presence of burrows (due to scabies), plate-like scaling (due to xerosis), and other lesions that will aid in the diagnosis should be performed.
2. If no obvious skin cause is found, examination of the abdomen (to look for hepatosplenomegaly) and the peripheral lymph nodes is necessary.

C. Diagnostic tests. If the history and physical examination fail to reveal the likely cause of the patient's pruritus, then blood tests [e.g., a **complete blood count** (CBC) with platelets, **bilirubin, alkaline phosphatase, thyroid-stimulating hormone** (TSH), and **creatinine** levels] and a **chest radiograph** should be considered. Biopsy of the skin should also be considered for patients with persistent symptoms without an obvious cause.

IV. TREATMENT of the specific cause is, of course, the optimal management.

A. Discontinue medications, if possible, that may cause the release of histamine (e.g., opiates, nonsteroidal anti-inflammatory drugs).

B. Consider antihistamines. Hydroxyzine (25–50 mg orally every 4–6 hours) or loratadine (10 mg orally daily) may provide symptomatic relief.

C. If the cause of the pruritus is not evident, try **empirically treating for xerosis** with a 2-week course of emollients (e.g., Aquaphor) and the use of a mild soap (e.g., Dove).

REFERENCES

Bergasa N. Update on the treatment of the pruritus of cholestasis. Clin Liver Dis 2008;12:219–234.

Braun M, Lowitt MH. Pruritus. Adv Dermatol 2001;17:1–27.

Narita I, Iguchi S, Omori K, et al. Uremic pruritus in chronic hemodialysis patients. J Nephrol 2008;21:161–165.

Clubbing

I. INTRODUCTION. A curious relationship exists between certain systemic disorders and the shape of the fingertips: some diseases cause the tips of the phalanges to become enlarged, or "clubbed."

A. Clubbing is a bulbous enlargement of the connective tissue in the distal phalanges of the fingers and toes.

B. Hypertrophic osteoarthropathy is a more advanced stage of clubbing that is characterized by:

1. Periosteal new bone formation (especially of the long bones)
2. Symmetric arthritis-like changes in various joints
3. Neurovascular changes of the hands and feet (leading to paresthesias, erythema, or sweating)
4. Excess vascular endothelial growth factor release is hypothesized to be the etiologic agent of clubbing.

II. CLINICAL MANIFESTATIONS OF CLUBBING

A. The **thumb** and **index finger** are typically affected first.

B. Clubbing is **usually symmetric;** however, it may be unilateral in certain vascular disorders (e.g., aortic arch anomalies, subclavian artery aneurysms, patent ductus arteriosus).

C. Clubbing is usually a **gradual, painless process;** however, some patients will complain of a **dull aching** in the fingertips. In general, there are **three stages** in clubbing:

1. During the initial stage, the most difficult stage to appreciate, the nail bed becomes spongy.

The best way to assess whether a patient's nail bed is spongy is to compare it with your own nail of the same finger.

2. During the next stage, the angle made by the nail and the dorsum of the distal phalanx increases (when viewed from the side). Normally, this angle is less than 180°, but in patients with clubbed fingers, the angle exceeds 180°. **Schamroth's sign** can be helpful in confirming this increased angle. In patients without clubbing, when the

dorsal surfaces of distal digits of similar fingers are placed together, a diamond-shaped opening appears at the bases of the nails. Schamroth noted that in patients who have mild clubbing, this opening is obliterated.

3. During the final stage, the overall shape of the digit is visibly altered.

III. COMMON CAUSES OF CLUBBING

A. Acquired

1. **Pulmonary disease.** Approximately 75% of patients with acquired clubbing have pulmonary disease.
   a. **Lung abscess**
   b. **Bronchiectasis**
   c. **Cancer** (usually primary lung cancer)
2. **Cardiac disease.** Approximately 10% of patients with acquired clubbing have cardiac disease.
   a. **Congenital cyanotic heart disease**
   b. **Subacute bacterial endocarditis**
3. **Gastrointestinal disease.** Approximately 10% of patients with acquired clubbing have gastrointestinal disease.
   a. **Inflammatory bowel disease**
   b. **Cirrhosis**
   c. **Colon** or **esophageal cancer**
4. **Miscellaneous causes**
   a. **Hyperthyroidism**
   b. **Hemoglobinopathies**
   c. **Local vascular diseases** (leading to unilateral clubbing)

B. Hereditary. Clubbing caused by hereditary factors is indistinguishable morphologically from clubbing caused by acquired disease. However, hereditary clubbing generally **develops during childhood** and persists for life. There is usually a family history of clubbing.

Patients of African-American descent may also exhibit mild clubbing unrelated to any pathologic process.

IV. APPROACH TO THE PATIENT.

For patients with **acquired clubbing,** an exhaustive search for the underlying causes is unnecessary; however, looking for potentially treatable and reversible diseases is worthwhile. If the patient gives a history compatible with hereditary clubbing, no further evaluation is usually necessary.

A. Patient history. The history should focus on eliciting information about pulmonary symptoms; constitutional symptoms (e.g., fever, weight loss, night sweats); signs (e.g., bloody diarrhea, jaundice, nervousness, tremulousness); alcohol and tobacco use; and family history.

B. Physical examination. The examination should be focused on finding evidence of pulmonary, cardiac, gastrointestinal, or thyroid disease.

C. Diagnostic tests. A complete blood count (CBC), a chest radiograph, an electrocardiogram (ECG), blood gas analysis, serum thyroid-stimulating hormone (TSH) levels, and stool samples (to search for occult blood) may be useful. Additional tests may also be necessary.

V. TREATMENT usually entails treatment of the underlying cause and pain relief with nonsteroidal anti-inflammatory medications if necessary. Preliminary studies have suggested that bisphosphonates may also be helpful in refractory pain.

REFERENCES

Dickenson, CJ. The aetiology of clubbing and hypertrophic osteoarthropathy. Eur J Clin Invest 1993;23(6):330–338 [Classic article].

Marrie T, Brown N. Clubbing of the digits. Am J Med 2007;120:940–941.

Martinez-Lavin M, Vargas A, Rivera-Vinas M. Hypertrophic osteoarthropathy: a palindrome with a pathogenic connotation. Curr Opin Rheumatol 2008;20:88–91.

Myers KA, Farquhar DR. The rational clinical examination. Does this patient have clubbing?. JAMA 2001;286(3):341–347 [Classic article].

Alcohol Intoxication and Withdrawal

I. INTRODUCTION. Alcohol use is important to consider in hospitalized patients for many reasons.

A. Although modest alcohol intake (i.e., up to one 14-g drink daily) may have cardioprotective effects, heavier use contributes to multiple medical conditions including hypertension, cardiomyopathy, cardiac arrhythmias, encephalopathy, peptic ulcer disease, pancreatitis, cirrhosis, and nutritional deficiency.

B. Alcohol has a potent immunosuppressive effect. Its use increases the frequency and mortality of infectious diseases such as bacterial pneumonia.

C. As opposed to patients withdrawing from opiates, patients with severe alcohol withdrawal (delirium tremens) are at a significant risk of death if not treated properly.

II. ALCOHOL INTOXICATION. Tolerance occurs with chronic alcohol consumption. Thus, higher serum alcohol levels are needed to cause intoxication in long-term, heavy drinkers compared with first-time drinkers.

A. Clinical manifestations of alcohol intoxication. Alcohol is a central nervous system (CNS) depressant. Alcohol intoxication results in a wide variety of responses that may include slurred speech, euphoria, disinhibition, uncontrolled mood swings, violence, nausea, ataxia, stupor, altered mental status, and respiratory depression.

B. Approach to the patient

1. **Supportive care.** The clinical approach depends on the degree of CNS and respiratory depression. Supportive care may mean as little as observation until the patient is clinically sober or as much as intubation in a comatose patient if he or she is unable to protect his or her airway. The cervical spine should be protected if there is any history of trauma. Physical restraints should be used cautiously and only with frequent re-evaluation. Chemical restraints may worsen respiratory depression but may be necessary to prevent further harm to the patient as well as health care providers.

2. **Glucose.** Due to liver dysfunction, alcohol use without glucose intake may result in hypoglycemia. Rapid blood glucose assessment should be undertaken in all acutely intoxicated patients with altered mental status.
3. A **blood alcohol level** (BAL) of 500 mg/dl is fatal to 50% of adults. Tolerant individuals may, however, present with significantly higher levels. An altered mental status with a low alcohol level or one that fails to improve with time should prompt further evaluation, which may include a head computed tomography (CT) scan, lumbar puncture, or further toxicologic assessment (see Chapter 82).
4. Toxic alcohol ingestion (e.g., methanol or ethylene glycol) should always be considered if an anion gap acidosis (see Chapter 42) is accompanied by an osmolar gap.
5. Patients with isolated alcohol intoxication typically do not require admission to the hospital unless they have a comorbid condition or develop concerning signs of moderate to severe withdrawal. Those with evidence of mild withdrawal can potentially be treated as outpatients with the appropriate medications.

III. ALCOHOL WITHDRAWAL

A. Pathogenesis. Alcoholics may drink continually to avoid the discomfort of alcohol withdrawal. As physiologic tolerance develops, more alcohol is needed to avoid withdrawal. When something occurs to keep the alcoholic from drinking, such as an illness or hospitalization, withdrawal may develop.

B. Clinical manifestations of alcohol withdrawal. As the blood alcohol level decreases, symptoms and signs develop that are generally opposite in nature to the primary CNS depressant effects of the drug (i.e., generalized CNS arousal and hyperactivity). In chronic alcoholics, symptoms of withdrawal usually begin well before the BAL is zero. There are **four alcohol withdrawal syndromes** that may have differing time courses and clinical manifestations; however, substantial overlap may occur. If only one sign of withdrawal appears, consider other diagnoses.

1. **"The shakes."** Symptoms may appear within 3–12 hours of the patient's last drink. Early symptoms include jitters or shakes, an intense craving for alcohol, anxiety, weakness, diaphoresis, nausea, and myalgias. The patient is often agitated, irritable, and hypervigilant. Common signs also include tachycardia, hypertension, and a coarse tremor of the hands or tongue.
2. **Seizures.** Withdrawal seizures are typically diffuse tonic-clonic seizures that peak 12–24 hours after the patient's last drink. Single seizures occur 50% of the time, with short bursts being most common when multiple seizures

occur. The postictal period is often short, and status epilepticus is rare. Many alcoholics, however, have other reasons for seizing, and it is important to look for these, especially if the patient is febrile, has head trauma, has prolonged seizure activity, or if the seizures begin more than 48 hours after the last drink.

3. **Hallucinations.** Hallucinations are classically visual or tactile (e.g., bugs crawling on the wall), but can be auditory. Patients may become fearful or paranoid, which may further increase agitation. Hallucinations typically occur 24–48 hours after the last drink.
4. **Delirium tremens** is characterized by hallucinations, profound confusion, diaphoresis, fever, and tachycardia. Typically, delirium tremens begin 2–3 days after the patient's last drink, peak on day 4, and may last 1–2 weeks. If not treated appropriately, DT's can be fatal.
5. **Other illnesses** to consider in the setting of the autonomic hyperactivity that defines alcohol withdrawal are sepsis, thyrotoxicosis, heat stroke, hypoglycemia, intracranial hemorrhage, and cocaine intoxication.

When managing a patient who appears to be withdrawing from alcohol, always ask yourself: is this patient septic?

C. Approach to the patient

1. Alleviate withdrawal symptoms.
   a. **Supportive measures.** Keep the patient in a quiet room. Restraining the patient may worsen paranoia and agitation. Restraints should be used only when necessary. The patient's status must be monitored frequently for changes in vital signs as well as neurologic function.
   b. **Pharmacologic therapy**
      (1) **Benzodiazepines** are the drugs of choice. They, like alcohol, act at the γ-aminobutyric acid (GABA) receptor to sedate the patient. Lorazepam (1–2 mg intravenously every 30 minutes until symptoms resolve) is the preferred agent, especially in the elderly, because of its short half-life and fast onset of action. The **barbiturate** phenobarbital is another possibility. If outpatient treatment is desired, lorazepam, diazepam, phenobarbital, or chlordiazepoxide may be used in a tapering dose over 3–5 days.
      (2) **β-blockers** and **central α_2 agonists** (e.g., clonidine) block the hypertension and tachycardia of withdrawal but should not be used alone as therapy as they do not

treat the underlying autonomic derangement, thus potentially masking delirium tremens.

(3) **Phenytoin** should be used only to treat seizures *not* entirely attributable to alcohol.

2. **Correct metabolic deficiencies.**
   a. **Fluid deficit** should be replaced initially with normal saline, with appropriate adjustment in volume for renal insufficiency or heart failure.
   b. **Thiamine** (100 mg intravenously) should be administered before infusing glucose to prevent the development of Wernicke's encephalopathy. Other vitamins, including folic acid, can also be given.
   c. **Glucose** may be infused as 50% dextrose or as part of the intravenous fluid rehydration [D5 normal saline (D5NS)], or as a good meal.
   d. **Potassium, magnesium,** and **phosphorus** tend to be low in chronic alcoholics and should be repleted.
   e. **Vitamin K** may be administered if the prothrombin time (PT) is prolonged.
3. **Manage associated medical conditions.** Perform a complete history and physical examination to look for associated medical conditions and to rule out other causes of altered mental status and autonomic hyperactivity. A head CT, chest radiograph, and lumbar puncture are often necessary in patients with fever, persistent altered mental status, seizures, or abnormal neurologic examination findings.
4. **Attempt rehabilitation.** The patient should be referred to an alcohol rehabilitation center, Alcoholics Anonymous, or an outpatient mental health center.

IV. ALCOHOLISM. Alcohol plays a roll in over 100,000 deaths and costs the U.S. economy approximately $170 billion annually. Every $1 invested in treatment saves an estimated $7. Men at risk for alcohol abuse are defined as individuals consuming 14 drinks per week or 4 drinks per occasion. Women at risk are those consuming 7 drinks per week or 3 drinks per occasion.

A. Detection. Screening recommendations include asking patients about whether they drink beer, wine, liquor, or distilled spirits. The CAGE questions—In the last 12 months, have you ever felt that you should ***c***ut down on your drinking? Have people ever ***a***nnoyed you by criticizing your drinking? Have you ever felt bad or ***g***uilty about your drinking? Have you ever had a drink first thing in the morning to steady your nerves or get rid of a hangover (an ***e***ye-opener)?—have a sensitivity of 75% and specificity of 88% for at-risk drinkers when one or more responses are positive for women and two or more are positive for men.

B. Approach to the patient

1. **Brief negotiated interview (BNI).** The BNI is a short method by which the practitioner attempts to facilitate awareness and change in the drinker. The process consists of **five steps.**
   a. Establish rapport with the patient.
   b. Ask the patient's permission and then discuss the pros and cons of alcohol use.
   c. Summarize what the patient has said.
   d. Ask the patient to describe (e.g., from 1 to 10) his or her readiness to change.
   e. Negotiate with the patient based on the perception of readiness. If the patient is ready, approaches to quitting might be brainstormed; if the patient is unsure, then pros and cons might be further explored.
2. **Medications** used in alcohol treatment include disulfiram (Antabuse), which induces symptoms of a hangover when patients drink alcohol, and naltrexone, which curbs the urge to drink.
3. In all cases, the patient should be provided a list of **resources and referrals.** If the patient is ready to accept referral, a hospital staff member may be able to assist in arranging an appointment or entry into a treatment program.

V. ALCOHOLIC KETOACIDOSIS (AKA)

A. Pathogenesis. AKA typically occurs after a period of heavy drinking associated with "relative starvation" when vomiting or limited food intake has reduced the amount of glucose available for metabolism. In response, the body produces ketones as an alternative source of energy.

B. Clinical manifestations. No physical findings point definitively to AKA. Most commonly, patients complain of nausea, vomiting, and abdominal pain and are found to be tachycardic and tachypneic, with mild, diffuse abdominal tenderness. An **increased anion gap** must be present to diagnose AKA. Other simultaneous conditions such as fever or contraction alkalosis may produce a mixed acid-base disorder and thus may mask acidosis. Testing urine for **ketosis** may be of limited value as β-hydroxybutyrate, which most urine dipsticks do not demonstrate, is far more abundant than acetoacetate. **Blood glucose** is often slightly elevated but less than 300 mg/dl.

C. Approach to the patient

1. **Fluid rehydration and glucose administration.** Patients typically are not hyperosmolar, and fluid resuscitation can be undertaken with less concern for cerebral edema than exists with diabetic ketoacidosis. Typically, normal saline containing dextrose (D5NS) can be used to replete volume

and promote endogenous insulin secretion, thus inhibiting ketogenesis.

2. **Repletion of vitamins and electrolytes.** Thiamine (100 mg) should be given before glucose-containing fluids. A multivitamin may be needed, and magnesium, potassium, or phosphorous repletion may be indicated.
3. **Search for concurrent illness.** The development of AKA may be associated with an underlying illness that led the patient to stop drinking. Pancreatitis, gastrointestinal bleeding, withdrawal, and infection should all be considered.

REFERENCES

McGuire LC, Cruickshank AM, Munro PT. Alcoholic ketoacidosis. Emerg Med J 2006;23:417–420.

McKeon A, Frye MA, Delanty N. The alcohol withdrawal syndrome. J Neurol Neurosurg Psychiatry 2008;79:854–862.

The National Institutes of Health National Institute on Alcohol Abuse and Alcoholism. http://www.niaaa.nih.gov

94 Toxicologic Emergencies

I. INTRODUCTION. Drug overdose is common in medical practice and, if not managed expediently and appropriately, can be lethal. Over 4,000,000 poisonings were estimated to have occurred in the United States in 2006, accounting for more than 1200 deaths. Analgesics (acetaminophen and aspirin), antidepressants, stimulants (including many street drugs), opioids, and cardiovascular medications are the most commonly fatal classes of medication.

II. GENERAL APPROACH TO THE OVERDOSE PATIENT

A. ABCs. Initial attention should focus on **a**irway, **b**reathing, and **c**irculatory system management. Intravenous catheterization, supplemental oxygen, and cardiac monitoring are usually required. Serial monitoring of vital signs and respiratory and mental status allows one to follow the progress of intoxication.

B. Patient history. The patient history is of critical importance and should be obtained from the patient, friends, caregivers, and paramedics. Pill counts and attention to empty bottles found at the site are useful.

C. Physical examination. Areas of focus include the patient's vital signs with pulse oximetry, mental status, pupillary size and responsiveness, skin moisture, and bowel sounds. Table 94-1 summarizes physical examination findings for four of the major types of overdoses.

D. Testing

1. **Electrocardiography.** An electrocardiogram (ECG) is indicated for all patients with ingestion to rule out any potential cardiac effects of ingested drugs. Particularly notable are dysrhythmias and widening of the QRS.
2. **A chest radiograph, complete blood count (CBC), serum electrolytes, blood glucose,** and **renal panel** are useful for evaluating possible concomitant disease or toxicologic effects.
3. **Drug levels** and **toxicologic screens.** Drug-specific urine and serum analysis may be useful in the management of ingestion patients. A positive qualitative urinalysis screen, which can remain positive for days and provides no quantitative information, should not be relied on to explain a change in mental status. Most commonly, serum acetaminophen and salicylate levels are requested when an

TABLE 94-1

CLINICAL MANIFESTATIONS OF COMMON OVERDOSES

Type of Overdose	Vital Signs	Mental Status	Pupils	Bowel Sounds
Opioid	↓ RR, ↓ BP	Varies from euphoria to obtundation	Constricted	Decreased
Adrenergic agonist (stimulant)	↑ HR, ↑ RR, ↑ BP	Hypervigilance	Dilated	Variable
Cholinergic agonist	↓ HR	Restless, confused	Constricted	Increased
Cholinergic antagonist*	↑ HR, ↑ temperature	Irritability, delusions	Dilated	Decreased

BP = blood pressure; *HR* = heart rate; *RR* = respiratory rate.
*In patients with clinical manifestations of an anticholinergic syndrome, tricyclic overdose should be considered.

unknown ingestion has occurred, but a more extensive serum analysis can be performed if clinically indicated.

E. Gut decontamination

1. **Activated charcoal** (50 g by mouth or nasogastric tube, typically with sorbitol) is the preferred agent for limiting absorption of acute ingestions. It works best when **given within 1 hour of ingestion.** It should never be given to a patient who cannot protect his or her airway unless that patient is intubated, as aspiration of charcoal can have dire pulmonary consequences. Some toxins (e.g., theophylline, carbamazepine, phenobarbital) may require multiple intermittent doses of activated charcoal.
2. **Gastric lavage** has no clear evidence supporting a clinical benefit, has concerning risks including aspiration and esophageal injury, and should only be considered within 1 hour of a massive or life-threatening ingestion.
3. **Emetics** (e.g., syrup of ipecac) are of no benefit compared with activated charcoal alone and are best **avoided.**
4. **Whole bowel irrigation** with polyethylene glycol (2 L/hr until stools run clear) may be indicated for some ingestions such as iron, lithium, or sustained-release preparations.

F. Antidotes. The first goal in clinical toxicology is treating the patient symptomatically, providing respiratory and cardiovascular support as needed. There are occasions, however, when an antidote may be both indicated and available [e.g., N-acetylcysteine in the setting of acetaminophen overdose, glucagon for β-blocker overdose, or digoxin Fab (Digibind) for digoxin overdose].

III. SPECIFIC TOXIC SYNDROMES ("TOXIDROMES")

A. Opioid receptor agonists include **morphine** and related narcotic substances such as heroin and oxycodone. Acute toxicity can result from both clinical overdose in the hospitalized patient and accidental overdose in the intravenous drug user.

1. **Clinical manifestations of opioid overdose.** These patients are typically lethargic and have constricted pupils. There may be needle marks or other paraphernalia suggesting intravenous drug use. A memory aid for the opioid toxidrome may be derived from the street term for heroin, "DOPE."

MNEMONIC **Clinical Manifestations of Opioid Agonist Overdose ("DOPE")**

Decreased respiratory drive
Obtundation
Pinpoint pupils
Euphoria

2. **Major concerns**
   a. **Respiratory depression** is the major clinical concern and may lead to hypoventilation, hypoxemia, and death. In the setting of persistent hypoxemia, consider noncardiogenic pulmonary edema. **Seizures** may occur with some opioid compounds including meperidine.
   b. **Hypotension** may also complicate opioid overdose.
3. **Treatment.** The establishment of a patent airway and adequate ventilation are critical first steps. The opioid antagonist **naloxone** (0.2–2 mg intravenously repeated every 2–3 minutes if no response, up to a total dose of 10–20 mg; lasts 20–60 minutes) may produce dramatic reversal of some of the acute symptoms of opioid overdose including respiratory depression. However, the effects of the opioid often outlast the effects of naloxone, mandating frequent monitoring and repeat naloxone doses in some patients.

B. Stimulants include **cocaine** and **amphetamines** (e.g., **ecstasy, speed**).

1. **Clinical manifestations of stimulant overdose.** The clinical syndrome results primarily from stimulation of adrenergic receptors, leading to tachypnea, tachycardia, vasoconstriction, and psychostimulation including hyperactivity.
2. **Major concerns** include **tachycardia**, **hypertension,** and **vasospasm of the coronary arteries.** The last may lead to myocardial infarction even with otherwise normal coronary arteries.
3. **Treatment** in the acute setting is primarily supportive.

a. **Benzodiazepines** reduce agitation and often effectively treat hypertension and tachycardia. Persistent hypertension may be treated with a peripheral vasodilator such as nitroprusside.
b. **Chest pain** should be treated as any acute coronary syndrome with aspirin, nitrates, and oxygen. Benzodiazepine use should be liberal, but **β-blockers should be avoided in cocaine toxicity** as they may generate unopposed α-adrenergic effects and actually worsen hypertension.

C. Cholinergic agonists. Organophosphate and carbamate **insecticides** inhibit acetylcholinesterase and are a common cause of a pure cholinergic syndrome. They may be ingested, inhaled, or absorbed through the skin. The resulting toxidrome is primarily seen in farm workers. The chemical warfare agents Sarin and VX work through the same mechanism.

1. **Clinical manifestations of cholinergic agonist toxicity** typically begin within 1–2 hours. Sustained stimulation of acetylcholine (ACh) receptors causes muscarinic effects (nausea, vomiting, urinary incontinence, diarrhea, sweating, bradycardia); nicotinic effects (tremor, respiratory muscle paralysis); and central nervous system (CNS) effects (agitation to seizure or coma). Many of the important features can be remembered using the mnemonic "SLUDGE."

MNEMONIC **Clinical Manifestations of Cholinergic Agonist Toxicity ("SLUDGE")**

Salivation
Lacrimation
Urination
Defecation
Gastrointestinal upset
Emesis

2. **Major concerns** include **respiratory muscle paralysis** with subsequent **hypoxemia, bronchospasm, seizures,** and **hypotension** secondary to **dehydration.**
3. **Treatment**
   a. **Supportive measures.** Contaminated clothing should be removed and the patient washed thoroughly with soapy water. Respiration and blood pressure should be maintained. Intubation may be needed. Benzodiazepines should be given for seizures.
   b. **Atropine,** repeated frequently, is administered to block the action of ACh at the receptor until oral secretions are controlled.

c. **Pralidoxime (2-PAM)** is the specific antidote to organophosphates, reversing effects at all receptors. Ideally, it is given within 24–36 hours.

D. **Anticholinergic agents** antagonize the activity of ACh at muscarinic and CNS receptors. Many common drugs including atropine, antihistamines, phenothiazines, and tricyclic antidepressants produce anticholinergic effects. Exposure to deadly nightshade (*Atropa belladonna*) or jimsonweed may also cause toxicity.

1. **Clinical manifestations of cholinergic antagonist toxicity** include the following:
   a. Restlessness, irritability, and delusions ("mad as a hatter")
   b. Dilation of cutaneous blood vessels ("red as a beet")
   c. Decreased apocrine and salivary gland secretion, most easily checked at the axilla ("dry as a bone")
   d. Mydriasis and cycloplegia ("blind as a bat")
   e. Tachycardia ("fast as a rabbit")
   f. Decreased gastrointestinal motility with decreased bowel sounds ("slow as a mule")
   g. Increased bladder sphincter tone ("tight as a drum")
2. **Treatment**
   a. **Supportive treatment.** Respiratory and circulatory support may be necessary. Cardiac monitoring will provide warning of arrhythmias. Benzodiazepines can be used for agitation.
   b. **Decontamination** with activated charcoal is appropriate. Hemodialysis and hemoperfusion are not effective.
   c. **Physostigmine** may be used in the setting of pure anticholinergic toxicity, but it carries the risks of cardiac arrhythmias and seizures, and should only be used for severe toxicity.

E. **Acetaminophen** is the most commonly reported drug overdose.

1. **Clinical manifestations** of acetaminophen toxicity can be divided into four stages.
   a. In the first 24 hours, patients may be asymptomatic or have mild nausea and malaise.
   b. From 24–48 hours, hepatic necrosis begins and patients develop right upper quadrant pain and tenderness, as well as transaminitis.
   c. Fulminant hepatic failure with coagulopathy and encephalopathy occurs by days 3–4.
   d. Recovery, if the patient survives, takes place over the ensuing week.
2. **Treatment** is based on acetaminophen serum levels with the first level drawn at 4 hours after ingestion.

a. **N-acetylcysteine (NAC)** works by replenishing glutathione, an essential component in the metabolism of acetaminophen. It is best given early but has beneficial effects out to 24 hours from ingestion, and possibly longer.
b. **Supportive care** includes monitoring for coagulopathy, renal failure, and hepatic encephalopathy. These may indicate a need for liver transplantation.
c. **Activated charcoal** should be given for decontamination, if the patient is awake and compliant.

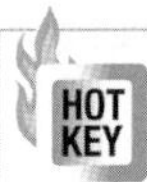

When given within 8 hours of acetaminophen ingestion, NAC will completely prevent hepatic failure.

F. Salicylate is most commonly found in **aspirin** but is also contained in many topical preparations.
1. **Clinical manifestations** are numerous.
   a. **Respiratory alkalosis** occurs secondary to direct stimulation of the respiratory centers of the brain.
   b. **Anion gap metabolic acidosis** can lead to a compensatory respiratory alkalosis.
   c. **Tinnitus** may occur either with acute or chronic ingestions.
   d. Arrhythmias, pulmonary edema, coma, seizures, and acute renal failure may also occur.
2. **Treatment** must be instituted early for maximal benefit.
   a. **Sodium bicarbonate** aids with elimination of salicylate in the urine and should be given to maintain a urine pH of 7.5–8.
   b. **Dialysis** is effective when levels are greater than 100 mg/dl in acute ingestions, or with severe acidosis or toxic effects.

G. Tricyclic antidepressants (TCAs)
1. **Clinical manifestations**. TCA overdose may produce any of **three syndromes.** Symptoms often begin within 30 minutes of ingestion.
   a. **Anticholinergic effects** include dry skin, dilated pupils, urinary retention, tachycardia, and myoclonic jerking.
   b. **Cardiovascular effects** result from both TCA blockade of the myocardial fast sodium channel (similar to a type Ia antiarrhythmic) and blockade of α_1-adrenergic receptors. Effects include decreased myocardial contractility, bradycardia, and hypotension.
   c. **Seizures** may result in rhabdomyolysis, brain damage, and death.
2. **Approach to the patient.** Rapid diagnosis is imperative and is made on the basis of the patient history; physical

examination findings; and ECG findings (e.g., QRS prolongation > 100 ms, R wave in avR, rightward shift of the terminal 40 ms of the QRS complex).

3. **Treatment**
   a. **Supportive measures** include supporting respiration and circulation as needed.
   b. **Activated charcoal** should be given for gut decontamination. Hemoperfusion and hemodialysis are ineffective.
   c. **Seizures** should be treated with benzodiazepines.
   d. **Cardiac effects** as demonstrated by hypotension or QRS prolongation may be reversed through **sodium bicarbonate** infusion with a goal serum pH of 7.45–7.55.

H. Phenothiazines include both antipsychotics (clozapine, haloperidol) and antiemetics (prochlorperazine, promethazine).

1. **Clinical manifestations of phenothiazine overdose.** Like tricyclic antidepressants, phenothiazines have multiple pharmacologic effects and produce a similar clinical syndrome.
   a. At low doses, **anticholinergic effects** may predominate including dry mouth, tachycardia, and urinary retention.
   b. **Cardiac effects** may include QRS or QT interval prolongation.
   c. **Extrapyramidal dystonic effects** from dopamine receptor antagonism include torticollis, jaw muscle spasm, and oculogyric crisis. Akathisia is a condition of motor restlessness.
   d. **Neuroleptic malignant syndrome (NMS)** is an idiosyncratic and occasionally fatal reaction comprising lead-pipe rigidity, altered mental status, and autonomic instability including high fever, diaphoresis, and tachycardia.
2. **Treatment**
   a. **Supportive care** includes respiratory and cardiovascular support as well as cooling of fever.
   b. Decontamination with **multiple-dose activated charcoal** may be beneficial.
   c. **Diphenhydramine** can be used to treat dystonic reactions.
   d. **Benzodiazepines** can be used to treat seizures and musculoskeletal rigidity.
   e. **Dantrolene,** a skeletal muscle relaxant, and **bromocriptine** can be used in the management of NMS.

REFERENCES

The American Association of Poison Control Centers. http://www.aapcc.org

Erickson TB, Thompson TM, Lu JJ. The approach to the patient with an unknown overdose. Emerg Med Clin North Am 2007;25:249–281.

Greene S, Harris C, Singer J. Gastrointestinal decontamination of the poisoned patient. Pediatr Emerg Care 2008;24:176–186.

Appendix: Procedures

Procedures are an essential part of taking care of a patient. This section provides an overview of the most common procedures a clinician is likely to perform as a student or house officer. Table A-1 describes some essential steps that apply to the majority of the procedures described in this section.

I THORACENTESIS

A. Definition: removal of pleural fluid

B. Indications

1. **Diagnostic:** to determine the etiology of a pleural effusion
2. **Therapeutic:** to relieve dyspnea due to a pleural effusion

C. Contraindications: none (but a coagulopathy or severe thrombocytopenia should ideally be corrected prior to the procedure)

D. Complications: pneumothorax, hemothorax

E. Before the procedure

1. Obtain decubitus chest radiographs to confirm that fluid is free-flowing (i.e., forms a layer along the lateral chest wall).
2. Consider ultrasound localization of the pleural fluid.

F. Patient positioning: seated at the edge of the bed, with arms resting on a bedside table

G. Locating the point of entry

1. Identify the highest point of the effusion by percussion and move one or two interspaces below.
2. Mark the skin at the superior aspect of the inferior rib of the interspace. Use a pen or the indentation of a needle hub.
3. Alternatively, mark the location of the pleural effusion with ultrasound guidance.

H. Technique

1. Clean the entry point with povidone-iodine solution.
2. Palpate the superior aspect of the inferior rib of the previously marked interspace.
3. Anesthetize the skin at the mark with 1% lidocaine, using a 25-gauge needle.
4. Anesthetize the subcutaneous tissue and the periosteum of the rib's superior aspect using a 22-gauge needle. Note

TABLE A-1

ESSENTIAL STEPS TO CONSIDER WHILE PERFORMING PROCEDURES

Before the Procedure

Obtain informed consent from the patient.
Inform the nurse of the procedure and enlist his or her assistance.
Prepare all equipment. An extra set of equipment is often helpful.
Remove your pager, stethoscope, and "lab" coat; sign out pager if necessary.
Comfortably position yourself and the patient.
Always wash hands and observe universal precautions.
Wear a mask for all procedures.
Review procedure technique and pertinent anatomy.

After the Procedure

Dispose of all sharps in the sharps container.
Carry important or hard-to-obtain specimens to the laboratory yourself.
Write a procedure note, including the procedure name and indication, a one-line description of the procedure, any medications used (e.g., lidocaine), any complications, and follow-up studies ordered.
Always wash hands after a procedure.

that the planned trajectory is *above* the rib, avoiding the neurovascular bundle that courses *below* the rib.

5. Advance the needle over the rib while withdrawing. Inject anesthetic if there is no return of fluid. Appearance of pleural fluid in the syringe signifies entry into the pleural space (i.e., between the visceral and parietal pleura).
6. Remove the needle, noting the site of insertion and trajectory.
7. Insert a 14- or 16-gauge catheter-over-needle apparatus along the same path, carefully advancing over the rib.
8. Use the nondominant hand to stabilize the needle. Use the dominant hand to apply negative pressure to the syringe as you slowly advance.
9. With the return of pleural fluid into the syringe, stop advancing and withdraw 30–60 ml of fluid (for diagnostic studies). (See Figure A-1.)
10. If therapeutic drainage is anticipated, advance the catheter-over-needle apparatus slightly farther inward.
11. While maintaining the position of the syringe and needle with the dominant hand, use the nondominant hand to advance the catheter into the pleural space; then pull the needle out.
12. Quickly attach the end of the catheter to the extension tubing, which is then connected to vacuum drainage bottles. Alternatively, the catheter-over-needle apparatus

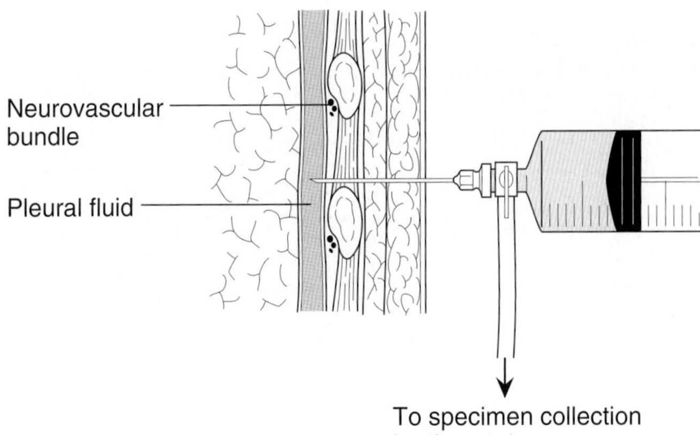

FIGURE A-1

can be attached to a three-way stopcock, initially opening to the syringe and then switching over to preattached extension tubing connected to vacuum drainage bottles. (See Figure A-2.)

13. Once the desired amount of fluid is removed, remove the catheter and quickly apply a bandage.
14. Consider performing a chest radiograph to rule out a pneumothorax. This is not always necessary if the thoracentesis has proceeded smoothly (i.e., without excessive pain or shortness of breath during fluid removal).

I. Fluid analysis (see Chapter 24)

II PARACENTESIS

A. Definition: removal of peritoneal fluid

B. Indications

1. **Diagnostic:** to determine the cause of ascites, to diagnose or exclude peritonitis
2. **Therapeutic:** to relieve abdominal pain or dyspnea due to ascites

C. Contraindications: surgical scar or hernia at the site of needle entry. Note that **coagulopathy is not a contraindication.**

D. Complications

1. Bowel perforation, persistent leakage of peritoneal fluid, abdominal wall hematoma
2. Hypotension (after large-volume paracentesis)

E. Before the procedure

1. Have the patient empty his or her bladder; alternatively, insert a Foley catheter. (This step avoids the very rare complication of puncture of the bladder.)

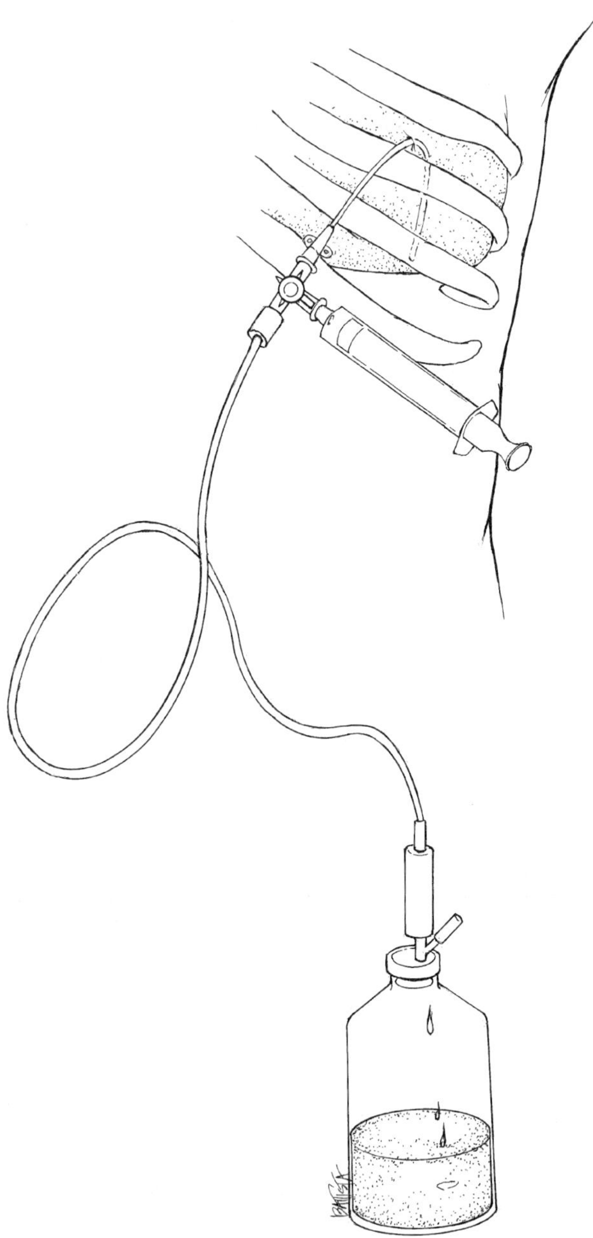

FIGURE A-2

F. Patient positioning: semi-recumbent

G. Locating the point of entry

1. Choose one of the following entry sites (the preferred site is not universally agreed on):
   a. At the midline, 2–3 cm below the umbilicus
   b. In either of the lower quadrants, lateral to the rectus abdominus muscle and below the level of the umbilicus (i.e., at the anterior superior iliac spine)
2. Localize the fluid by percussion or by ultrasound.
3. Mark the skin with a pen or the indentation of a needle hub.

H. Technique

1. Clean the entry site with povidone-iodine and apply the sterile drape.
2. Anesthetize the skin at the mark with 1% lidocaine, using a 25-gauge needle.
3. Inject additional anesthetic into the subcutaneous tissue and anterior abdominal wall.
4. Keep the needle perpendicular to the skin and aspirate while advancing, both to avoid entry into a vessel and to detect peritoneal fluid (typically straw-colored).
5. With the return of peritoneal fluid, withdraw the needle, noting the site of insertion and trajectory.
6. Choose the needle for the next puncture.
   a. For **diagnostic paracentesis:** 22-gauge 1.5-inch needle attached to a 30-ml or 60-ml syringe
   b. For **therapeutic paracentesis:** 16-gauge catheter-over-needle apparatus (or 15-gauge multihole blunt needle with removable trocar) with an attached syringe
7. For large-volume (therapeutic) paracentesis, a "Z" technique is recommended. Before insertion, pull the skin 1 inch to the side and then insert the needle. When the procedure is completed and the needle is withdrawn, the intact skin will slide back over the hole created in the abdominal wall, preventing a persistent track that can leak.
8. Slowly advance the needle along the same track. Aspirate after each small advancement. If there is no fluid (or blood), release negative pressure on the syringe and advance farther.
9. Withdraw 30–60 ml of peritoneal fluid into the syringe (for diagnostic studies).
10. After diagnostic paracentesis, withdraw the needle and apply a bandage.
11. For therapeutic paracentesis, use the nondominant hand to stabilize the catheter position, and use the dominant hand to slowly pull back and remove the syringe and attached needle.

12. Quickly attach tubing to the end of the catheter.
13. Insert the needle attached at the other end of the tubing into vacuum drainage bottles.
14. Drain up to 6 L of peritoneal fluid.
15. If fluid return decreases unexpectedly, gently manipulate the position of catheter, turn the patient, or both.
16. Once all desired fluid is removed, remove the catheter and apply a bandage.

I. Fluid analysis (see Table 32-1)

III LUMBAR PUNCTURE

A. Definition: removal of cerebrospinal fluid (CSF)

B. Indications: diagnosis of various neurologic diseases (e.g., meningitis, subarachnoid hemorrhage, tertiary syphilis)

C. Contraindications

1. Infection at the site of lumbar puncture
2. Increased intracranial pressure secondary to a mass lesion
3. Coagulopathy or platelets less than 50,000/ml

D. Complications: postprocedure headache, local hematoma (rare), infection (rare), tonsillar herniation (rare)

E. Before the procedure

1. Rule out elevated intracranial pressure with funduscopic and neurologic examinations.
2. If papilledema or a focal neurologic deficit is present, obtain a computed tomography (CT) scan of the brain to rule out a mass lesion.

F. Patient positioning

1. Lateral decubitus position, with the neck, back, hips, and knees all maximally flexed, putting the patient into the "fetal position"
2. Alternatively, the patient can be seated leaning over a bedstand. With this technique, opening pressure measurements are not accurate.

G. Locating the point of entry

1. Find the intersection of a line formed by the spinous processes and a line formed between the superior iliac crests; this marks the L3–L4 interspace. (See Figure A-3).
2. Feel between the spinous processes for the site of entry, and mark the skin here with a pen or the indentation of a needle hub.

H. Technique

1. Clean the area with povidone-iodine solution (this is often provided in the lumbar puncture tray) and then apply the sterile drape.
2. Anesthetize the skin at the mark with 1% lidocaine, using a 25-gauge needle.

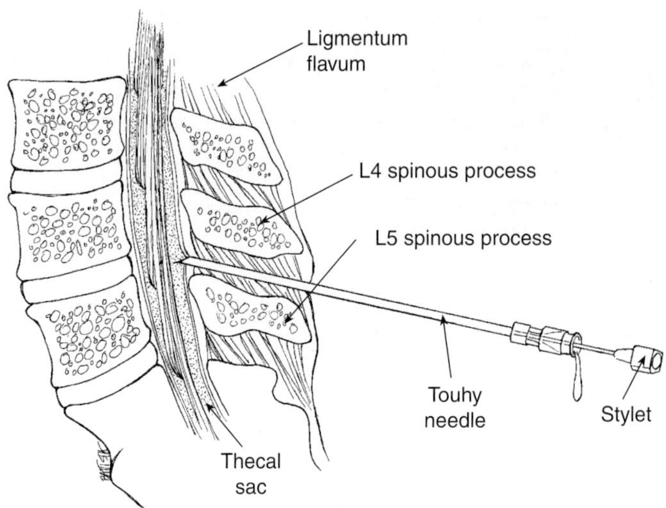

FIGURE A-3

3. Anesthetize the subcutaneous tissues with 1% lidocaine, using a 22-gauge needle, injecting in the intended track of the lumbar puncture (i.e., slightly toward the head and parallel to the midline).
4. Introduce the spinal needle (with the bevel upward, facing the ceiling) in the interspace along the same track.
5. Slowly advance the needle, frequently stopping to remove the stylet and check for the return of CSF.
6. If there is no CSF, replace the stylet and advance the needle slightly, then check again; a "pop" or giving-way is felt as the needle penetrates the dura.
7. With the return of fluid, attach the pressure manometer and measure the opening pressure. The patient must be relaxed and in the lateral decubitus position in order to obtain an accurate measurement.
8. Collect 2–3 ml in each of the four collecting tubes (see Figure A-4, bottom).
9. Replace the stylet in the needle and withdraw the needle.
10. Apply a bandage over the entry site.

I. Fluid analysis (see Chapter 88)

IV ARTHROCENTESIS

A. Definition: removal of synovial fluid from a joint

B. Indications

1. **Diagnostic:** to determine the etiology of a joint effusion or arthritis

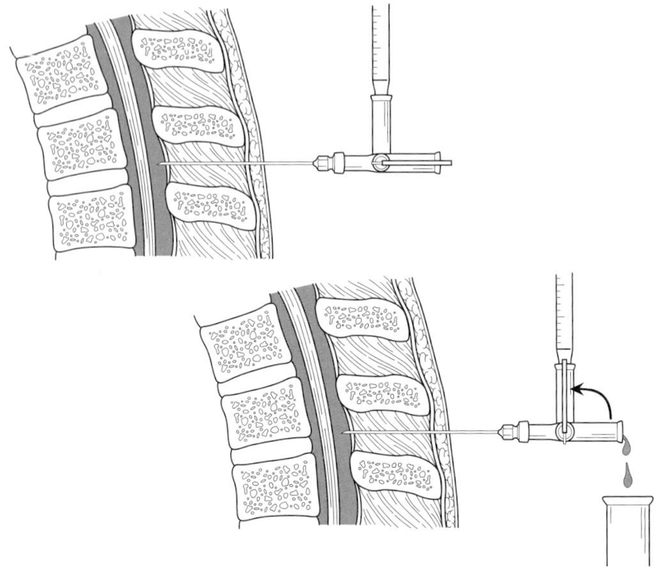

FIGURE A-4

2. **Therapeutic:** to drain large, hemorrhagic, or purulent effusions, or to inject medication into a joint

C. **Contraindications**
   1. Infection overlying the arthrocentesis site
   2. Prosthetic joint (procedure should be performed by an orthopedic surgeon)

D. **Complications:** septic joint (very rare), bleeding at injection site or into joint (very rare)

E. **Patient positioning (knee):** supine with the knee slightly flexed; place a roll under the knee

F. **Locating the point of entry (knee)**
   1. Confirm the presence of an effusion (ballottable patella, lateral or medial fluid bulge around the patella).
   2. The needle will be injected midway between the top (rostral) and bottom (caudal) of the patella, just under the inferior aspect of the patella (Figure A-5).

G. **Technique (knee)**
   1. OPTIONAL: use sterile gloves instead of standard gloves.
   2. Clean the entry point with povidone-iodine solution.
   3. OPTIONAL: anesthetize the entry site with 1% lidocaine.
   4. Advance a 1.5-inch 18-gauge needle (attached to a 30–60-ml syringe) rapidly through the entry point, directed at the center of the joint.

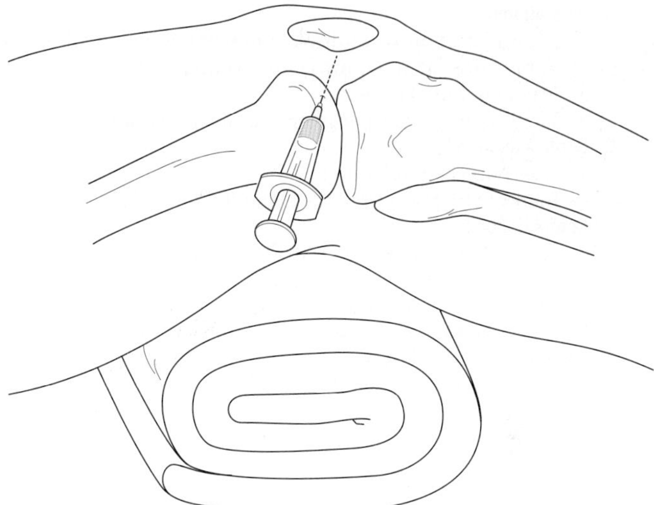

FIGURE A-5

5. Apply negative pressure on the syringe as you advance the needle.
6. Once synovial fluid enters the syringe, do not advance any farther.
7. Stabilize the position of the needle with the nondominant hand and continue to withdraw fluid by applying negative pressure on the syringe with the dominant hand.
8. To attach another syringe to either withdraw more fluid or inject a medication, secure the position of the needle with a sterile hemostat.
   a. Remove the first syringe and carefully attach a second syringe to the needle.
   b. Inject or withdraw.
9. Withdraw the needle and apply a bandage

H. Fluid analysis (see Table 74-1)

V FEMORAL LINE PLACEMENT. Femoral vein cannulation is the easiest central venous procedure to learn and perform. (Though internal jugular and subclavian vein cannulation are preferred, these procedures have important anatomic considerations and are not outlined here.)

A. Definition: catheterization of the central venous circulation via the femoral vein

B. Indications

1. Administration of multiple intravenous medications or medications that require central venous delivery
2. Frequent blood draws
3. Inability to place a peripheral intravenous catheter

C. Contraindications

1. Overlying skin infection
2. Inability to leave leg in the extended position

D. Complications

1. Arterial puncture with or without local hematoma
2. Retroperitoneal hemorrhage
3. Infection or thrombosis of the line

E. Patient positioning: recumbent

F. Locating the point of entry

1. Palpate the femoral pulse
2. Locate the point of entry into the femoral vein, 2–3 cm below the inguinal ligament and 1 cm medial to the femoral arterial pulsation (Figure A-6).
3. Alternatively, one may use bedside ultrasonographic localization of femoral artery and vein.

G. Technique

1. Sterilize the entry site and a wide field with chlorhexidine gluconate solution.
2. Anesthetize the overlying skin with 1% lidocaine using a 25-gauge needle.
3. Anesthetize the underlying subcutaneous tissue with 1% lidocaine using a 20-gauge needle.
4. With the nondominant hand palpating the femoral artery, use the dominant hand to insert an 18-gauge needle on a syringe at a 45° angle aiming cephalad and slightly medially (Figure A-7).
5. While applying negative pressure to the syringe, slowly advance the needle forward until blood enters the syringe.
6. If there is no blood return, slowly withdraw the needle, watching for a flash of blood that may occur if the vein was completely punctured on the first pass.
7. When good blood flow is achieved, maintain the position of the needle with the nondominant hand, which is braced on the patient's skin.
8. Lower the angle of the needle and aspirate to confirm good flow (i.e., that the needle remains in the vessel).
9. With the position of the needle secured with the nondominant hand, remove the syringe from the needle with the dominant hand.
10. Assess the flow of blood (via the needle), which should be dark and steady but not bright red or pulsatile (which would suggest femoral artery puncture).

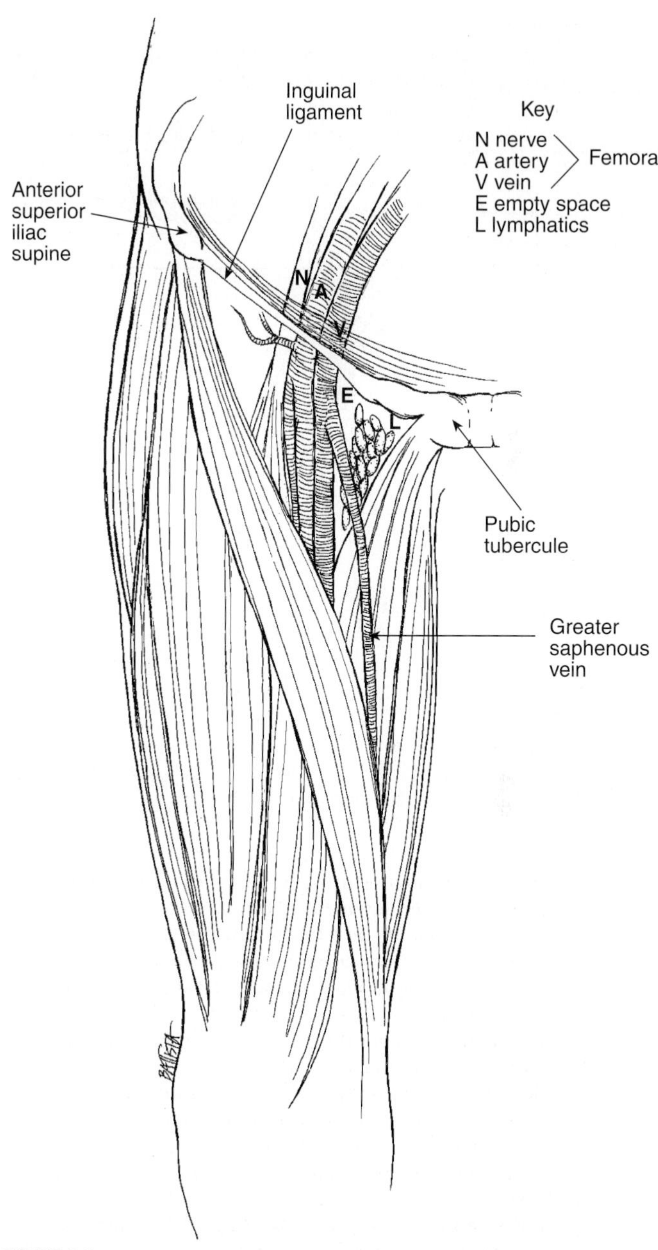
Inguinal
ligament
Key
N nerve
A artery
V vein
Femoral
E empty space
L lymphatics
Anterior
superior
iliac
supine
N
A
V
E
L
Pubic
tubercule
Greater
saphenous
vein

FIGURE A-6

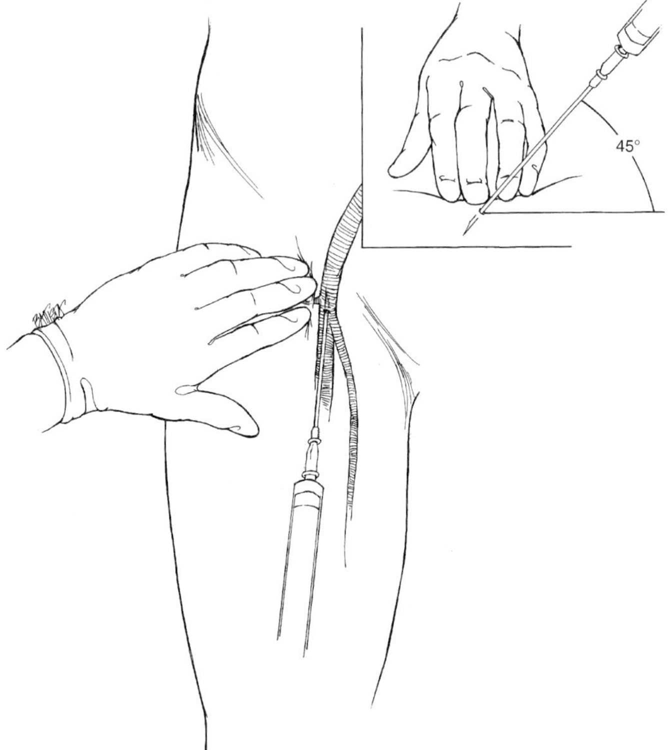

FIGURE A-7

11. Feed the guidewire through the needle. Be sure to have control of the guidewire at all times.
12. Remove the needle over the guidewire.
13. Make an incision in the skin at the entry of the guidewire. The scalpel should penetrate both the skin and the subcutaneous tissue.
14. Pass the dilator over the guidewire, dilating down to the subcutaneous tissue.
15. With the dominant hand, pass the triple-lumen catheter (distal port uncapped) over the guidewire.
16. When the end of the catheter nearly reaches the skin, advance the guidewire **backward,** until it just exits the distal port.
17. Grab this end of the guidewire, and then advance the entire catheter over the guidewire into the vein.

18. Remove the guidewire.
19. Aspirate blood from each port, and flush with saline.
20. Sew the catheter into place, and apply a sterile dressing.

VI ARTERIAL LINE PLACEMENT

A. Definition: introduction of a catheter into the (radial) artery

B. Indications

1. Continuous monitoring of heart rate and blood pressure
2. Frequent arterial blood gas measurement

C. Contraindication: digital ischemia

D. Complications

1. Hematoma at the insertion site
2. Arterial pseudoaneurysm
3. Thrombosis or infection of the arterial line
4. Hand or digit ischemia or infarction

E. Technique

1. Place a roll under the dorsal surface of the wrist, leaving it in dorsiflexion. (See Figure A-8.)
2. Secure the fingers and forearm to an armboard.
3. Localize the radial artery pulsation proximal to the wrist crease.
4. Sterilize the entry site with povidone-iodine or chlorhexidine gluconate solution.
5. OPTIONAL: anesthetize the skin at the entry site with 1% lidocaine.

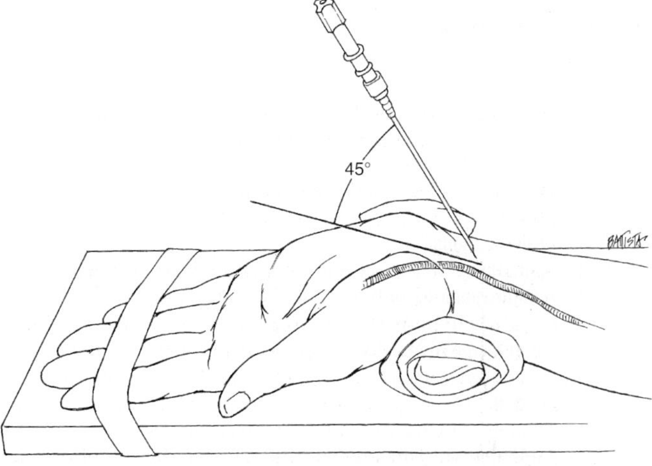

FIGURE A-8

6. Advance a 20-gauge catheter-over-needle apparatus at a 45° angle while gently palpating the radial artery proximal to the site of insertion (too much pressure will occlude the pulse).
7. Stop when bright red blood appears in the hub of the needle; this signifies entry of the **needle** into the artery.
8. Slowly lower the entire apparatus, making a more acute angle with the skin.
9. Advance the entire apparatus approximately 2 mm; this places **the catheter,** as well as the needle, into the lumen of the artery.
10. While resting the dominant hand against the skin to stabilize the position of the needle (do not pull back on the needle), slowly advance the catheter with the nondominant hand until the hub is at the skin (Figure A-9).
11. With compression applied proximal to the catheter insertion site, remove the needle with the dominant hand.
12. Release compression; the return of pulsatile, bright blood signifies the presence of successful arterial cannulation.
13. If there is no blood return, then the catheter is not within the artery lumen.
    a. Remove the catheter and apply pressure for 5 minutes.
    b. Repeat the process at a more proximal entry site.
14. Attach the catheter to the flush system and sensors, and check for an adequate arterial waveform on the monitor.
15. Secure the catheter with a suture and/or sterile dressing and remove the arm board.

VII ARTERIAL BLOOD GAS

A. Definition: sampling of (radial) arterial blood

B. Indications

1. Measurement of pH
2. Measurement of partial pressures of oxygen and carbon dioxide (PO_2, PCO_2)
3. Assessment of methemoglobinemia and carboxyhemoglobinemia

C. Contraindications: none

D. Complications: insertion point hematoma, arterial thrombosis

E. Patient positioning: patient seated or recumbent with the wrist in a slightly hyperextended position

F. Locating the point of entry: palpate the radial artery at the proximal wrist crease.

G. Technique

1. Clean the overlying skin with an alcohol swab.
2. OPTIONAL: anesthetize the skin with 1% lidocaine using a 25-gauge needle.

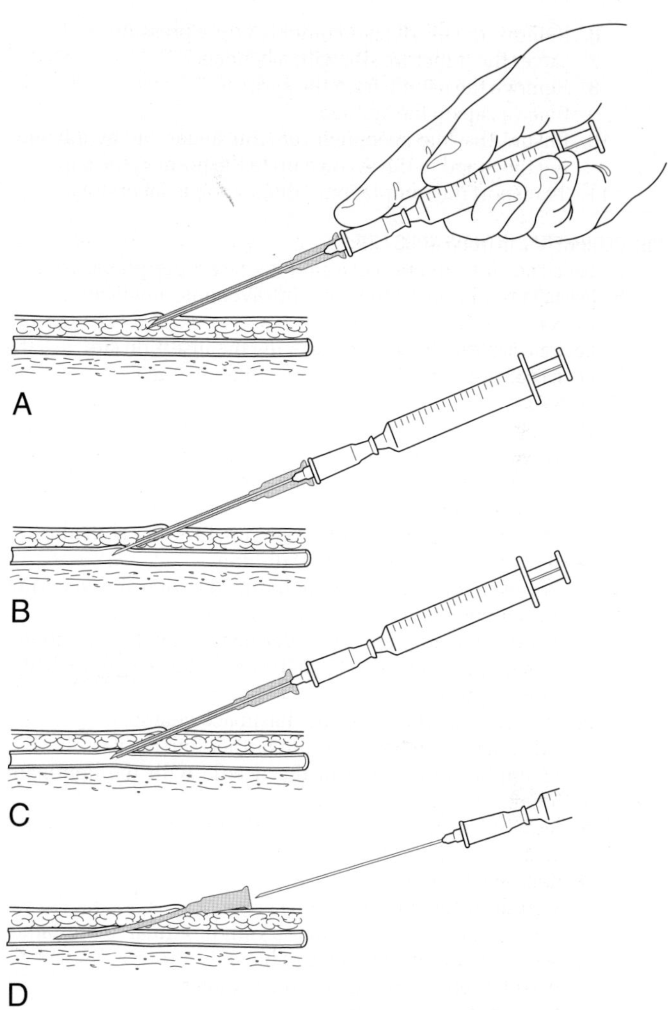

FIGURE A-9

3. Flush the blood gas needle and syringe with heparin, and leave 1 ml of air in the syringe.
4. With your nondominant hand lightly palpating the artery, enter the artery at a 45° angle. The return of briskly flowing bright red blood signifies arterial puncture.
5. Keep the needle in the same position, collecting 2–3 ml of blood.

6. Remove the needle, and quickly apply pressure.
7. Cover the puncture site with a bandage.
8. Remove the needle from the syringe.
9. Place a cap on the syringe.
10. Ensure that the specimen remains anaerobic by advancing the blood in the syringe up to the point of the cap.
11. Transport the sample immediately to the laboratory.

VIII PERIPHERAL INTRAVENOUS LINE

A. **Definition:** introduction of a catheter into a peripheral vein

B. **Indication:** administration of intravenous medications or fluids

C. **Contraindication:** infection overlying the insertion site

D. **Complications:** infection, bleeding, or hematoma

E. **Technique**

1. Locate the vein with inspection and palpation, preferably in the upper extremity at a point of vein bifurcation.
2. Apply a tourniquet proximal to insertion point, allowing the vein to engorge.
3. Clean the overlying skin at the puncture site with alcohol or chlorhexidine gluconate solution.
4. Apply slight pressure distal to the insertion site, securing the vein position.
5. Insert a 20-gauge catheter-over-needle apparatus into the vein at an acute angle (as flat as possible), with the bevel facing upward.
6. Stop when blood enters the flashback chamber.
7. Advance the apparatus 1 mm farther into the vessel.
8. Maintain the position of the needle with the dominant hand.
9. Slowly advance the catheter into the lumen of the vessel with the nondominant hand.
10. Remove the tourniquet.
11. Withdraw the needle.
12. Quickly apply pressure to the vein proximal to the catheter, interrupting the return of blood.
13. Attach tubing and fluids to the catheter.
14. Apply a sterile dressing.

Index

B

C

D

E

F

I

N

O

P

Q

W

X

Y

Z